Obesity in Europe

ou may renew this

SPORT SCIENCES INTERNATIONAL

Edited by Herbert Haag (University of Kiel)
Dieter Hackfort (University of Munich)
Ken Hardman (University of Worcester)
Manfred Lämmer (German Sport University, Cologne)
Roland Naul (University of Duisburg-Essen)
Maurice Pieron (University of Liège)
George H. Sage (University of Northern Colorado, Greeley)
Robert W. Schutz (University of British Columbia, Vancouver)
Daryl Siedentop (Ohio State University, Columbus)

Vol. 4

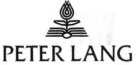

PETER LANG

Frankfurt am Main · Berlin · Bern · Bruxelles · New York · Oxford · Wien

Wolf-Dietrich Brettschneider
Roland Naul
(eds.)

Obesity in Europe

Young people's physical activity and sedentary lifestyles

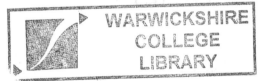
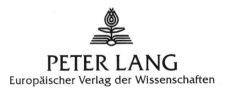

PETER LANG

Europäischer Verlag der Wissenschaften

Bibliographic Information published by the Deutsche Nationalbibliothek
The Deutsche Nationalbibliothek lists this publication in the Deutsche Nationalbibliografie; detailed bibliographic data is available in the internet at <http://www.d-nb.de>.

ISSN 0939-3706
ISBN 978-3-631-56469-1

© Peter Lang GmbH
Europäischer Verlag der Wissenschaften
Frankfurt am Main 2007
All rights reserved.

Printed in Germany 1 2   4 5 6 7

www.peterlang.de

SPORT SCIENCES INTERNATIONAL

Despite the term Science being narrowly associated in some countries and cultures with medicine, biomechanics and other disciplines representing the natural science paradigm, Sport Science today, however, is becoming a globally accepted term, which embraces a variety of disciplines and areas of study related to a range of physical activities, including sport.

Thus, whilst hitherto, international research and cross-cultural exchange in Sport has largely been fostered through text books drawing mainly from natural science disciplines, increasing attention is being paid to the considerable contributions that Social/Behavioural Sciences and Humanities make to the academic study of sport and related phenomena.

Sport Sciences International is a book series which will make a significant contribution to the global exchange of knowledge and research findings in the fields of Social/Behavioural Sciences and Humanities in Sport. Scholars, who are internationally renowned for their expertise in the fields of Sport History, Sport Pedagogy, Sport Philosophy, Sport Psychology and Sport Sociology have been brought together to edit an international series of books serving to promote the cause of Sport Science in a more comprehensive manner.

Table of Contents

Introduction

Wolf-Dietrich Brettschneider & Roland Naul

Recently there have been increasing reports in the media that focus on adolescents and depict them as a high-risk group: they are allegedly becoming fatter and fatter, supposedly because they eat too much, particularly too much fat and too much sugar, spend too much time sitting in front of the computer and of the television, fail to take enough exercise in their daily life and are less physically fit than any generation before them. To find out whether this scenario represents a distorted view or an accurate picture of the reality is not an easy task. Though we find almost identical and equally alarming reports in the media of all European countries, science has not been able to offer a clear answer. What data is available within Europe on the prevalence of overweight and obesity in children and young people is generally just as inconsistent as that relating to nutrition, media consumption, physical activity and fitness, and in some cases shows considerable variance.

This observation holds true in spite of considerable endeavours on the part of international institutions. In particular we can cite the activities of the World Health Organisation (WHO) and the International Obesity Task Force (IOTF), who are making increasing efforts, firstly, to promote research into the question, and secondly, to establish common guidelines for diagnostics, prevention and therapy.

It was in this context that the EU Commission, Directorat for Education and Culture, in 2003 commissioned a "Study on young people's lifestyles and sedentariness and the role of sport in the context of education and as a means of restoring the balance". In order to answer this array of questions a research consortium of experts from different European countries and representing academic disciplines in the areas of bio-medicine, social science, physical education and sport sciences was formed.[1]

---

[1] The project "Study on young people's lifestyles and sedentariness and the role of sport in the context of education and as a means of restoring the balance" (AZ DG EAC/33/03) was awarded to the University of Paderborn under the leadership of Prof. Dr. Wolf-Dietrich Brettschneider, University of Paderborn, and Prof. Dr. Roland Naul, University of Duisburg-Essen. Also involved as cooperation partners were: Prof. Dr. Neil Armstrong (GBR), Prof. Dr. José Alvez Diniz (POR), Prof. Dr. Karsten Froberg (DEN) and Prof. Dr. Lars Bo Andersen (NOR), Prof. Dr. Lauri Laakso and Prof. Dr. Risto Telama (FIN), Prof. Dr. Skaiste Laskiene (LHT), Prof. Dr. Göran Patriksson (SWE), Prof. Dr. Antonin Rychtecky (CZE), Prof. Dr. Willem van Mechelen (NED) and Prof. Dr. Bart Vanreusel (BEL).
In addition valued input was made by Prof. Dr. Viera Bebcáková (SVK), Dr. Damina Herman (POL), Prof. Dr. Paolo Parisi (ITA), Prof. Dr. Janko Strel (SLO), Andrea Bünemann and Dirk Hoffmann (GER).

The purpose of this study was to compile an intercultural comparative analysis of adolescents' lifestyles within the EU with the emphasis on lack of physical exercise (sedentariness). This analysis was based on international and national studies from the areas of epidemiology, cardiology, paediatrics, physiology, nutrition, psychology, sociology and sport sciences dealing with physical activity, fitness and motor abilities. This approach made it possible to use not only results from different scientific disciplines but also studies that had, in many cases, previously been available only in the language of the country, particularly from southern and eastern Europe.

In addition to these state-of-the-art reports on young people's lifestyles as well as their determinants and outcomes from the perspectives of specific disciplines and cultural contexts valuable information was given by experts form ministries and companies in the media, food & beverage, and electronic devices industries.

In some important areas, especially those concerning family and school-based nutrition and physical intervention studies to prevent sedentary lifestyles European findings are limited. Therefore relevant US findings were integrated into the study.

Our report therefore falls into three parts:

In part I the focus is on active and sedentary lifestyles and their correlates. N. Armstrong reviews the newest literature on habitual physical activity and aerobic fitness in European teenagers and concludes that the evidence linking these two categories is not very compelling. His findings show an emerging polarization with the difference between active and inactive as well as fit and unfit European youth increasing in the course of the last decades.

The contribution of L.B. Andersen, K. Froberg and their co-authors focus on linking physical inactivity and low fitness to metabolic disorders and cardiovascular disease risk factors including obesity. They show that risk factors cluster in the population of children and that this clustering is strongly related to low physical activity and fitness. They emphasize the potential of increased physical activity for primary prevention of CVD and obesity.

P. Parisi refers to the motto of the European Year of Education through Sport (2004) "Move your body, stretch your mind" and looks at the relation of health and lifestyle from an integral perspective on young people's development. In this context sport appears to play a major role, not only as a measure to keep the balance between energy intake and energy expenditure, but as a fundamental source in stimulating the body's physical and emotional expressions.

B. Vanreusel and B. Meulders argue that sedentariness is part of a "risk society" and refer to the paradox that today's young people is the first generation in Europe to grow up in societies that at the same time provide the determinants for sedentary behaviour and produce the risk factors associated with such a lifestyle. They offer an integrated framework for increasing health promoting physical activity and reducing the risks of sedentariness.

The American group around J. Elder refers to the finding that a number of physical activity or dietary change programs exist, some of which have successfully achieved behaviour change in specific areas, but none of the changes has been effective to prevent childhood obesity. The authors argue and produce empirical evidence that only comprehensive strategies incorporating both behaviour change and the creation of supportive and stimulating changes in children's home, school and community environments may help to combat the obesity epidemic.

In part II the prevalence of obesity and the prevention programs launched by the ministries and conducted by research groups are in the fore. A. Niederhaus describes the efforts of the German government to slow the overweight and obesity development. Special attention is paid to the national "Platform for Nutrition and Physical Activity" (PEB) as well as to the nation-wide competition "Eat better and be more active" (Besser essen – mehr bewegen) which initiate campaigns to improve food and meals at home and increase physical activity in the daily lives of young people.

S. Danielzik et al. refer to a prospective study, the so-called "Kiel Obesity Prevention Study" (KOPS), and its potential for prevention. Its findings show the strong effect of a low socio-economic status and its role as a limiting factor in any intervention program. In accordance with other findings the authors emphasize the necessity of complementing school and family based interventions by measures tackling the obesogenic environment.

This is also the message of H. Heseker's and Anke Oepping's contribution. Though they argues from the perspective of nutrition they strongly favours an approach characterised by an internal and external linking. The internal linking implies the increase of physical activity, the decrease of media consumption and the improvement of nutrition. The external linking means a networked strategy combining the activities of all individuals and institutions responsible for the development of children and youth.

C. Graf and S. Dordel refer to their school-based invention study "CHILT". They do not focus too much on childhood fatness, but rather on childhood fitness and activity. Their findings give evidence for a correlation of physical activity and fitness and specific aspects of cognition, though the causal relationship still remains undecoded.

Part III contains various state-of-the-art reports on young people's lifestyles and sedentariness written from the specific perspective of individual countries, respectively cultural contexts. The country reports by A. Rychtecký, S. Laskiene,

J. Strel and co-authors, R. Telema and co-authors and W.-D. Brettschneider, R. Naul and co-authors are taken as exemplars to show to which degree the prevalence rates of overweight and obesity in children and youth vary within the EU. They also show their changes over time and (with respect to Eastern Europe) especially in the context of the transformation processes after the fall of the iron curtain. The reports do not only agree in the decline of motor ability and physical fitness, but also in the increase of media consumption and physical inactivity in the daily lives of young people all over Europe.

The book provides a comprehensive state-of-the-art analysis concerning modern lifestyles of European teenagers with a special focus on the rising prevalence of childhood obesity and its determinants. It shows clearly the important role of physical activity and sport in the combat against the obesity epidemic.

Those readers who are interested in getting an overview of the physical activity and fitness level of European youth, the prevalence of childhood obesity, its risk factors and determinants and recommendations for intervention programs and prevention strategies, will receive a comprehensive tool with this volume of "Sport Science International".

Finally, we would like to thank all authors for their valued contributions to this project and our assistants Eva-Maria Natus, Paderborn, and Dirk Hoffmann, Essen, who are responsible for the layout of the book. We also express our gratitude to the Lang publishing house for its support to print the text book.

I.
Overweight and obesity in the context of young people's lifestyles

Chapter 1:
Obesity in Europe. Young people´s physical activity and sedentary lifestyle

Wolf-Dietrich Brettschneider & Roland Naul

Overweight and obesity: definition and prevalence

The difficulties associated with registering overweight and obesity and their causes and consequences begin with determining their symptomatology and specifying appropriate cut-off values.

Overweight and obesity are diagnosed on the basis of the proportion of fat in relation to body weight. This definition is generally agreed upon throughout Europe, but there are considerable differences as to the methods used to measure the various quantities. Among direct methods of measurement, skin fold thickness enjoys a certain popularity; body mass index (BMI) has achieved international acceptance not at least because it is easy to use, being calculated from the subject's weight and body length (kg/m^2), which are themselves measured with a set of scales and a tape measure or taken from statements made either by the children being surveyed or by their parents.

Without additional information, however, the BMI is not a great deal of use for children and young people, because the changes to body weight and physical form are associated with puberty and increasing height also produce age-related and sex-related changes to the BMI. For this reason such analyses generally introduce age-related and sex-related percentiles obtained from appropriate populations – usually local to the particular country. The values that are considered to mark the cut-offs for overweight and obesity vary from country to country. Many European countries take the 90th or 97th percentile as the threshold to overweight and obesity respectively for the investigated populations of adolescents, but since other percentile values are also used within Europe to classify overweight and obesity, and since there is no common reference population for European adolescents so that national reference populations often have to be used, the figures are, in some cases, extremely difficult to compare.

Different methods of assessment also influence the determined rates of prevalence of overweight and obesity in children and young people, as demonstrated by a comparison between European countries on the basis of a subjective survey (WHO) and objective measurements (IOTF) of body size and weight with the identical reference system (cf. Tab. 1).

Tab. 1:   Overweight and obese adolescents (in %): comparison of WHO data (Currie et al, 2004) and IOTF data (IOTF, 2004)

Country	Overweight/Adipositas of 13-year-old children (by WHO criteria)	Overweight/Adipositas of 15-year-old adolescents (by WHO cirteria)	Overweight/Adipositas of children aged 7 – 10 years (by IOTF criteria)
Malta	28.6	22.5	35
Spain	18.2	15.7	34
England	16.9	14.6	20
Italy	16.7	14.7	36
Greece	16.2	15.8	31
Germany	11.4	11.2	16
Austria	11.3	11.1	19
Belgien	10.9	10.7	18
Sweden	10.0	10.9	18
Czech Republic	9.4	9.3	17
Denmark	8.8	11.9	15
Poland	7.7	6.6	18
Netherlands	6.6	8.8	12

Although the established values vary depending on the method of assessment, and in some cases quite considerably, it is still possible to identify a corresponding pattern in the prevalence of overweight and obesity in European adolescents: The percentage of overweight children is highest in the countries of southern Europe, lowest in those of eastern Europe, with the Scandinavians and western European counties (apart from Great Britain) somewhere in the middle (cf. Fig. 1).

Independently of the currently varying prevalence figures, many national studies carried out in recent years report a common trend characterised by rapidly growing percentages of overweight and obesity in both boys and girls. We should, however, point out that the results of such national studies are often inconsistent, because generally no time series comparisons are given and the studies do not permit international comparisons within the EU because they were carried out over different time periods.

Causes of overweight and obesity

Although the actual mechanisms whereby the interaction of nutritional habits, lack of exercise and media consumption give rise to overweight and obesity in children and young people are as yet unresolved, there is general agreement with the assumption that genetic factors on the one hand and lifestyle variables on the

Fig. 1: 13 to 15-year-old European adolescents whose BMI showes them to be overweight or obese (compiled from data collected by Brettschneider & Naul, 2004)

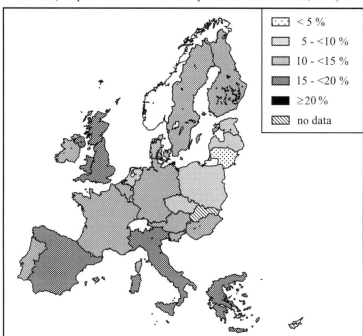

obesity. But since we can assume that the contents of the human gene pool have not changed substantially over the last few decades, a genetic predisposition cannot adequately explain the rapid spread of overweight over the last 20 years nor the steepness with which it has risen. It is far more reasonable to look for the cause in a change of lifestyle. More precisely: the increase in overweight in childhood and adolescence can be seen as the result of the persistent energy imbalance that occurs when the energy output is too low in comparison to the energy intake. Whereas food is available in abundance, many children's everyday lives are increasingly characterised by physical inactivity.

It therefore seems logical to analyse, firstly, adolescents' nutrition, and secondly, the reason for their physical (in)activity.

The nutritional behaviour of European adolescents

It is no easy task to report on the nutritional behaviour of European children and young people. There are no representative national studies available, nor has comprehensive data been gathered for all the member countries of the EU. But we will nonetheless examine a number of studies from various European regions and attempt to depict general tendencies in juvenile nutritional behaviour on that basis.

The DONALD study (Kersting, Alexy, Kroke & Lentze, 2004), which was carried out in Germany, was designed in the same way as similar studies in other European countries. It contains recommendations for the consumption of various groups of foodstuffs for particular age groups and gives desired values for the percentage distribution of energy-supplying foodstuffs. With this background information the empirically gathered data relating to the test persons' actual consumption is then described. In the case of the DONALD study the recommendations are summarised in the prevention concept "optimised mixed diet".

Figure 2 shows, on the one hand, that German children and young people consume too many fatty, protein-rich meat products, and on the other hand, that their consumption of high-carbohydrate products such as potatoes, pasta and rice is below the level recommended by the "optimised mixed diet" – a tendency that can also be found in other European countries such as Spain, Poland and Austria, indeed, the meat consumption of Austrian kindergarten and schoolchildren is three times the recommended value (Elmadfa, Freisling, König, et al., 2003).

The patterns exhibited by the consumption of vegetables and confectionery are also very similar within Europe: adolescents' actual consumption of vegetables is up to 50 % below the recommended level but, in contrast, they exhibit a considerable predilection for confectionery which they consume to a significantly greater extent than recommended. Fruit is the only group of foodstuffs whose consumption fails to exhibit a uniform trend throughout Europe. While Spanish adolescents eat sufficient fruit, and German adolescents' consumption of fruit and fruit juices is also adequate, Polish, Swedish and Austrian children and young people eat too few sources of vitamins, such as apples and other native fruits (Brettschneider & Naul, 2004, pp.52).

This representation of European adolescents' food consumption makes it clear that their nutritional behaviour possesses optimisation potential, and this is also shown by the distribution of energy-supplying foodstuffs (fat, carbohydrate and protein), which, throughout Europe, is characterised by a higher percentage of fat than recommended. For example, in Slovakia the fat in the diet provides between 36 % and 39.7 % of the daily energy intake, which is clearly much too high compared to the 27% recommended in that country. Only in Portugal is young people's actual consumption close to the national recommendation, namely between 31 % and 33 %.

Fig. 2: Consumption of meat, poultry and sausage (top) and potatoes, pasta and rice
(bottom) by 500 4 to 18-year-old test persons in the DONALD study (Kersting et al.,
2004)

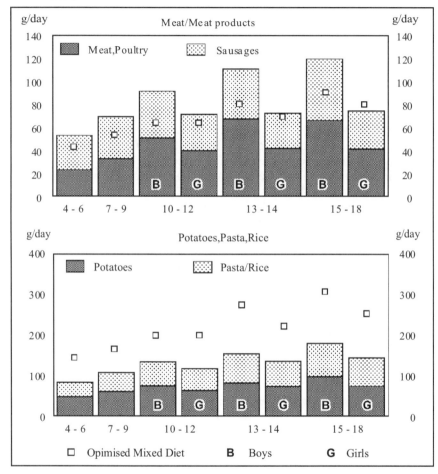

But the really interesting question for determining the potential cause of overweight and obesity is not so much which foodstuffs are consumed in which categories and quantities and how the energy supplied is distributed among those foodstuffs: the far more significant question is whether the overall energy intake exceeds the recommended level and might thereby contribute to a positive energy balance.

For six of the countries in the EU we are in a position to compare figures for the desired and actual energy intake. And we find that the energy intake of children and young people in Spain and Great Britain is within the recommended range, while in the remaining four countries the energy intake of children and young people is *below* the specific national recommendation. For Germany we do not have any precise figures, but the data for Slovakian, Swiss and Czech adolescents shows their energy intake to be around 10 % below the recommended level. We can therefore state that, in spite of the abundance of food available and contrary to popular assumptions, young people adolescents *do not eat too much* and their total energy intake has not increased over time.

For the question as to how much energy intake has changed over the last few years or decades we were able to find data from Germany, the Netherlands and Great Britain. While the energy intake in Germany has remained broadly unchanged over a period of 15 years (1985 and 2000), Dutch adolescents' overall energy intake shows a reduction over the ten years 1987/88 to 1997/98. And a British comparison of energy intake for 1930 and 1980 substantiates that the energy intake over those 50 years exhibited a downward trend (cf. Fig. 3). other both influence the development and dissemination of overweight and obesity. But since we can assume that the contents of the human gene pool have not changed substantially over the last few decades, a genetic predisposition cannot adequately explain the rapid spread of overweight over the last 20 years nor the steepness with which it has risen. It is far more reasonable to look for the cause in a change of lifestyle. More precisely: the increase in overweight in childhood and adolescence can be seen as the result of the persistent energy imbalance that occurs when the energy output is too low in comparison to the energy intake. Whereas food is available in abundance, many children's everyday lives are increasingly characterised by physical inactivity. It therefore seems logical to analyse, firstly, adolescents' nutrition, and secondly, the reason for their physical (in)activity.

Fig. 3:   Energy intake of 14 to 15-year-olds in Great Britain (Armstrong 2004)

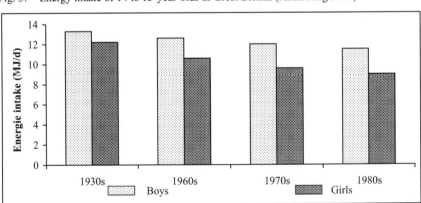

When we look at what potential determinants are influencing adolescents' nutritional behaviour we can register a polarisation: this indicates that adolescents in high-income groups, and children of better educated parents, have better eating habits than children and young people of the same age from uneducated and lower social strata. Migration of the family of origin, and being a member of the male sex, also have a negative effect on children's and young people's nutritional behaviour.

Discrepancies between recommended nutritional behaviour and the foodstuffs actually consumed cannot be the only factors responsible for the imbalance between energy intake and energy output. It follows that the positive energy balance is principally attributable to the insufficient expenditure of energy, i.e. inadequate physical activity. This explanation also applies if we consider not only the total energy intake but also the high energy density and low nutritional value of many foodstuffs. We therefore need to take a closer look at energy expenditure, specifically at the extent to which daily exercise, physical exertion and the associated leisure behaviour contribute to the energy imbalance. The first impression we get is irresistible: the younger generation's lifeworld today is characterised less by exercise than by physical inactivity.

Media consumption as a part of inactive leisure behaviour

At the present time, young Europeans' daily life is characterised to no little degree by their use of electronic media. In the "old" EU countries the principal such medium used has remained unchanged for years – the television, that almost every adolescent switches on every single day – as illustrated in Figure 4 by the data for German adolescents. While German adolescents' use of classic print media (books, magazines) has already been declining since 1999, and their use of radios since 2002, their use of computers has increased markedly since it was first measured in 1998 – an increase which, in 2005, has for the first time enabled "using the computer" to overtake "listening to the radio" as an adolescent leisure pursuit.

This reverse trend in the use of media in favour of the computer is also observed for Dutch adolescents, but a number of years earlier than in Germany. Similar developments are reported by investigations in Sweden, Denmark and Switzerland. In the "old" EU countries we can thus recognise a tendency towards greater consumption of modern communications media such as the computer, but contrary to expectations this move towards modern electronic media does not appear to be necessarily associated with an increase in the total number of hours per week for which media is used. The individual media that are actually consumed are in a state of flux, but the total duration remains constant (Biddle, Gorely & Stensel, 2004).

Fig. 4:   Media used by German 14 to 19-year-old adolescents (daily and several times per week) 1998 to 2005 (based on information from Brettschneider & Bünemann, 2004, compiled from data from the MPFS, 1998-2005)

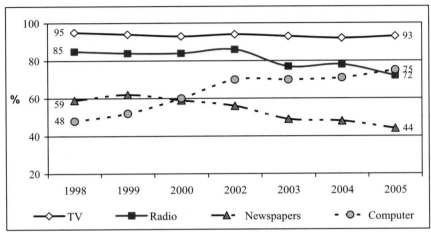

Unfortunately there is no data available regarding developments in the "new" EU countries, those that became member states in May 2004, but there are certainly studies in eastern Europe that rank the media consumed. While the same rankings are found for Polish adolescents and Czech boys as for west European adolescents, listening to music has a higher ranking with Czech girls and Slovakian children and young people than does the television, and those children and young people also consider printed media more significant than the computer, a difference which is probably not unconnected to the different economic income levels of the countries' private households.

Throughout the whole of Europe, however, most adolescents not only switch on the television most frequently, they also devote the most time to it. There are still sizeable differences between individual EU countries (cf. Tab. 2), but in attempting this comparison we again need to remember not only that there is almost no representative national data to be had, but that some of the random samples also feature differing age structures and were taken at different times.

While Swiss 9 to 16-year-olds spend on average 'only' one and a half hours per day in front of the television, schoolchildren from the Baltic states spend more than twice as long watching television. Austrian adolescents come in the centre of the scale with 126 minutes per day.

We do not yet have any comprehensive national data on the use of computers in the various countries of the EU, only isolated collections of data from local and regional studies that make use of different representations and therefore cannot

Tab. 2: Use of television by adolescents in various EU member countries (based on Brettschneider & Naul, 2004)

Country	Age class	Time spend on viewing TV	
		Original data for children and/or adolescents	Minutes/day
Baltic States	School-aged children	22,5 hours/week or 3,2 hours/day	192 min/day
Slovenia	11 to 14-year-olds	153 min/day*	153 min/day*
Portugal	Children & adolescents	Nearly $^2/_3$ > 2 hours/weekday Nearly ¼ of them > 4 hours/weekday ¾ > 2 hours/weekend-day on average a child watches 2 ½ hours/day	150 min/day
Italy	Children	82 % ~ 90 min/day + 18 % having watched a video for 66 min/day as a whole: 2½ hours/day	128 min/day
	Adolescents	88 % ~ 90 min/day + 16 % having watched a video for 14 min/day as a whole: 1¾ hours/day	
Slovakia	Adolescents	An average adolescent spends approx. 2 hours/day watching TV	120 min/day
Germany	3 to 13-year-olds	93 min/day	106 min/day
	14 to 19-year-olds	118 min/day	
Netherlands	12 to 15-year-olds	98 min/day	106 min/day
	16 to 18-year-olds	84 min/day	
Finland	3 to 8-year-olds	At least ½ hour a day	
Sweden	15 to 16-year-olds	80 % > 4 hours/week $^1/_3$ of this group > 10 hours/week	
Swiss	9 to 16-year-olds		91 min/day

really be compared. The only available source that can be used for a European comparison is the HBSC study (Currie et al., 2004), which established that 13.3 % of European adolescents spend an average of over three hours per weekday using their computer. At weekends this value rises to 23.8 %. Austrian adolescents are slightly below the European average for computer usage, with 12.2 % on weekdays and 22.9 % at weekends.

One factor that has decisive influence on media consumption is personal ownership of electronic equipment. Adolescents from lower social and educational strata and lower income levels own more televisions, video games and computer games and devote more time to them than do adolescents in families from higher social and educational strata, but the influence of social class and educational level is reversed when it comes to the ownership and creative use of computers. Compared by age, younger adolescents own and use video and computer games more frequently than older ones, as is clearly shown in Figure 5 for a sample of Austrian adolescents. And in both respects boys are more frequently addicted to such media than are girls.

Tab. 5: Possession of media by 14 to 19-year-olds Austrian adolescents (based on information from the Austrian Federal Ministry for Social Security and Generations, 1999)

	14-15	16-17	18-19
TV	48	49	52
Video recorder	23	17	33
Video camera	2	2	3
Hi-fi stereo system	58	64	59
Walkman/ portable CD	80	67	69
Minidiscs	15	7	7
Computer	33	31	37
Digital video games	40	22	19
Computer games	43	31	33

There are other differences that are not mirrored by personal ownership. Boys in general watch more television and use more computers than girls. Surfing the internet and the creative use of computers increases throughout Europe with the age of the adolescents. Only in relation to television consumption is there no uniform finding for age: in Italy, for example, children watch more television than do adolescents, but in Germany the proportions are reversed.

To summarise media use, we can say that modern media plays a very important role in European adolescents' daily life, whereby computers in particular are acquiring increasing significance to the detriment of traditional media. And although the time that adolescents spend at the computer is increasing, and their television consumption is high and in many EU countries is stable, it is apparently only media preferences that are changing – the total number of hours spent using media seems not to have increased significantly over the last few years.

It follows that the rapid increase in the prevalence of overweight over this period cannot simply be attributed to increased use of media, and nor can we apply the popular and simplistic argument "media consumption displaces sporting activity" – which, so stated, has also so far not been confirmed by any scientific study (Biddle, Gorely, Marshall, Murdey & Cameron, 2003) but still remains a popular assessment in the general public and within sport organisations.

Involvement in sport, physical performance and fitness

In almost every member state of the EU there are studies on children's and young people's involvement in sport and their fitness and motor performance. But even here, specific features of the various national school and sport systems, the different methods of gathering data, and the different questions and indicators that were included mean that it is barely possible to make direct comparisons between the various age-groups of children and young people over a number of EU countries. Even investigations that were carried out almost simultaneously in many EU countries and which all used the EUROFIT test on children and young people of matching age-groups (Kemper & van Mechelen, 1996) can be compared only with reservations, because some batteries of tests are incomplete and the individual tests were not carried out in the same way. There are also considerable differences between individual EU countries, because some of them (e.g. England, the Netherlands, Denmark, Finland, Poland and Slovenia) have for many years commissioned research institutes to carry out ongoing health and physical activity surveys of their adolescents (Kemper, 2004; Strel, Kovac & Jurak, 2004; Raczek, 2002) while other EU countries do not yet have any such monitoring systems or are still engaged in setting them up. There have, however, been numerous bi-national studies carried out in northern, western and eastern Europe that do make it possible to compare the individual countries' sport involvement using a series of indicators, including physical performance and motor fitness of populations in matched age-groups (Naul, Telama & Rychtecky 1997; Rychtecky, 2004; Jurimäe & Volbekiene, 1998).

To this day, however, we find hardly any instances of identically designed studies being carried out simultaneously in a number of EU countries, using identical investigation and testing methods on sufficiently contemporary sample groups, that have not only taken into account factors relating to the adolescents' sporting lifestyles but also empirically investigated their motor performance (Telama et al., 2002).

The two most frequently investigated indicators that have been dealt with by national studies on the sporting involvement of children and young people in Europe include the membership of a sports club (degree of organisation) and the daily or weekly time budget, measured as the hours or minutes of physical and sporting activity.

As indicated by the rates of participation in organised sport, European adolescents' involvement in sport remains high, and this applies regardless of whether the driving force for their sporting activity is the sports club, school, or community (cf. Tab. 3).

There is a remarkable level of agreement, showing that about two thirds of children and half of adolescents are engaged in organised sport, whereby social inequalities are still to be found – a point on which findings throughout Europe are equally in agreement: boys are more active than girls, and children from socially privileged families play more sports than adolescents at the bottom end of the social ladder.

Tab. 3:   The degree of organisation of children and young people in sports clubs in Europe (based on information from Brettschneider & Naul, 2004)

Country	Membership in sports clubs	
	Boys	Girls
Germany (12 – 18-year-olds)	ca. 50 %	ca. 35 %
Czech Republic(9 – 18-year-olds)	ca. 45 %	ca. 36 %
Polend (12 – 13-year-olds)	ca. 47 %	ca. 35 %
Belgium (12 – 18-year-olds)	ca. 60 %	ca. 40 %
Italy (12 – 18 -year-olds)	ca. 48 %	ca. 34 %
Sweden (12 – 16-year-olds.)	ca. 52 %	ca. 36 %
Finland (12 – 16-year-olds)	ca. 50 %	ca. 40 %

Enthusiasm for sport also leaves its traces in the area of informal activities. In almost all EU countries today, the popularity of non-organised sports increases at a remarkable rate with increasing social class.

Jogging, aerobics, skating and cycling plus football and basketball belong to the common sporting profile of adolescents in almost all EU countries (Telama et al., 2002, 52ff). Studies of their respective time budgets also show that the time spent on sport by the various age-groups of children and young people follow quite parallel contours in the different EU member states, regardless of how much or how little they are organised as members of sports clubs.

There are currently two ambivalent but contemporaneous developments emerging in almost all EU countries: the percentage of those who virtually never engage in any sports other than school sport is still growing (ca. 7 to 15 % depending on age and country), but so is the group of those who engage in active leisure pursuits almost every day (ca. 6 to 19 % depending on age and country) (cf. Fig. 6). This means that there are currently two contrary tendencies: the proportion of physically inactive children in an age group and the proportion of their peers that regularly engage in sports are both increasing. So it is not surprising that the spread of children's and young people's physical performance has been continually increasing for the last few years, nor that we observe some conflicting results between individual studies of motor and fitness, such as those that have been carried out in Germany (Kurz, 2001). While all discussions consider only average values, and the different extreme group distributions in individual survey populations are disregarded, we should not be surprised by contradictory findings for identical motor parameters in different contemporary populations.

Fig. 6:   Physical exercise sufficient to cause sweating (hours per week) taken by European young people from Belgium, Estonia, Finland, Germany and the Czech Republic (Telama et al., 2002)

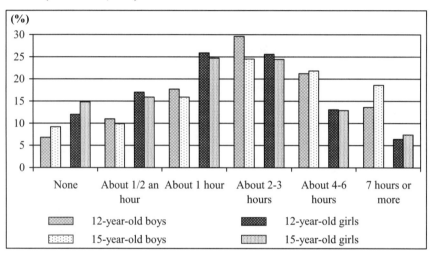

But it is a fact that in all EU countries there is at present a steadily increasing number of children and young people who are less physically active than was their age group 10 or 20 years ago. And it is also a fact that in all European conurbations, increasing urbanisation and the planning of building development and roads in and around their home environments have contributed to a marked reduction of children's and young people's day-to-day physical activities, running, playing, and walking or cycling to school. A British study found that the number of children whose parents drive them to school has almost doubled within 15 years from 16 % to 29 % (DETR, 1999). Similar results are reported for 6 to 9-year-old children in Switzerland (Swiss Federal Office for Spatial Development, Federal Statistical Office, 2001). For the problem group of physically inactive children and young people, the reduction in their leisure sporting activity is further reinforced in their daily life by their increasing use of motorised transport to school and to their leisure pursuits.

The consequences of this mounting physical inactivity are impossible to ignore.
European time series studies show that physical fitness has reduced by around 10
to 15 % over the last 25 years: this applies at varying rates almost everywhere in
Europe (Bös, 2003) and affects almost every basic motor ability (cf. Fig. 7).

Fig. 7: Differing motor ability of German children and young people measured in 1975 and
2000 (from Bös, 2003)

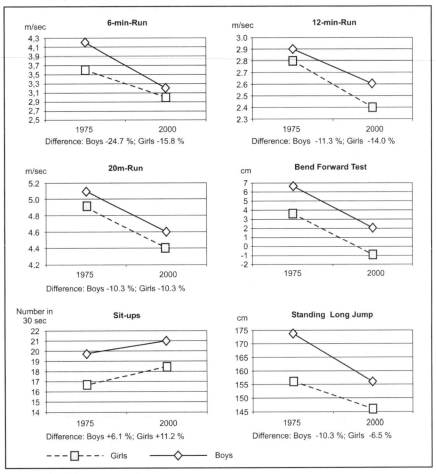

In addition, long-term trends indicate that health-related fitness is also receding:
throughout Europe. National cross-sectional and longitudinal studies all show a
downward trend in children's and young people's values for aerobic stamina
(VO_2 max) compared to earlier investigations with test subjects of the same age:

today's children and young people measure as much as 25 or 30 % below the critical standard values that represent a risk to their health, and this applies particularly to girls and boys in western and southern European countries (Brettscheider & Naul, 2004, pp.88). Whereas up until 15 or 20 years ago it was primarily the girls who stood out, since then we increasingly also find boys in the at-risk group, and the problem is affecting both boys and girls at an ever younger age.

Here, too, we still do not have any representative pan-European time series investigations, but there are some national findings that agree with similar results from other countries. British findings tell us:
Only 55 % of the boys and 39 % of the girls under 16 managed the requisite 60 minutes cumulated moderate physical activity per day, and 29 % of the boys and 43 % of the girls were physically active for less than 30 minutes per day (Prescott-Clarke & Primatesta, 1998).

In spite of the difficulty in using these datasets at the present time to establish valid figures for children's and young people's involvement in sport, their physically activity and their health-related fitness over a sufficiently large random pan-European sample, it does seem logical to assume a correlation between these two factors. Typical of between roughly a quarter and a third of all adolescents in the EU between ages 10 and 15 is a low level of involvement in leisure sport coupled with deteriorating everyday motor, plus a motor development status that must be considered critical – reaching values that represent a health risk. We must not omit to consider the role played by the school in this. Children spend most of their time at school sitting down. In addition, of the three lesson periods per week that for example he curriculum of the average federal German state allocates to sport, an average of just 70 to 75 % actually take place. And then, on average, cancellations due to situational factors put paid to a further 6 %, for half of which the children are given a free period and a further 30 % of which are replaced by tuition in some other subject (DSB, 2006). Since we also find that many German schoolchildren would prefer their school sport to be more physically strenuous than it currently is, it is clear that the motor demands made by sports lessons are not sufficiently intense (DSB, 2006).

There is some evidence that these Gernman findings are not unique compared to other EU countries as Hardman (2002) documented in his PE review on the status of PE time allocation at school and objektives of many national PE curricula across Europe (cf. Brettschneider & Naul, 2004, pp. 142). In his study the development of a „active lifestyle" and „physical fitness" ranked only seventh and eleventh among other objektives of school PE curricula.

In the context of PE and school sport we thus need to reconsider how to combine active exercise time with moderate physical exertion. And for this we can also find some pioneering examples within the EU, particularly in the Scandinavian countries (Pühse & Gerber 2005, Richter 2006).

There is in the EU at present insufficient representative evidence to prove the existence of a relationship between the increasing prevalence of overweight and obesity in childhood and adolescence and young people's reduced sporting and everyday physical activities, but there are increasing indications of inverse correlations between involvement in sport and physical activity on the one hand and overweight and obesity on the other. The statement that "physically active adolescents suffer less from overweight" therefore has some claim to plausibility, as do the relationships that individual studies have already established between the increased prevalence of overweight and the diminished fitness of the younger generation.

Consequences and recommendations

In spite of the difficulties we have mentioned in making clear statements about the correlation of overweight, nutritional behaviour, media consumption and physical activities in children and young people that will be applicable throughout Europe, it is possible to formulate a number of common features. There are differences in the design of the research projects, and the volume of investigated criteria in the various national studies is also non-uniform; the use of different investigative methods, and non-identical standards for the reference values used to measure overweight and obesity, also hinder comparisons between the various European studies (WHO, IOTF, and others). But from these international and national studies we can nonetheless draw a number of common conclusions for future research projects and formulate recommendations for intervention measures that could be enacted in order to avoid and prevent overweight and physical inactivity.

The negative and positive correlations that have been established in the many national and few European studies between nutritional behaviour and overweight, between passive leisure habits and motor development, and between an active lifestyle with involvement in sports and a healthy diet, are almost all based on bivariate associations. But since it is always the interplay between varying combinations of a number of these factors that are the cause of this increase in overweight, the conclusion is as follows: In future we will need to develop more ambitious research designs for studies in order to empirically investigate the complex fabric of operationalised and multivariate factor relationships.

It is equally obvious that in order to carry out comparative studies in the EU we need to use datasets that really are comparable as well as identical standards and criteria. These should then rely less on subjective self-assessments, such as are used for instance in WHO studies, but rather on objectively verifiable methods and procedures. If we hope to fulfil these requirements it would be advisable to set up a network of research institutes that regularly conducts an integrated system of pan-European surveys of children and young people using agreed criteria. In view of the large number of factors whose interaction leads to overweight, passive leisure behaviour, and sedentariness in children and young people, such surveys should in future be planned only with an interdisciplinary design and implemented only by corresponding teams of experts.

Corresponding conclusions should be drawn for interventive and preventive measures for children and young people. Where individual factors reinforce one another in their tendency to cause and encourage overweight and sedentariness, it is the combination of these factors that must be the object of such measures. They should include both education about the basics of nutrition, with appropriate nutrient parameters for each age-group, and the encouragement of an active lifestyle with plenty of exercise, games and sport, preferably for at least one hour per day (see also the undated publication of the European Economic and Social Committee). In particular, we need to exploit every possible means of consistently increasing children's and young people's everyday physical activity. These include more opportunities for exercise during the school day and an "active school route", whether walking, skating or cycling. Such efforts often fail because parents consider their little dears' school route to be unsafe or positively dangerous and prefer to take them to school by car. On the other hand, the studies and reports we have cited show that, where the surroundings offer appropriate conditions for school routes, or where such conditions can be brought about, an "active school route" can have numerous positive effects not only on children's and young people's weight problems, but possibly also on their ability to concentrate and their cognitive performance at school.

The task of giving children a better diet and more exercise calls for cooperation between all those involved and all those affected: family, school, sports clubs and communities (cf. Fig. 8). Only such a setting approach, combining all the necessary measures into one communal network, is likely to effectively counter the complex structure of contributing factors to overweight and lack of exercise.

Promotion of an active lifestyle calls for mutual support from all these partners. School sport and club sport must also reinforce one another by means of joint programmes, as must parents, teachers and partners from the various municipal departments (public health, youth welfare, education authority, planning department) who are responsible for providing an exercise-friendly infrastructure (school yards, public parks, paths and roads). The present tasks and objectives of school sport and the associated timetables and guidelines all need to be reconsidered in the light of the problem illustrated by the rapidly escalating prevalence values. In many European countries the various forms of "all-day school" now offer a broad basis for targeted offers (lunch, exercise periods) in order to promote both healthy eating and more exercise and sport.

Fig. 8:   Socio-cultural structure of a communal network for an active lifestyle for children and young people

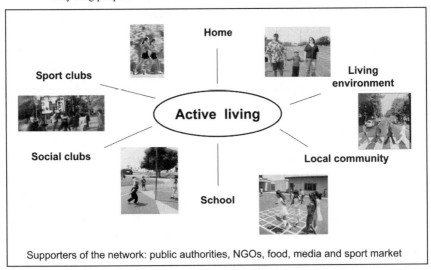

Supporters of the network: public authorities, NGOs, food, media and sport market

However, what is really crucial is for those children and young people who are already overweight and sedentary to accept the help they are offered in their various settings, and a purely cognitive explanation of the health risks and consequences given in formal lessons will not suffice. Affected children and young people are often socially excluded by their classmates, also and particularly during sports lessons, and simply withdraw from their peer groups. They want the teasing to stop ("fatty", large but not great) and are weary of continually being confronted by their own motor and psycho-social inadequacy. They often believe themselves capable of less than they really are. Here we need an intervention strategy that takes into account not only children's and young people's cognitive appreciation of the problem of "overweight" but also the emotional and social side of the problem, in order to promote and support their own acceptance of a change in their lifestyle.

Eventually, in view of the available results and developments regarding "overweight and sedentariness", it will be unavoidable for both existing and future education and training of sports teachers to broaden and intensify the job profile to include professional, methodical, practical, and sport-pedagogic and didactic training in order to impart the additional specialist teaching skills needed for the changed requirements of overweight and obese children.

References

Armstrong, N. (2004). Physical fitness and physical activity patterns of European youth. United Kingdom: University of Exeter.

Biddle, S., Gorely, T., Marshall, S. J., Murdey, I. & Cameron, N. (2003). Physical activity and sedentary behaviours in youth: issues and controversies. *The Journal of the Royal Society for the Promotion of Health, 124 (1),* 29-33.

Biddle, S., Gorely, T., & Stensel, D. J. (2004). Health-enhancing physical activity and sedentary behaviour in children and adolescents. *Journal of Sports Sciences, 22,* 679-701.

Bös, K. (2003). Motorische Leistungsfähigkeit von Kindern und Jugendlichen. In W. Schmidt, I. Hartmann-Tews & W.-D. Brettschneider (Eds.), *Erster Deutscher Kinder- und Jugendsportbericht* (pp 85-107). Schorndorf: Hofmann.

Brettschneider, W.-D. & Bünemann, A. (2004). *National report "Young people's lifestyles and sedentariness. Germany"*. Paderborn: University of Paderborn.

Brettschneider, W.-D. & Naul, R. (2004). *Study on young people's lifestyles and sedentariness and the role of sport in the context of education and as a means of restoring the balance – Final report.* Accessed on 3 February 2005 from http://europa.eu.int/comm/sport/documents/lotpaderborn.pdf

Austrian Federal Ministry for Social Security, Generations and Consumer Protection (Ed.) (1999). 3. Bericht zur Lage der Jugend in Österreich. Vienna.

Currie, C., Roberts, C., Morgan, A., Smith, R., Settertobulte, W., Samdal, O. et al. (2004). *Young People's Health in Context. Health Behaviour in School-aged Children (HBSC) study: international report from the 2001/2002 survey (Health Policy for Children and Adolescents, No. 4).* Copenhagen: World Health Organization Regional Office for Europe.

DETR (Department of the Environment, Transport and the Regions) (1999). *National Travel Survey 1996/98.* London: DETR.

DSB (Ed.) (2006). *Die SPRINT-Studie.* Aachen: Meyer & Meyer.

Elmadfa, I., Freisling, H., König, J. et al. (2003). *Österreichischer Ernährungsbericht 2003. Vienna: Institute of Nutritional Science.*

European Economic and Social Committee (Ed.) (undated). *Civil Society on the Move for a Healthier Europe!.* Bruxelles: EESC.

Gogoll, A., Kurz, D. & Menze-Sonneck, A. (2003). Sportengagements Jugendlicher in Westdeutschland.In W. Schmidt, I. Hartmann-Tews & W.-D. Brettschneider (Eds.), *Erster Deutscher Kinder- und Jugendsportbericht* (pp 145-165). Schorndorf: Hofmann.

HEA (Health Education Authority) (1998). *Young and Active? Policy framework for young people and health-enhancing physical activity.* London: HEA.

Hoffmann, D. (2004). *Young people's lifestyles and sedentariness. The case of Switzerland and Austria.* Essen: University of Duisburg-Essen.

IOTF (2004). *International Obesity Task Force data, based on population weighted estimates from published and unpublished surveys, 1990-2002 (latest available) using IOTF recommended cut-offs for overweight and obesity.*

Junrimäe, T. & Volbekiene, V. (1998). Eurofit test results in Estonia and Lithuania for 11 to 17-year-old children: a comparative study (abstract). *European Journal of Physical Education, 3 (2)*, 178.

Kemper, H.C.G. (Ed.) (2004). *Amsterdam growth and health longitudinal study*. Basle: Karger.

Kemper, H. C. G. & Van Mechelen, W. (1996). Physical fitness testing of children. A European perspective. *Pediatric Exercise Science, 2*, 359-371.

Kersting, M., Alexy, U., Kroke, A. & Lentze, M. J. (2004). Kinderernährung in Deutschland. Ergebnisse der DONALD-Studie. *Bundesgesundheitsblatt – Gesundheitsforschung – Gesundheitsschutz, 47*, 213-218.

Knop, P. de, Engström, L.M. & Skirstad, B. (Eds.) (1996). *Worldwide Trends in Youth Sport*. Champaign/Ill.: Human Kinetics.

Kurz, D. (2001). Bewegen sich Kinder und Jugendliche heute weniger als früher? In Club of Cologne (Ed.) (2001), *Special edition from the Second Conference of the Club of Cologne*, 25 Sept. 2001.

MPFS (Medienpädagogischer Forschungsverbund Südwest) (1998-2005). *JIM-Studien*. Accessed on 1 March 2006 from http://www.mpfs.de/studien/jim/

Naul, R., Telama, R. & Rychtecky, A. (1997). Physical Fitness and Active Lifestyle of Czech, Finnish and German Youth. *Kinanthropologica, 33 (2)*, 5-15.

Prescott-Clarke, P. & Primatesta, P. (ed.) (1998). *Health survey for England: The health of young people 1995-1997*. Vol. 1. London: The stationery office.

Pühse, U. & Gerber, M. (2005) (Ed.). *International Comparison of Physical Education. Concepts – Problems – Prospects*. Aachen: Meyer and Meyer.

Raczek, J. (2002). Entwicklungsveränderungen der motorischen Leistungsfähigkeit der Schuljugend in drei Jahrzehnten (1965-1995). *Sportwissenschaft, 32 (2)*, 201-216.

Richter, Ch. (2006). *Konzepte für den Schulsport in Europa. Bewegung, Sport und Gesundheit*. Aachen: Meyer & Meyer.

Rychtecky, A. (2004) *Study on young people's lifestyles and sedentariness and the role of sport in the context of education and as a means of restoring the balance. Czech, Polish, Slovak and Slovenian cases*. Prague: Charles University of Prague.

Strel, J., Kovac, M., & Jurak, G. (2004). *Study on young people's lifestyles and sedentariness and the role of sport in the context of education and as a means of restoring the balance*. Case of Slovenia. Ljubljana: University of Ljubljana.

Swiss Federal Office for Spatial Development, Federal Statistical Office (2001). *Mobilität in der Schweiz. Ergebnisse des Mikrozensus 2000 zum Verkehrsverhalten*. Berne and Neuenburg: BBL.

Telama, R., Naul, R., Nupponen, H., Rychtecky, A. & Vuolle, P. (2002). *Physical fitness, sporting lifestyles, and Olympic ideals: cross-cultural studies on youth sports in Europe*. Schorndorf: Karl Hofmann.

Chapter 2:
Physical fitness and physical activity patterns of European youth

Neil Armstrong

Physical activity and physical fitness are often used interchangeably but they are not synonymous and before proceeding the terms require clarification. Physical activity is a complex set of behaviours that encompass any bodily movement produced by skeletal muscles that results in energy expenditure (Casperson, Powell, & Christenson, 1985). Physical activity is therefore a component of total energy expenditure, which also includes resting metabolism, growth and the thermic effect of food.

Physical fitness is a complex phenomenon that is difficult to define in the context of health It can be conceived as a set of attributes that people have or achieve and that relate to the ability to perform physical activity (Casperson et al., 1985). Thus defined, physical fitness includes discrete components such as aerobic (or cardiorespiratory) fitness, muscle strength, muscle power, flexibility, agility, balance, reaction time and body composition. The physical fitness component most frequently associated with health is aerobic fitness and this review, although acknowledging the importance of other components of physical fitness, will therefore focus on aerobic fitness.

Relevant studies for review were located through computer searches of Medline, Sport Discus and personal databases supplemented with an extensive search of bibliographies of accessed studies and through personal contacts with colleagues in other European countries. Where data from specific countries were sparse embassies were requested to provide departmental contacts.

Aerobic Fitness

Aerobic fitness depends upon the pulmonary, cardiovascular and haematological components of oxygen delivery and the oxidative mechanisms of the exercising muscle. Maximal oxygen uptake (VO_2 max), the highest rate at which an individual can consume oxygen during exercise, limits the capacity to perform aerobic exercise and is widely recognized as the best single measure of adults' aerobic fitness (American College of Sports Medicine, 1995). The conventional criterion for the attainment of VO_2 max during a progressive exercise test is a levelling-off or plateau of VO_2 but it is well-documented that the majority of young people can exercise to exhaustion without demonstrating a true VO_2 max plateau (Armstrong, Kirby, McManus, & Welsman, 1995). The appropriate term to use with children and adolescents is therefore peak oxygen uptake (peak VO_2), the highest oxygen uptake observed during an exercise test to exhaustion, rather than VO_2 max which conventionally implies the existence of a VO_2 plateau (Armstrong & Davies, 1984). If the determination of peak VO_2 is rigorously monitored it can be regarded as a maximal index of young people's aerobic fitness (Armstrong, Welsman, & Winsley, 1996) and it will therefore be used as the criterion measure of aerobic fitness in this review.

In the laboratory, peak VO_2 has been shown to be a reliable measure of aerobic fitness (Welsman, Bywater, Farr, Welford, & Armstrong, 2005) but scores may differ according to the ergometer used in the exercise protocol. Treadmills engage a larger muscle mass during exercise than cycle ergometers and the peak VO_2 obtained is less likely to be limited by local muscle fatigue. Treadmill scores are therefore consistently 8-10 % higher than those determined during cycle ergometry (Boileau, Bonen, Heyward, & Massey, 1977) and in any comparison of fitness levels this needs to be taken into account.

The laboratory assessment of peak VO_2 requires technical expertise and sophisticated apparatus (Armstrong & Welsman, 2000a) and as a result a number of performance tests have been developed to estimate aerobic fitness, with the 20 m shuttle run (20mSRT) emerging as the most popular test (Leger & Lambert, 1982). It has been demonstrated that a large part of the variability in the 20mSRT can be explained by variability in peak VO_2 (Tomkinson, Leger, Olds, & Cazonla, 2003) but factors other than peak VO_2 also contribute to 20mSRT performance. These factors include running efficiency, body mass and composition, anaerobic capacity, environmental differences, clothing, running surfaces, test familiarisation, and motivation (Armstrong & Welsman, 1994). With young children attention spans, motor skills and cognitive ability may affect 20mSRT scores but even in laboratory determinations of peak VO_2 data from children of less than 8 years of age need to be evaluated cautiously (Armstrong & Welsman, 1994). Although there is no real substitute for a laboratory determination of peak VO_2 this review will use 20mSRT or similar performance test data as an estimate of aerobic fitness if no, or limited, peak VO_2 data have been located in a European Union (EU) member state.

The aerobic fitness of European youth has been documented since Åstrand's (1954) pioneering studies of Swedish young people over 50 years ago. Studies of aerobic fitness have emerged from France (Falgairette, Bedu, Fellmann, Van Praagh, & Coudert, 1991; Flandrois, Grandmontagne, Mayet, Favier, & Frutoso, 1982), the Netherlands (Binkhorst, Van't Hof, & Saris, 1992; Saris, Noordeloos, Ringnalda, Van't Hof, & Binkhorst, 1985), Sweden (Ekelund, Poortvleit et al., 2001; Sunnegardh & Bratteby, 1987), Poland (Prezewada & Dobosz, 2003; Wilczewski, Sklad, Krawczyk, Saask, & Majle, 1996), United Kingdom (Armstrong et al., 1995; Armstrong et al., 1991), Belgium (Van Gerven &

Vanden Eynde, 1987; Weymans, Reybrouck, Stijns, & Knops, 1986), Estonia (Raudsepp & Jurimae, 1996; Sallo & Viru, 1996), Lithuania (Jurimae & Volbekiene, 1998), Hungary (Farkas, Petrekanits, MészáRos, & Mohács, 1992; Szabó & Pápai, 1997), Czechoslovakia (Macek & Vavra, 1971; Seliger et al., 1971), Czech Republic (Telema, Naul, Nupponen, Rychtecky, & Vualle, 2002; Bunc, 2000), Denmark (Hansen, Froberg, Hydlebrandt, & Nielsen, 1991; Hasselstrom, Hansen, Frobert, & Andersen, 2002), Greece (Koutedakis & Bouziotas, 2003; Maniôs, Kafatos, & Codrington, 1999), Germany (Mocellin, Lindemann, Rutenfranz, & Sbreny, 1971; Rychtecky, Naul, & Neuhaus, 1996), Italy (Ceretelli, Aghemo, & Rovelli, 1963; Cilia & Bellucci, 1993), Ireland (Watson & O'Donovan, 1976), Austria (Gaisl & Buchberger, 1977), Latvia (Aberberga-Augskalne, 2002), Portugal (Guerra, Ribeiro, Coita, Duarte, & Mota, 2002; Mota et al., 2002), Slovenia (Kovaĉ, Jurak, Strel, & Bednarik, 2003; Kovaĉ & Strel, 2000), Finland (Sundberg & Elovainio, 1982), and Spain (Sainz, 1996). No data have been located from Luxembourg, Slovakia, Cyprus or Malta. Longitudinal studies are sparse but data on Dutch (Kemper, 1995), German (Rutenfranz, Andersen, Seliger, Klimmer, Berndt et al., 1981) and British (Armstrong & Welsman, 2001; Armstrong, Williams, Balding, Gentle, & Kirby, 1991) children and Czech boys (Sprynarova, Parizkova, & Bunc, 1987) have been published and longitudinal studies of trained children from the United Kingdom (Baxter-Jones, Goldstein, & Helms, 1993) and Poland (Beunen, Rogers, Woynarowska, & Malina, 1997) are available.

No data are available on randomly selected groups of children although one study provides data on a sample representative of Danish 16 to 19 year olds (Andersen, Henckel, & Saltin, 1987). Some studies have defined their sample in relation to the population (Armstrong, et al., 1995; Armstrong et al., 1991) but participants are volunteers and selection bias cannot be ruled out, as relatively few participants are likely to be drawn from the markedly sedentary or overweight sections of the population. Few studies have defined the maturity status of their participants and this confounds direct comparisons between studies. Sample sizes are generally small, particularly in those studies which measured peak VO_2 directly, and not necessarily representative of any country or region. This prevents valid comparisons of youth peak VO_2 across countries although some studies using the 20mSRT have been carried out (Jurimae & Volbekiene, 1998; Telema, Naul, Nupponen, Rychtecky, & Vualle, 2002). Nevertheless, both cross-sectional and longitudinal studies provide a consistent picture of the aerobic fitness of European youth.

Aerobic Fitness and Age

Cross-sectional data from EU countries indicate that boys' peak VO_2 demonstrates a progressive increase in relation to chronological age. Girls' data demonstrate a similar but less consistent trend with a tendency for peak VO_2 to level-off from about 13-14 years of age.

Longitudinal studies provide a more secure analysis of aerobic fitness in relation to age but only four studies of untrained children and adolescents from EU states have been published. Studies of German and Dutch children and Czech boys were initiated in the 1970s. Rutenfranz et al (1981) determined the peak VO_2 of 28 boys and 24 girls on a cycle ergometer annually from the age of 12.7 to 17.8 years. Sprynarova et al. (1987) determined the peak VO_2 of 90 Czech boys from age 11 to 15 years and then followed 36 of the boys for a further 3 years. The Amsterdam Growth and Health Study (Kemper, 1985, 2004) is a 23 year follow-up study of young people aged 13 at the start of the project and it provides annual peak VO_2 data on about 80 boys and 97 girls from the age of 13 to 16 years. More recently in the United Kingdom, Armstrong et al. (1999) reported annual peak VO_2 measures on about 90 boys and 90 girls from ages 11 to 13 years and then re-tested 37 of the boys and 26 of the girls at age 17.0 years (Armstrong & Welsman, 2001).

The boys' data are consistent and the two longer studies (Sprynarova et al 1987; Armstrong and Welsman, 2001) show peak VO_2 to double over the age range 11 to 17/18 years. The largest annual increase occurred between 13 and 14 years in all studies covering this age range. Dutch boys showed a 38 % increase in peak VO_2 between 13 and 16 years of age. Girls' data are less clear and peak VO_2 appears to progressively rise from 11 to 13 years and then level-off from about age 14 years. The British girls exhibited about a 45 % increase in peak VO_2 from 11 to 17 years whereas the German girls' aerobic fitness declined from 14.7 years and by 15.7 years mean values were below those at 12.7 years with a continuing decline through to 17.8 years. This fall in aerobic fitness amongst German girls might have been an artefact of the motivation of the participants as the authors noted that some of the girls aged 16 and 17 years refused to take part in the tests at that age. Dutch girls observed from 13 to 16 years exhibited a levelling-off, but not a reduction, in peak VO_2 with only a 2 % increase (2.60 to 2.65 L·min^{-1}) from 14 to 16 years. This is generally consistent with findings from cross-sectional studies.

The increase in aerobic fitness with age during childhood and adolescence may be explained by examining the components of peak VO_2. Minute ventilation at peak VO_2 seldom exceeds values greater than 70 % of maximal voluntary ventilation (Armstrong, Kirby, McManus, & Welsman, 1997) and although there are age, growth, maturation and sex differences (Rowland, 2000a) in exercise ventilation and its constituents, tidal volume and respiratory frequency, ventilation does not limit the peak VO_2 of healthy children and adolescents.

Peak VO_2 is a function of cardiac output and arteriovenous oxygen difference but our understanding of cardiac output is clouded by the methodological limitations of measuring it during maximal exercise (Driscoll, Staats, & Beck, 1989). Nevertheless, the few data that are available consistently indicate that cardiac output at peak VO_2 increases with age in both sexes (Rowland, 2000b). The components of cardiac output are heart rate and stroke volume and although maximal heart rate is subject to wide individual variations it is independent of both age and sex (Rowland, 2000b). The increase in cardiac output at peak VO_2 with age is therefore wholly due to stroke volume, which increases parallel to left ventricular size (Rowland, 2000b).

Arteriovenous oxygen difference at peak VO_2 is calculated from measurements of peak VO_2 and estimates of the related cardiac output via the Fick equation (oxygen uptake = cardiac output x arteriovenous oxygen difference) and therefore few secure data are available. Evidence is equivocal with some authors reporting age-related increases in arteriovenous oxygen difference (Rowland, Popowski, & Ferrone, 1997) and others observing no relationship with age (Yamaji & Miyashita, 1977). Although data showing an age-related increase in arteriovenous oxygen difference must be treated cautiously the lower blood haemoglobin concentration in children than adults (Dallman & Siimes, 1979) supports the premise that adults have a greater arterial oxygen content and therefore potentially a higher arteriovenous oxygen difference. However, children can at least partially compensate for their lower blood haemoglobin as they have been observed to have a greater facility than adults for unloading oxygen at the tissues (Cassels & Morse 1962) and this may be influenced by the decline in 2,3 diphosphoglycerate with age (Kalafoutis, Paterakis, Koutselinis, & Spanos, 1976).

The rise in peak VO_2 with age during childhood and adolescence appears to be primarily due to an increase in stroke volume and therefore cardiac output. Arteriovenous oxygen difference may increase with age, but additional insights into oxygen delivery and subsequent oxidative metabolism at peak VO_2 are dependent on technological advances in non-invasive methodology.

Aerobic Fitness and Growth

Peak VO_2 is strongly related to body size with correlation coefficients describing its relationship with body mass or stature typically exceeding $r = 0.70$ (Armstrong & Welsman, 1994). Thus, much of the age-related increase in peak VO_2 reflects the overall increase in body size during the transition from childhood through adolescence. As most physical activities involve moving body mass from one place to another, to compare the aerobic fitness of young people who differ in body mass, peak VO_2 is conventionally expressed in relation to mass as millilitres of oxygen per kilogram body mass per minute (ie $mL \cdot kg^{-1} \cdot min^{-1}$).

When peak VO_2 is expressed in ratio with body mass, a different picture emerges from that apparent when absolute values ($L \cdot kg^{-1}$) are used. Boys' mass-related peak VO_2 remains remarkably stable with values approximating 48-50 $mL \cdot kg^{-1} \cdot min^{-1}$ whereas girls' values show a tendency to fall with increasing age, from about 45 $mL \cdot kg^{-1} \cdot min^{-1}$ to 39 $mL \cdot kg^{-1} \cdot min^{-1}$ (Armstrong & Welsman, 1994). Individual longitudinal studies generally confirm the stability of boys' mass-related peak VO_2 with age although there are reports of both an increase (Sprynarova et al., 1987) and a decrease (Rutenfranz et al., 1981) in mass-related peak VO_2 between 12 and 14 years of age. Longitudinal studies of girls' mass-related peak VO_2 show unequivocally a progressive decline with age (Rutenfranz et al., 1981; Van Mechelen & Kemper, 1995). Boys demonstrate higher mass-related peak VO_2 than girls throughout childhood and adolescence, the sex difference being reinforced by the greater accumulation of body fat by girls during puberty (Armstrong & Welsman, 2000a).

Although the expression of peak VO_2 in ratio with body mass is the conventional method of partitioning out the influence of body mass compelling arguments have been presented to question the validity of using simple ratio scaling to remove the influence of body size from size dependent performance measures such as peak VO_2. The theoretical and statistical principles involved are beyond the scope of this review but we have discussed them in detail elsewhere (Welsman & Armstrong, 2000a, 2000b).

Several studies have produced findings that illustrate how inappropriate scaling using ratio standards can lead to misplaced interpretation of physiological mechanisms. For instance, Williams, Armstrong, Winter and Crichton (1992) used a linear regression model to investigate changes in peak VO_2 with chronological age in two groups of boys aged 10 and 15 years. The mean values for mass-related peak VO_2 in the two groups were, as expected, not significantly different. However, the regression lines for the relationship between peak VO_2 and body mass described two clearly different populations and led to the conclusion that for a given body mass, older boys have a significantly higher peak VO_2 than younger ones. The same group (Welsman, Armstrong, Kirby, Nevill, & Winter, 1996) used both ratio and allometric (log-linear analysis of covariance) scaling to remove the effects of body size from peak VO_2 in groups of prepubertal boys and girls, circumpubertal boys and girls, and adult men and women. In males, the conventional ratio analyses were consistent with the extant literature and demonstrated no significant differences between the groups. In contrast, the allometric analyses revealed significant, progressive increases in peak VO_2 across groups, indicating that relative to body mass peak VO_2

increases with growth rather than remaining static. Analysis of the females' data also challenged conventional findings. Mass-related peak VO_2 followed the expected pattern with no change from prepuberty to circumpuberty but a significant decrease from circumpuberty to adulthood. The allometrically scaled data demonstrated that, relative to body mass, female's peak VO_2 increases into puberty and is then maintained into young adulthood.

Despite the differences in the patterns of change in peak VO_2 with age revealed with body size controlled by allometric scaling, studies which have concurrently examined sex differences have shown that these remain when allometric scaling models are applied (Armstrong et al., 1995; Welsman et al., 1996).

The application of allometry to longitudinal data is complex, but the recent emergence of multilevel modelling techniques (Goldstein et al., 1998) has enabled body size, age and sex effects to be partitioned concurrently within an allometric framework. Armstrong and Welsman (2001) used multilevel modelling to analyse their longitudinal data and confirmed the cross-sectional findings of Welsman et al. (1996) that over the age range 11 to 17 years peak VO_2 increases with age in both boys and girls even with body mass and stature controlled. Peak VO_2 remained lower in girls than boys with sex differences increasing over the age range observed.

Aerobic Fitness and Maturation

As young people grow they also mature and the physiological responses of adolescents must be considered in relation to biological as well as chronological age. Relatively few studies have investigated the relationship between peak VO_2 and maturity, perhaps because of the difficulty in assessing maturity. In the exercise sciences, maturity is usually assessed using indicators of skeletal, sexual or somatic maturation or serum hormone concentrations. No single assessment gives a complete description of the tempo of maturation but there is a reasonably high concordance between them (Beunen, 1989).

Kemper and Verschuur (1981) used skeletal age as an indicator of maturity in 375 Dutch children aged 13 to 14 years. The skeletal age of the sample ranged from 9 to 16 years and a multiple regression analysis revealed that the increase in peak VO_2 with increasing skeletal age was completely due to the increase in body size. Welsman, Armstrong and Kirby (1994) observed that serum testosterone concentration made no significant contribution to the explained variance in the peak VO_2 of 12 to 16-year-old English boys beyond the 74 % accounted for by age, stature and mass.

In a study of 176 English 12-year-olds classified according to Tanner's indices for pubic hair, Armstrong, Welsman and Kirby (1998a) demonstrated in both boys and girls a significant effect of maturation on peak VO_2 independent of chronological age and body mass. Armstrong and Welsman (2001) used the same criteria of maturation in their longitudinal study of 11 to 17-year-olds and demonstrated, using multi-level modelling, an incremental effect of stage of maturation on peak VO_2 independent of age, body mass or fatness. The positive effect of maturation on aerobic fitness was consistent for both boys and girls.

There is some evidence from longitudinal studies of Canadian (Mirwald & Bailey, 1986) and Japanese (Kobayashi et al., 1978) children that the greatest increase in peak VO_2 is associated with the attainment of peak height velocity (PHV) in both boys and girls. However, Beunen and Malina (1988), in their critical review of research concerning peak VO_2 and the adolescent growth spurt, commented that the available data should be interpreted with caution, and concluded that the evidence suggests a spurt in peak VO_2 in boys, which reaches a maximum gain at the time of PHV. Secure data are insufficient to offer any generalization for girls.

Aerobic Fitness and Sex

Boys' peak VO_2 values are consistently higher than those of girls by late childhood and the sex difference becomes more pronounced as young people progress through adolescence. Sex differences during childhood and adolescence have been attributed to a combination of factors including habitual physical activity, body composition and blood haemoglobin concentration.

Boys are more physically active than girls (Armstrong, 1998; Armstrong & VanMechelen, 1998) but the evidence relating habitual physical activity to young people's peak VO_2 is weak (Armstrong, Balding, Gentle, Williams, & Kirby, 1990a; Morrow & Freedson, 1994) and the issue is confounded by problems with accurately assessing children's and adolescents' physical activity patterns (Armstrong & Welsman, 1997; Trost, 2001). The nature of young people's daily physical activity is not conducive to the promotion of aerobic fitness (see later in this review) and habitual physical activity is therefore unlikely to contribute to sex differences in peak VO_2.

Muscle mass increases through childhood and although boys generally have more muscle mass than girls, marked sex differences do not become apparent until the adolescent growth spurt. Girls experience an adolescent spurt in muscle mass but it is less dramatic than that of boys. Between 5 and 16 years boys' relative muscle mass increases from 42 to 54 % of body mass whereas in girls muscle mass increases from 40 to 45 % of body mass between 5 and 13 years and then, in relative terms, it declines due to an increase in fat accumulation during adolescence. Girls have slightly more body fat than boys during childhood but during the adolescent growth spurt, girls' body fat increases to about 25 % of body mass while boys' declines to about 12 to 14 % (Malina & Bouchard, 1991). These dramatic changes in body composition during puberty are highly likely to contribute to the progressive increase in sex differences in peak VO_2 over this period. Boys' greater muscle mass will not only facilitate the use of oxygen during exercise but will also supplement the venous return to the heart and therefore augment stroke volume (Rowland & Lisowski, 2001).

During puberty there is a marked increase in blood haemoglobin concentration and hence oxygen-carrying capacity in boys whereas girls' values plateau around 13 years of age (Dallman & Siimes, 1979). The difference in haemoglobin concentration between boys and girls, which is about 11 % at 16 years, is likely to be a contributory factor to the sex difference in peak VO_2 and by the midteens boys' superior haemoglobin concentration augments their greater muscle mass in attaining higher peak VO_2 than girls.

Prior to puberty there are small sex differences in muscle mass and haemoglobin concentration is independent of sex until 12 years of age yet prepubertal boys have higher levels of aerobic fitness than prepubertal girls. For example, Armstrong et al. (1995) determined the aerobic fitness of 164 11-year-old prepubertal children (ie Tanner stage one for pubic hair and either breast or genitalia rating) and reported a 22 % higher peak VO_2 in the boys. With the removal of the influence of body mass using allometry the boys' peak VO_2 remained significantly higher (16 %) than the girls' despite there being no sex differences in either skinfold thickness or haemoglobin concentration. There is no evidence to indicate sex differences in either heart rate or arteriovenous oxygen difference at peak VO_2 and prepubertal boys' higher peak VO_2 has been attributed to a greater stroke volume (Vinet et al., 2003).

Are Young People Fit?

There is no consensus about levels of optimal aerobic fitness for children and adolescents. Nevertheless, an expert group drawn from the European Group of Pediatric Work Physiology suggested that it may be possible to express a lower limit of peak VO_2 that, in the absence of other health-related problems may represent a "health risk" (Bell, Macek, Rutenfranz, & Saris, 1986). They proposed 35 $mL \cdot kg^{-1} \cdot min^{-1}$ for boys and 30 $mL\ kg^{-1} \cdot min^{-1}$ for girls. They also suggested levels greater than 40 $mL\ kg^{-1} \cdot min^{-1}$ for boys and 35 $mL\ kg^{-1} \cdot min^{-1}$ for girls may be used as "health indicators". The European Group of Pediatric Work Physiology agreed these recommendations but no empirical evidence was provided in support of the thresholds.

Few studies have reported their results in sufficient detail to estimate the number of young people falling below these levels of peak VO_2. Kemper and Verschuur (1990) analysed data from 200 participants in the Amsterdam Growth Study and reported that the percentage of males "at risk" increased from 1 to 8 % over the age range 13 to 17 years and the percentage of females falling into this category rose from 3 to 17 % over the same time span. The higher percentage of females "at risk" was partly explained by the extra gain in body mass caused by the sex-specific increase in body fat during puberty. A re-working of Armstrong et al. (1991) data on 220 11 to 16-year-old British children revealed that 3 % of the boys and 3 % of the girls could be classified as "at risk". A study of a representative sample of 164 English 11-year-old prepubertal children (Armstrong et al. 1995) reported that all children had values of peak VO_2 above the "health risk" threshold. All girls demonstrated a level of aerobic fitness above the "health indicator" threshold only two boys had peak VO_2 values below 40 $mL·kg^{-1}·min^{-1}$. Much of the variation in the three studies can be attributed to the use of the ratio standard ($mL· kg^{-1}·min^{-1}$) in the expression of peak VO_2 as heavier (usually older) children are penalised and lighter (usually younger) children are favoured by this method of scaling.

The aerobic fitness of European children and adolescents compares favourably with that of young people from elsewhere (Armstrong, 1995; Armstrong & Welsman, 1994). Scrutiny of published values of peak VO_2 reveals that the "health risk" threshold is at least a standard deviation below mean values suggesting that relatively few young people fall into this category.

Secular Trends in Aerobic Fitness

Observation of the results of studies over the last 50 years suggests a consistency over time in young people's peak VO_2 (Armstrong and Welsman, 1994; Armstrong and Van Mechelen, 1998) but no study involving direct determinations of the peak VO_2 of European youth has specifically addressed the issue of secular trends in aerobic fitness. Published values of peak VO_2 are not population-representative values and the data could be interpreted as the peak VO_2 of young people volunteering for exercise studies has not changed much over the last five decades.

Several studies have investigated secular trends using performance tests (Strel, Kovač & Jurak, 2004; Westerstahl, Barnekow-Bergkvist, Hedberg, & Jansson, 2003; Przeweda & Dobosz, 2003) to predict peak VO_2. Tomkinson et al. (2003) reviewed 55 studies of the 20mSRT in 11 countries, including 9 current EU member states, over the period 1980-2000. There was a great deal of variability between countries in the magnitude of secular changes in performance ranging, in EU countries, from an increase of 0.5 % per year in Greek girls to a decrease of 1.4 % per year in Greek boys. When sample-weighted mean rates of change were calculated for age-groups rather than for countries, a more consistent trend was revealed with a reduction in aerobic fitness of 0.5 to 0.3 % per year in children and 1 % per year in adolescents. The authors noted, however, that performance fitness in running can be reduced by lower aerobic fitness or increased body fatness or both and that children and adolescents were fatter in 2000 than in 1980.

Two recently published studies from Scandanavia (Ekblom, Oddson, & Ekblom, 2004; Wedderkop, Froberg, Hansen, & Andersen, 2004) used laboratory-based tests to predict peak oxygen uptake (mL· kg^{-1}·min^{-1}). Ekblom et al. (2004) used the Åstrand-Ryhming normogram to predict the peak VO$_2$ (mL· kg^{-1}·min^{-1}) of Swedish 10, 13 and 16-year-olds in 1987 and 2001. The initial study included 538 boys and 415 girls and the second observation involved 503 boys and 408 girls. The boys' aerobic fitness was reported to decline by 12 % from 1987 to 2001 but no significant change was observed in girls' predicted peak VO$_2$.

In the only published study to use a maximal laboratory-based test of aerobic fitness, Wedderkop et al. (2004) analysed secular trends through two cross-sectional surveys performed 12 years apart on representative samples of 9-year-old children from Odense, Denmark. In 1985-86, 670 girls and 699 boys participated in the study and in 1997-98 310 girls and 279 boys participated. On both occasions fitness was determined by a maximal work test (watt-max test) which involved the children exercising to exhaustion on a cycle ergometer. The data were then used to predict peak VO$_2$ in mL·kg^{-1}·min^{-1}. The boys in 1997-98 had a lower predicted mass-related peak VO$_2$ and a higher fat percentage than those in 1985-86, whereas no overall differences in peak VO$_2$ or fatness were found between girls in 1997-98 or 1985-86. The percentage of children who exceeded internationally accepted BMI thresholds of obesity was significantly greater in 1997-98 than in 1985-86.

Wedderkopp et al. (2004) split their sample into deciles and noted that in 1997-98, the most fit boys had the same level of fitness as in 1985-86, and the most fit girls had a significantly higher level of fitness in 1997-98 than in 1985-86. Both the girls and boys with the poorest fitness level in 1997-98 had a significantly lower level of fitness than the poorest fitness levels of girls and boys from 1985-86 respectively. The authors observed that the difference between the least fit and the most fit increased over time in both boys and girls. In boys, the difference between the top 10 % and the lowest 10 %, in aerobic fitness expressed in relation to body mass, was 38 % in 1985-86 and 45 % in 1997-98. The same polarization was found in girls, with a difference between the top 10 % and the lowest 10 % of 37 % in 1985-86 and 44 % in 1997-98. However, the decrease in predicted peak VO$_2$ (mL· kg^{-1}·min^{-1}) from 1985-86 to 1997-98 in the least fit was partly explained by a higher body mass.

Data examining secular trends in aerobic fitness are sparse and although predictions of peak VO$_2$ indicate a decrease in aerobic fitness the methodology used in published studies suggests that it may be a reflection of the rise in paediatric obesity throughout Europe over the last 20 years (Livingstone, 2001) rather than a true reduction in peak VO_2. Nevertheless, Wedderkopp et al's (2004) report indicates an emerging polarisation with the difference between fit and unfit young people increasing over time. Furthermore, it appears that the secular increase in body mass is not being accompanied by a proportional increase in aerobic fitness with the inevitable result that in activities which involve moving body mass young people's maximal performance is declining.

Physical Activity Guidelines

The habitual physical activity of children and adolescents is difficult to interpret but two major conferences have provided guidelines or recommendations for young people's activity in the context of promoting health. In 1993, an International Consensus Conference on Physical Activity Guidelines for Adolescents (ICC) was convened in California "to develop empirically based guidelines that can be used by clinicians in their counselling, as well as by policy makers with responsibility for youth health promotion" (Sallis, Patrick, & Long, 1994). The literature was systematically reviewed to provide an evidence base (Sallis & Patrick, 1994) and two guidelines were propsed: i) all adolescents should be physically active daily or nearly every day, as part of play games, sports, work, transportation, recreation, physical education or planned exercise, in the context of family, school, and community activities; and ii) adolescents should engage in three or more sessions per week of activities that last 20 minutes or more at a time and that require moderate to vigorous levels of exertion. Moderate to vigorous activities were defined as those that require at least as much effort as brisk or fast walking. The ICC guidelines informed youth physical activity studies throughout the 1990s.

In 1998 in England, the Health Education Authority (HEA) hosted a similar conference based on a series of reviews of the scientific paediatric literature which updated those of the ICC (Biddle, Sallis, & Cavill, 1998). The primary recommendation to emerge was that all young people should participate in physical activity of at least moderate intensity for one hour per day and that young people who currently do little activity should participate in physical activity of at least moderate intensity for at least half an hour per day. The secondary recommendation was that at least twice a week, some of these activities should help to enhance and maintain muscular strength and flexibility and bone health (Biddle et al., 1998).

The HEA's primary recommendation shifted the emphasis from vigorous to moderate intensity physical activity, and from sustained periods of activity to activity accumulated over a day. The recommendation was intended to take into account the current physical activity patterns and lifestyles of young people, so that it represented an attainable goal. However, the evidence that health benefits might be gained from accumulating moderate intensity activity in short bouts over a day has been challenged (Barinaga, 1997; Hardman, 1999). Nevertheless, this recommendation has been influential in the conclusions drawn from recent studies of young people's physical activity.

Physical Activity of European Youth

More than 30 methods of estimating physical activity have been identified but the reliability, objectivity and validity of many of these methods have not established with young people. Methodological issues have been discussed at length elsewhere (Sirard & Pate, 2001; Trost, 2001, Armstrong & Van Mechelen, 1998; Armstrong & Welsman, 1997) and will not be addressed further here. For the purpose of this review I will focus on data generated through self-report, direct observation, heart rate monitoring and accelerometry.

Self-Report

Self-report is the widely used method in epidemiological research due to ease and low costs of implementation. Self-report methods include retrospective questionnaires, interview-administered recall, activity diaries and mail surveys. Proxy reports by parents and/or teachers have been employed in studies with children and some studies have estimated level of physical activity through self-report of surrogate measures such as sports participation. The use of self-report techniques is common in studies of children's physical activity but in anything but large studies with high statistical power the data need to be interpreted cautiously. Studies of non-representative samples of young people are widely available and data have emerged from Belgium (Deforce et al., 2003; Guillaume, Lapidus, Bjorntorp, & Lambert, 1997), Ireland (Hussey, Gormley, & Bell, 2001; O'Sullivan, 2002), Austria (Currie, Hurrelmann, Settertobulte, Smith, & Todd, 2000; King & Coles, 1992), United Kingdom (Riddoch, 1990; Heartbeat Wales,1986), Italy (Marella, Colli, & Faina, 1986; Currie, Roberts, Morgan, Smith, Settertobulte, Samda, & Barnekow-Rasmussen, 2004), Spain (Cantera-Garde & Devís-Devís, 2000; King & Coles, 1992), Finland (Silvennionen, 1984; Telama et al., 1985), Hungary (Currie et al., 2000; King & Coles, 1992), Greece (Bouziotas & Koutedaiks, 2003; Maniôs, Kafatos, & Markakis, 1998), France (Deheeger, Rolland-Cachera, & Fontvielle, 1997; Vermorel, Vernet, Bitar, Fellman, & Coudert, 2002), Sweden (Engstrom, 1980; Sunnegardh, Bratteby, Sjolin, Hagman, & Hoffstedt, 1985), Poland (Currie et al., 2000; King & Coles, 1992), Germany (Fuchs et al., 1988; Rutenfranz, Berndt, & Knauth, 1974), Portugal (Guerra, Duarte, & Mota, 2001; Ribeiro et al., 2003), Denmark (Andersen & Schelin, 1994; Hasselstrom, Hansen, Froberg, & Andersen, 2002) , Lithuania (Currie et al., 2000; King, Wold, Tudor-Smith, & Harel, 1996), Cyprus (Loucaides, Chedzoy, Bennett, & Wolshe, 2004), Latvia (Aberberga-Augskalne, 2002; Currie et al., 2000), Czechoslovakia (Seliger, Trefny, Bartenkova, & Pauer, 1974), the Czech Republic (Naul, Telema, & Rychtécky, 1997; Telema et al., 2002), Malta (Currie et al., 2004), Slovenia (Jurak, Kovaĉ, & Strel, 2003; Jurak, Kovaĉ, Strel, & Stara, 2003), Slovakia (King et al., 1996) and Estonia (Raudsepp, Liblik, & Hannus, 2002; Sallo & Viru, 1996). There are no data on young people from Luxembourg. Levels of physical activity cannot be confidently compared across studies, but age and gender-related data are consistent and I will use a recent, large World Health Organisation (WHO) study to illustrate trends across Europe.

The 2001/02 WHO survey (Currie et al., 2004) involved 22 EU countries and 115,981 young people aged 11, 13 or 15 years. The national sample sizes varied from 1,980 in Malta to 14,372 in the United Kingdom. The German sample of 5,650 participants was regional and selected from Berlin, Hessen, North Rhine-Westphalia and Saxony. The data were collected from October 2001 to June 2002.

The participants were provided with a definition of physical activity as,' any activity that increases your heart rate and makes you out of breath some of the time. Physical activity can be done in sports, school activities, playing with friends, or walking to school. Some examples of physical activity are running, brisk walking, rollerblading, biking, dancing, skateboarding, swimming, soccer, basketball, football and surfing" (Currie et al., 2004, p 91).

The methodology was informed by the UKHEA physical activity guidelines and the participants were asked to, "add up all the time you spend in physical activity each day". About a third of young people met the UKHEA guidelines on physical activity. There were, however, wide variations across countries and although cross-country comparisons must be made cautiously Austria, Finland, Malta, Wales, Greece, Hungary, Latvia, Estonia, Portugal, Germany, Italy, Belgium and France were showed to have fewer than 20 % of 15-year-old girls reported to meet the recommendation. Comparisons within countries are more secure and in all countries more boys than girls reported being physically active for 60 minutes a day at least five times a week although the gender differences were small in some countries (eg among 15-year-olds, 1 % in the Netherlands and 5 % in Italy) but marked in others (eg among 15-year-olds, 25 % in Malta and 22 % in Wales). In all countries except boys in France and the Czech Republic, fewer 15-year-olds than 11-year-olds met the HEA criterion and in France and the Czech Republic more 13-year-olds than 15-year-olds met the guideline. Overall, the data are remarkably consistent across Europe and show that physical activity declines with age, at least through the teen years, and that girls are less likely to be physically active than boys. There is no evidence to indicate major differences in the level of physical activity of youth living in Europe in comparison to those living in North America (Currie et al., 2000, 2004).

Direct Observation

Sleap and Warburton's (1996) studies of English children are the most comprehensive observational studies of the physical activity of European youth. They observed 93 girls and 86 boys aged 5-11 years, on separate occasions, during school break times, lunch times and physical education lessons. Further observations were undertaken on one weekday evening and one 4 hour period on either a weekend or during a school vacation. In total each child was observed for an average of 418 min. During this time children were engaged in moderate to vigorous physical activity (MVPA) for 29.3 % of total time observed. Twenty one percent of children recorded at least one sustained 20 min period of MVPA. Ninety five percent of children engaged in at least one 5 min period of MVPA and no significant differences in MVPA were observed between boys and girls. Sleap and Warburton (1996) concluded that their results were disturbing since preadolescent children appeared to be engaging in very little sustained, playful physical activity during their free time outside of school.

Heart Rate Monitoring

Heart rate studies are over 30 years old and Bradfield, Chan et al., (1971) appear to have been the first to continuously monitor the heart rates of European boys. They reported the mean energy expenditure of 54 7 to 10-year-old boys as 9.2 kJ·min^{-1} during lunchtime and play periods. Seliger et al. (1974) monitored the heart rates of 11 12-year-old Czech boys for 24 h and reported that heart rates >150 beats·min^{-1} were rare and only fleetingly encountered. They noted that "the daily activity heart rate response implied that very little circulation response was required to support the daily activity" (p 57), but they did not describe their method of monitoring in any detail.

By the end of the 1980s heart rate monitoring technology had advanced to the point where unobtrusive telemetry systems allowed monitoring over several days. Data covering at least three days of monitoring have been reported from the United Kingdom (Armstrong, Balding, Gentle, & Kirby, 1990b; Armstrong & Bray, 1991), Estonia (Sallo & Silla,1997), France (Falgariette, Bedu, Fellmann, Van Praagh, & Coudert, 1991; Gavarray, Bernard, Giacomoni, Seymat, Euzet, & Falgarette, 1998), Greece (Manios, Kafatos, & Markakis, 1998) and Sweden (Ekelund Poortvleit, Nilsson, Yngve, Homberg, & Sjostrom, 2001). The data from these studies show boys to be more physically active than girls and boys to engage in moderate and vigorous, sustained periods of physical activity more often than girls, although this type of activity is not characteristic of European youth's physical activity patterns. Heart rate monitoring studies clearly and consistently demonstrate a decline in physical activity with age (Armstrong, 1998; Armstrong et al., 2000).

Accelerometry

The most comprehensive study of European children's physical activity using accelerometry was carried out by Riddoch and his colleagues (2004) as part of the European Youth Heart Study. They collected data from well-defined populations from four countries and 2,185 children 9 and 15-year-old children had their physical activity assessed over either four days (70 %) or three days (30 %).

The results confirmed significant gender differences in physical activity with 9-year-old boys 21 % more active than girls and 15-year-old boys 26 % more active than similarly aged girls. Gender differences in time spent in activity of at least moderate intensity were even more marked (20 % and 36 % difference respectively). Similarly, 9-year-olds of both genders were considerably more active than 15-year-olds (27 % more active in boys, 32 % in girls). The age difference was even more marked with time spent in moderate activity (94 % more active in boys, 129 % more active in girls).

Riddoch et al. (2004) commented on the remarkable consistency of the results across Denmark, Portugal, Estonia and Norway. Physical activity levels and age and gender differences were mirrored across the four countries despite the wide differences in geography, socio-economic circumstances, culture and climate.

Studies involving accelerometry monitoring over at least three days have also been reported from Estonia (Raudsepp & Pall, 1998), Sweden (Skalik, Fromel, Sigmund, Vasendova, & Wirdheim, 2001; Nilsson, Ekelund, Yngve, & Sjostrom, 2002), Portugal (Guerra, Santos, Ribeiro, Duarte, & Mota, 2003; Mota, Guerra, Leandro,Pinto, Ribeiro, & Duarte 2002), the Czech Republic (Skalic et al., 2001), the United Kingdom (Mallam, Metcalfe, Kirby, Voss, & Witkin, 2003) and Poland (Skalic et al., 2001) and the data are consistent with Riddoch et al.'s findings.

Secular Trends in Physical Activity

Historical data from the period 1930 to 1980 have been provided by Durnin (1992). He pooled energy intake data collected over a 50 year period from 1930 and demonstrated a progressive decrease in the energy intake of adolescents in the United Kingdom. As body mass had not decreased over this period Durnin concluded that the only conceivable explanation for the very marked reduction in energy intake, which must reflect diminished energy expenditure, is that adolescents' physical activity decreased radically over the period surveyed. Although Durnin's (1992) data are persuasive they were collected through adolescents' self-report and therefore must be interpreted cautiously.

Objective techniques of assessing young people's physical activity have only been in use for about 15 years and only one study appears to have examined secular trends in the physical activity patterns of European youth. In the late 1980s, Armstrong and his colleagues (1990b) continuously monitored the heart rates of 11 to 16 year-olds over three weekdays and a weekend day (see table 2). Ten years later the same research team (Welsman & Armstrong, 2000b) re-visited the same communities as their original study. They used identical methodology and interpretation techniques and reported remarkable consistencies between the findings of the two studies, particularly with reference to the percentage of children achieving sustained periods of physical activity and gender and age differences in these measures. Although they found sedentary lifestyles were common they concluded that a positive outcome of the study was that a notable decline in habitual physical activity over the last decade had not been observed in this population, which was derived from stable communities which had been shown to be representative of the South of England. They tentatively suggested that several of the major environmental factors which have been implicated in the reduction of young people's physical activity since the 1970s may have already had their biggest impact on youth physical activity.

Aerobic Fitness and Physical Activity

In 1994, Morrow and Freedson (1994) identified 17 published papers which had investigated the relationship between aerobic fitness and habitual physical activity. They included studies which used performance measures and predictions of peak VO_2 from submaximal data as criterion measures of aerobic fitness and concluded that the majority of reports suggested no relationship between habitual physical activity and aerobic fitness. The median correlation from all reviewed studies was $r = 0.17$ ($r^2 < 0.03$).

Several studies involving European children and adolescents in which directly determined peak VO_2 has been used as the measure of aerobic fitness have been reported. Seliger et al. (1974) found no significant relationship between physical activity and aerobic fitness. Saris (1982) grouped his prepubescent subjects into low, middle and high activity groups, and concluded that children with different levels of maximal aerobic power do not differ substantially in their daily physical activity. Andersen, Ilmarinen et al. (1984) analysed their longitudinal data and concluded that peak VO_2 was statistically unrelated to variations in "annual sport activity score", derived from retrospective recall. Sunnegardh and Bratteby (1987) reported low but significant correlations between peak VO_2 and questionnaire-determined physical activity in 8-year-old boys ($r = 0.41$) and 13-year-old boys and girls ($r = 0.48$) but not in 8-year-old girls. The one day accelerometer scores tended to be higher in children with a higher peak VO_2 than in those with a lower one, but the differences were not statistically significant.

More recent investigations have utilized three day heart rate monitoring to estimate physical activity. In a series of studies of relatively large numbers of young people, Armstrong and his colleagues (Armstrong, et al., 1990a; Armstrong, McManus, Welsman, & Kirby, 1996; Armstrong, Welsman, & Kirby, 1998b) reported no significant relationships between measures of moderate and vigorous physical activity and peak VO_2. In a study of 11 to 16-year-olds (Armstrong, et al., 1990a) they reported non-significant correlation coefficients ranging from $r = 0.01$ to -0.26 (median $r = 0.10$). With 12-year-olds (Armstrong et al., 1998b) the non-significant correlations between peak VO_2 and measures of physical activity ranged from $r = -0.13$ to 0.16 in boys and from $r = -0.02$ to 0.04 in girls. Their study of prepubescent children (Armstrong, et al., 1996) revealed non-significant correlation coefficients ranging from $r = -0.15$ to 0.09. In 14 to 15-year-olds, Ekelund et al. (2001) reported no significant relationships between MVPA (min·day^{-1}) and peak VO_2 in either boys ($r = -0.07$) or girls ($r = 0.25$) but noted significant correlations between AEE and peak VO_2 in both boys ($r = 0.30$) and girls ($r = 0.45$). However, after controlling for body fat and maturity level, none of the physical activity variables were significantly related to peak VO_2 in boys. Moreover when the highly active boys were compared to the rest of the boys no significant differences were observed in peak VO_2.

Dencker et al. (2006) estimated the habitual activity of 101 girls and 127 boys, aged 8-11 years, using accelerometry over 3 to 4 days. They reported no relationship between cycle ergometer-determined peak VO_2 and moderate physical activity but found a weak but significant correlation ($r = 0.27$ to 0.30) between peak VO_2 and vigorous physical activity. However, a major limitation of this study is the likely under-estimation of the aerobic fitness of many children. Only 71 % of children reached even 85 % of predicted maximal heart rate before voluntarily ending the exercise test. With such low end-exercise heart rates the data need to be interpreted cautiously.

Kemper et al. (2001) tested the hypothesis that habitual physical activity over a period of 15 years was beneficial to aerobic fitness in young male and female participants (13 to 27 years) in the Amsterdam Growth and Health Longitudinal Study (AGHLS). With 83 male and 98 female participants, they found a significant relationship between habitual physical activity, determined by standardized interview, and treadmill-determined peak VO_2 in the same individuals over the 15 year time span. They initially concluded that the development of aerobic fitness is independently and positively related to daily physical activity but the functional implications are small. For example, a relatively high increase in the physical activity score of 30 % over a period of 15 years resulted in a 2-5 % increase in aerobic fitness. In a subsequent publication reporting the same data, Kemper (2004) therefore concluded that, "data from the AGHLS population does not fully support the hypothesis that physical activity effects VO_2 max" (p 153).

In a study of British children, Armstrong, et al. (2000) used multilevel modelling to examine age, gender and maturity changes in moderate and vigorous physical activity in a longitudinal study of 104 boys and 98 girls, from the ages of 11 to 13 years. They investigated peak VO_2 as an additional explanatory variable of physical activity once age, gender and maturity had been controlled for and reported that a non-significant parameter estimate was obtained. They commented that this was not an unexpected finding because the habitual physical activity of children and adolescents typically lacks the intensity and duration which has been shown necessary to improve young people's aerobic fitness (Armstrong & Welsman, 1997).

On balance, the evidence does not support the premise that habitual physical activity is related to aerobic fitness during childhood and adolescence. This is not surprising as sustained exercise of the intensity and duration needed to improve aerobic fitness is rarely experienced in the daily physical activities of European youth.

Summary and Conclusions

The aerobic fitness of European children and adolescents has been documented for over 50 years and data are available from the vast majority of EU member states. No data are available on randomly selected samples of children who are representative of the population but data on peak VO_2 are generally consistent across studies, across countries and over time.

Young people demonstrate a progressive increase in peak VO_2 with age although some longitudinal data indicate that girls' values level off from about age 14 years. Over the age range 8-18 years girls' and boys' peak VO_2 rise by 80 % and 150 % respectively. The increase in aerobic fitness with age is strongly correlated with body size and inappropriate analyses have clouded our understanding of the independent contributions of age and maturation to the growth of peak VO_2. Traditional analyses using the ratio standard ($mL \cdot kg^{-1} \cdot min^{-1}$) have reported mass-related peak VO_2 to be unchanged in boys over the age range 8 to 16 years, whereas girls' values steadily decline. Studies using allometric techniques to remove the influence of body size have demonstrated that boys' peak VO_2 improves during growth rather than remaining static, whereas girls' peak VO_2 increases into puberty and then levels off into young adulthood. Maturation induces increases in peak VO_2 independent of those explained by body size, body fatness and age. Boys' peak VO_2 is higher than girls' at least from late childhood and there is a progressive divergence in boys' and girls' values during the teen years.

The aerobic fitness of European youth compares favourably with that of young people from elsewhere. There is no convincing evidence to suggest that low levels of aerobic fitness are common amongst European children and adolescents. Published values of peak VO_2 suggest that the aerobic fitness of young people who volunteer to have their peak VO_2 determined has remained consistent over five decades. Recent data indicate an emerging polarization with the difference between fit and unfit young people increasing over time. On a population basis, aerobic fitness is not increasing in line with the secular increase in body mass and therefore maximal performance in activities which involve moving body mass is declining.

Self-report of physical activity is the most widely used method of assessment but data from children need to be interpreted cautiously. Data are available from all European countries except Luxembourg. Of the more objective estimates of physical activity heart rate monitoring and, more recently, accelerometry have allowed valuable insights into young people's physical activity patterns although sample sizes tend to be small and non-representative of populations. Data are available from several EU countries, principally Estonia, Sweden, France, Portugal, the Netherlands and the United Kingdom and they are very similar. Boys of all ages participate in more physical activity than girls and the gender difference is more marked when moderate to vigorous physical activity is considered. The physical activity levels of both genders are higher during childhood and decline as young people move through their teen years. Physical activity patterns are sporadic and sustained periods of moderate to vigorous physical activity are seldom experienced by many children and adolescents.

The number of children who experience physical activity of the duration, frequency and intensity recommended by expert committees decreases with age but accurate estimates of how many girls and boys are inactive are clouded by methodological inconsistencies. For example, the two most informative recent contributions to the European physical activity literature are the studies led by Riddoch (2004) and Currie (2004). Both studies were rigorously designed and executed with large well-defined samples and data were collected from the same four countries at the same time. Riddoch et al. (2004), using accelerometry, reported 82 % of 15-year-old boys and 62 % of girls to satisfy the UKHEA guidelines whereas Currie et al. (2004), using self-report methods, noted only 28 % and 19 % of 15-year-old boys and girls respectively to satisfy the same criterion.

Self-report of energy intake indicates that young people's energy expenditure and therefore physical activity decreased over the period 1930 to 1980 but limited objective data tentatively suggest that the impact of the environmental factors implicated in the reduction of physical activity over time might have declined in the last 10 to 15 years.

The evidence linking habitual physical activity with aerobic fitness during youth is not compelling and young people with different levels of aerobic fitness do not necessarily differ in their daily physical activity. The explanation probably lies in the fact that the habitual physical activity of European youth lacks the intensity and duration necessary to promote increases in peak VO_2 .

References

Aberberga-Augskalne, L. (2002). Individual growth patterns and physical fitness in Riga schoolchildren. *Acta Medico-Historica Rigensia, 25*, 65-76.

American College of Sports Medicine. (1995). *ACSM's guidelines for exercise testing and prescription.* Baltimore: Williams and Wilkins.

Andersen, K. L., Ilmarinen, J., Rutenfranz, J., Ottman, W., Berndt, I., Kylian, H. & Ruppel, M. (1984). Leisure time sport activities and maximal aerobic power during late adolescence. *European Journal of Applied Physiology, 52*, 431-436.

Andersen, L. B., Henckel, P. & Saltin, B. (1987). Maximal oxygen uptake in Danish adolescents 16-19 years of age. *European Journal of Applied Physiology, 56*, 74-82.

Andersen, L. B. & Schelin, B. (1994). Physical activity and performance in a random sample of adolescents attending school in Denmark. *Scandinavian Journal of Medicine and Science in Sports, 4*, 13-18.

Armstrong, N. (1998). Young people's physical activity patterns as assessed by heart rate monitoring. *Journal of Sports Science, 16*, 9-16.

Armstrong, N., Balding, J., Gentle, P., Williams, J. & Kirby, B. (1990a). Peak oxygen uptake and habitual physical activity in 11 to 16-year-olds. *Pediatric Exercise Science, 2*, 349-358.

Armstrong, N., Balding, J., Gentle, P. & Kirby, B. (1990b). Patterns of physical activity among 11 to 16 year old British children. *British Medical Journal, 301*, 203-205.

Armstrong, N. & Bray, S. (1991). Physical activity patterns defined by continuous heart rate monitoring. *Archives of Disease in Childhood, 66*, 245-247.

.Armstrong, N. & Davies, B. (1984). The metabolic and physiological responses of children to exercise and training. *Physical Education Review, 7*, 90-105.

Armstrong, N., Kirby, B. J., McManus, A. M. & Welsman, J. R. (1995). Aerobic fitness of pre-pubescent children. *Annals of Human Biology, 22*, 427-441.

Armstrong, N., Kirby, B. J., McManus, A. M. & Welsman, J. R. (1997). Prepubescents' ventilatory responses to exercise with reference to sex and body size. *Chest, 112*, 1554-1560.

Armstrong, N., McManus, A., Welsman, J. & Kirby, B. (1996). Physical activity patterns and aerobic fitness among pre-pubescents. *European Physical Education Review, 2*, 7-18.

Armstrong, N. & van Mechelen, W. (1998) Are young people fit and active ? In J. Sallis & N. Cavill (Eds.), *Young and active* (pp. 69-97). London: Health Education Authority.

Armstrong, N. & Welsman, J. (1994). Assessment and interpretation of aerobic function in children and adolescents. *Exercise and Sport Sciences Reviews, 22,* 435-476.

.Armstrong, N. & Welsman, J. R. (1997). *Young people and physical activity.* Oxford: Oxford University Press.

Armstrong, N. & Welsman, J. R. (2000a). Aerobic fitness. In N. Armstrong & W. Van Mechelen (Eds.), *Paediatric exercise science and medicine* (pp. 65-76). Oxford: Oxford University Press.

Armstrong, N. & Welsman, J. R. (2000b). Development of aerobic fitness during childhood and adolescence. *Pediatric Exercise Science, 12,* 128-149.

Armstrong, N. & Welsman, J. R. (2001). Peak oxygen uptake in relation to growth and maturation in 11-17 year old humans. *European Journal of Applied Physiology, 85,* 546-551.

Armstrong, N., Welsman, J. R. & Kirby, B. J. (1998a). Peak oxygen uptake and maturation in 12-year-olds. *Medicine and Science in Sport and Exercise, 30,* 165-169.

Armstrong, N., Welsman, J. & Kirby, B. (1998b). Physical activity, peak oxygen uptake and performance on the wingate anaerobic test in 12-year-olds. *Acta Kinesiologiae Universitatis Tartuensis, 3,* 7-21.

Armstrong, N., Welsman, J. R. & Kirby, B. J. (2000). Longitudinal changes in 11-13-year-olds' physical activity. *Acta Paediatrica, 89,* 775-780

Armstrong, N., Welsman, J. R., Nevill, A. M. & Kirby, B. J. (1999). Modeling growth and maturation changes in peak oxygen uptake in 11-13 year olds. *Journal of Applied Physiology, 87,* 2230-2236.

Armstrong, N., Welsman, J. R. & Winsley, R. J. (1996). Is peak VO$_2$ a maximal index of children's aerobic fitness? *International Journal of Sports Medicine, 27,* 356-359.

Armstrong, N., Williams, J., Balding, J., Gentle, P. & Kirby, B. (1991). The peak oxygen uptake of British children with reference to age, sex and sexual maturity. *European Journal of Applied Physiology, 62,* 369-375.

Åstrand, P. O. & Ryhming, I. (1954). A nomogram for calculation of aerobic capacity (physical fitness) from pulse rate during submaximal work. *Journal of Applied Physiology, 7,* 218-221.

Barinaga, M. (1997). How much pain for cardiac gain? *Science, 27,* 1324-1327.

Baxter-Jones, A., Goldstein, H. & Helms, P. (1993). The development of aerobic power in young athletes. *Journal of Applied Physiology, 75,* 1160-1167.

Bell, R. D., Macek, M., Rutenfranz, J. & Saris, W. H. M. (1986). Health indicators and risk factors of cardiovascular diseases during childhood and adolescence. In J. Rutenfranz, R. Mocellin & F. Klimt (Eds.), *Children and exercise xii* (pp. 19-27). Champaign, Illinois: Human Kinetics.

Beunen, G. & Malina, R. M. (1988). Growth and physical performance relative to the timing of the adolescent spurt. *Exercise and Sport Sciences Reviews, 16,* 503-540.

Beunen, G. P. (1989). Biological age in pediatric exercise research. In O. Bar-Or (Ed.), *Advances in pediatric sport sciences volume 3* (pp. 1-40). Champaign, Illinois: Human Kinetics.

Beunen, G. P., Rogers, D. M., Woynarowska, B. & Malina, R. M. (1997). Longitudinal study of ontogenetic allometry of oxygen uptake in boys and girls grouped by maturity status. *Annals of Human Biology, 24,* 33-43.

Biddle, S., Sallis, J. & Cavill, N. (1998). *Young and active?* London: Health Education Authority.

Binkhorst, R. A., Van't Hof, M. A. & Saris, W. H. M. (1992). *Maximum exercise in children: Reference values for 6-18-year-old girls and boys.* The Hague: Dutch Heart Association.

Boileau, R. A., Bonen, A., Heyward, V. H. & Massey, B. H. (1977). Maximal aerobic capacity on the treadmill and bicycle ergometer of boys 11-14 years of age. *Journal of Sports Medicine and Physical Fitness, 17,* 153-162.

Bouziotas, C. & Koutedaiks, Y. (2003). A three year study of coronary heart disease risk factors in Greek adolescents. *Pediatric Exercise Science, 15,* 9-18.

Bradfield, R. B., Chan, H., Bradfield, N. E. & Payne, R. R. (1971). Energy expenditures and heart rates of Cambridge boys at school. *American Journal of Clinical Nutrition, 24,* 1461-1466.

Bunc, V. (2000). Standards of cardiovascular fitness in Czech children and adolescents. *Acta Universitatis Carolinae Kinanthropologica, 36* (2), 51-57.

Cantera-Garde, M. A. & Devís-Devís, J. (2000). Physical activity levels of secondary school Spanish adolescents. *European Journal of Physical Education, 5,* 28-44.

Casperson, C. J., Powell, K. & Christenson, G. (1985). Physical activity, exercise and physical fitness: Definitions and distinctions of health-related research. *Public Health Reports, 100,* 126-131.

Cassels, D. E. & Morse, M. (1962). *Cardiopulmonary data for children and young adults.* Springfield, Illinois: Thomas.

Ceretelli, P., Aghemo, P. & Rovelli, E. (1963). Morphological and physiological observation of schoolchildren in Milan. *Medicina Dello Sport, 2,* 109-121.

Cilia, G. & Bellucci, M. (1993). *Eurofit tests: Europei di attitudine fisica.* Roma: Instituto Superiore Statale di Educazione Fisica.

Currie, C., Hurrelmann, K., Settertobulte, W., Smith, R. & Todd, J. (2000). *Health and health behaviour among young people.* Copenhagen, Denmark: World Health Organisation.

Currie, C., Roberts, C., Morgan, A., Smith, R., Setertsbulte, W., Samda, O. & Barnekow-Rasmussen, V. (Eds.) (2004). *Young people's health in context.* Copenhagen, Denmark: World Health Organisation.

Dallman, P. R. & Siimes, M. A. (1979). Percentile curves for hemoglobin and red cell volume in infancy and childhood. *Pediatrics, 94,* 26-31.

Deforce, B., Lefevre, J., De Boudeaudhuig, I., Hills, A. P., Duquet, W. & Bouckaert, J. (2003). Physical fitness and physical activity in obese and non-obese Flemish youth. *Obesity Research, 11,* 434-441.

Deheeger, M., Rolland-Cachera, M. F. & Fontvielle, A. M. (1997). Physical activity and body composition in 10 year old French children: Linkages with nutritional intake? *International Journal of Obesity, 21,* 372-379.

Dencker, M., Thorsson, O., Karlsson, M. K., Linden, C., Svensson, J., Wollmer, P. & Andersen, L. B. (2006). Daily physical activity and its relation to aerobic fitness in children aged 8-11 years. *European Journal of Applied Physiology*, 96, 587-592.

Driscoll, D. J., Staats, B. A. & Beck, K. C. (1989). Measurement of cardiac output in children during exercise: A review. *Pediatric Exercise Science, 1,* 102-115.

Durnin, J. V. G. A. (1992). Physical activity levels past and present. In N. Norgan (Ed.), *Physical activity and health* (pp. 20-27). University Press: Cambridge.

Ekblom, O., Oddson, K. & Ekblom, B. (2004). Health-related fitness in Swedish adolescents between 1987-2001. *Acta Paediatrica, 93,* 681-686.

Ekelund, U., Poortvleit, E., Nilsson, A., Yngve, A., Holmberg, A. & Sjostrom, M. (2001). Physical activity in relation to aerobic fitness and body fat in 14-to-15 year-old boys and girls. *European Journal of Applied Physiology, 85,* 195-201.

Engstrom, L.-M. (1980). Physical activity of children and youth. *Acta Paediatrica Scandinavica, 283*, 101-105.

Falgairette, G., Bedu, M., Fellmann, N., Van Praagh, E. & Coudert, J. (1991). Bioenergetic profile in 144 boys aged from 6 to 15 years with special reference to sexual maturation. *European Journal of Applied Physiology, 62*, 151-156.

Farkas, A., Petrekanits, M., Mészáros, J. & Mohács, J. (1992). Chronological and morphological age related physiological variables of adolescent boys. In I. Szmodis, T. Szabó & J. Mészáros (Eds.), *Proceedings of the international round-table conference on sport physiology* (pp. 95-108). Budapest: Magyar Testnevelesi Egyetem.

Flandrois, R., Grandmontagne, M., Mayet, R., Favier, R. & Frutoso, J. (1982). La consommation maximale d'oxygene chez le jeune francais sa variation avec l'age le sexe et l'entrainement. Journal of Physiology (Paris). Cited by Krahenbuhl, G.S., Skinner, J.S. & Korht, W.M. (1985). Developmental aspects of maximal aerobic power in children. *Exercise and Sport Sciences Reviews*, 13, 503-538.

Fuchs, R., Semmer, N. K., Lippert, P., Powell, K. E., Dwyer, J. H. & Hoffmeister, H. (1988). Patterns of physical activity among German adolescents: The Berlin-Bremen study. *Preventative Medicine, 17*, 746-763.

Gaisl, G. & Buchberger, J. (1977). The significance of stress acidosis in judging the physical working capacity of boys aged 11 to 15. In H. Lavallee & R. J. Shephard (Eds.), *Frontiers of activity and child health* (pp. 161-168). Quebec: Pelican.

Gavarry, O., Bernard, T., Giacomoni, M., Seymat, M., Euzet, J. P. & Falgairette, G. (1998). Continuous heart rate monitoring over 1 week in teenagers aged 11-16 years. *European Journal of Applied Physiology, 77*, 125-132.

Goldstein, H., Rasbash, J., Plewis, I., Draper, D., Browne, W., Yang, M., Healy, M. Woodhouse, G. Langford, I. & Lewis, T. (1998). *A user's guide to MLWin.* London: University of London, Institute of Education.

Guerra, S., Duarte, J. & Mota, J. (2001). Physical activity and cardiovascular disease risk factors in schoolchildren. *European Physical Education Review, 7*, 269-281.

Guerra, S., Ribeiro, J. C., Coita, R., Duarte, J. & Mota, J. (2002). Relationship between cardiorespiratory fitness, body composition and blood pressure in schoolchildren. *Journal of Sport Medicine and Physical Fitness, 42*, 207-213.

Guerra, S., Santos, P., Ribeiro, J. C., Duarte, J. A. & Mota, J. (2003). Assessment of children's and adolescent's physical activity levels. *European Physical Education Review, 9*, 75-85.

Guillaume, M., Lapidus, L., Bjorntorp, P. & Lambert, A. (1997). Physical activity, obesity and cardiovascular risk factors in children. The Belgium Luxembourg child study II. *Obesity Research, 5*, 549-556.

Hansen, H. S., Froberg, K., Hydlebrandt, N. & Nielsen, J. R. (1991). A controlled study of eight months of physical training and reduction of blood pressure in children: The Odense schoolchild study. *British Medical Journal, 303*, 682-685.

Hardman, A. E. (1999). Accumulation of physical activity for health gains: What is the evidence? *British Journal of Sports Medicine, 33*, 87-92.

Hasselstrom, H., Hansen, S. E. Frobert, K. & Andersen, L. B. (2002). Physical fitness and physical activity during adolescence as predictors of cardiovascular disease risk in young adulthood. Danish youth and sports study. An eight year follow-up. *International Journal of Sports Medicine, 23*, 27-S31.

Heartbeat Wales. (1986). *Welsh youth health survey 1986.* Cardiff: Heartbeat Wales.

Hussey, J., Gormley, J. & Bell, C. (2001). Physical activity in Dublin children aged 7-9 years. *British Journal of Sports Medicine, 35,* 268-273.

Jurak, G., Kovač, M. & Strel, J. (2003a). How Slovenian primary school pupils spend their Summer holidays. In G. Jurak (Ed.), *Sports activities of Slovenian children and young people during their Summer holidays* (pp. 23-38). Ljubljana, Slovenia: University of Ljubljana.

Jurak, G., Kovač, M., Strel, J. & Stara, G. (2003b). How Slovenian secondary school children spend their Summer holidays. In G. Jurak (Ed.), *Sports activities of Slovenian children and young people during their Summer holidays* (pp. 39-58). Ljubljana, Slovenia: University of Ljubljana.

Jurimae, T. & Volbekiene, V. (1998). Eurofit test results in Estonian and Lithuanian 11 to 17-year-old children. *European Journal of Physical Education, 3,* 178-164.

Kalafoutis, A., Paterakis, S., Koutselinis, A. & Spanos, V. (1976). Relationship between erythrocyte 2, 3-diphosphoglycerate and age in a normal population. *Clinical Chemistry, 22,* 1918-1919.

Kemper, H. C. G. (1995). *The Amsterdam growth study.* Champaign, Illinois: Human Kinetics.

Kemper, H. C. G. (2004). *Amsterdam growth and health longitudinal study.* Basel, Switzerland: Karger.

Kemper, H. C. G., Twisk, J. W. R., Koppes, L. L. J., Van Mechelen, W. & Post, B.G. (2001). A 15-year physical activity pattern is positively related to aerobic fitness in young males and females (13-27 years). *European Journal of Physiology, 84,* 395-402.

Kemper, H. C. G. & Verschuur, R. (1981). Maximal aerobic power in 13 and 14 year old teenagers in relation to biological age. *International Journal of Sports Medicine, 2,* 97-100.

Kemper, H. C. G. & Verschuur, R. (1990). Longitudinal study of coronary risk factors during adolescence and young adulthood – the Amsterdam growth and health study. *Pediatric Exercise Science, 2,* 359-371.

King, A. J. C. & Coles, B. (1992). *The health of Canada's youth.* Canada: Ministry of Health and Welfare.

King, A., Wold, B., Tudor-Smith, C. & Harel, Y. (Eds.) (1996). *The health of youth – A cross national survey.* Copenhagen, Denmark: World Health Organisation.

Kobayashi, K., Kitamura, K., Miura, M., Sodeyama, H., Murase, Y., Miyashita, M. & Matsui, H. (1978). Aerobic power as related to body growth and training in Japanese boys: A longitudinal study. *Journal of Applied Physiology, 44,* 666-672.

Koutedakis, Y. & Bouziotas, C. (2003). National physical education curriculum: Motor and cardiovascular health related fitness in Greek adolescents. *British Journal of Sports Medicine, 37,* 311-314.

Kovač, M., Jurak, G., Strel, J. & Bednarik, J. (2003). Comparison of motor development of boys and girls aged 11, 13, 15 and 17. *Journal of Human Kinetics, 10,* 63-75.

Kovač, M. & Strel, J. (2000). Motor development of girls, aged from 10 to 18 years. *Acta Universitatis Carolinae Kinanthropologica, 36,* 39-50.

Leger, L. & Lambert, J. (1982). A maximal multistage shuttle run test to predict VO$_2$ max. *European Journal of Applied Physiology, 49,* 1-5.

Livingstone, M. B. E. (2001). Childhood obesity in Europe: A growing concern. *Public Health Nutrition, 4,* 109-116.

Loucaides, L. A., Chedzoy, S. M., Bennett, N. & Wolshe, K. (2004). Correlates of physical activity in a Cypriot sample of sixth-grade children. *Pediatric Exercise Science, 16,* 25-36.

Macek, M. & Vavra, J. (1971). Cardiopulmonary and metabolic changes during exercise in
    children 6-14 years old. *Journal of Applied Physiology, 30*, 200-204.
Malina, R. M. & Bouchard, C. (1991). *Growth, maturation and physical activity*. Champaign,
    Illinois: Human Kinetics.
Mallam, K. M., Metcalf, B. S., Kirby, J., Voss, L. D. & Witkin, T. J. (2003). Contribution of
    timetabled physical education to total physical activity in primary schoolchildren:
    Cross-sectional study. *British Medical Journal, 327*, 592-593.
Maniôs, Y., Kafatos, A. & Codrington, C. (1999). Gender differences in physical activity and
    physical fitness in young children in Crete. *Journal of Sports Medicine and Physical
    Fitness, 39*, 24-30.
Maniôs, Y., Kafatos, A. & Markakis, G. (1998). Physical activity of 6-year-old children:
    Validation of two proxy reports. *Pediatric Exercise Science, 10*, 176-188.
Marella, M., Colli, R. & Faina, M. (1986). Evaluation of de l'aptitude physique: Eurofit,
    batterie experimentagl. Romes scuola dello sport. The fitness and physical activity of
    adolescents. *The Medical Journal of Australia, 148*, 513-521.
Mirwald, R. L. & Bailey, D. A. (1986). *Maximal aerobic power*. London, Ontario: Sports
    Dynamics.
Mocellin, R., Lindemann, H., Rutenfranz, J. & Sbreny, W. (1971). Determination of W170
    and maximal oxygen uptake in children by different methods. *Acta Paediatrica
    Scandinavica, 217*, 13-17.
Morrow, J. R. & Freedson, P. S. (1994). Relationship between habitual physical activity and
    aerobic fitness in adolescents. *Pediatric Exercise Science, 6*, 315-329.
Mota, J., Guerra, S., Leandro, C., Pinto, A., Ribeiro, J. C. & Duarte, J. A. (2002). Association
    of maturation, sex and body fat in cardiorespiratory fitness. *American Journal of
    Human Biology, 14*, 707-712.
Naul, R., Telema, R. & Rychtécky, A. (1997). Physical fitness and active lifestyle of Czech,
    Finnish and German youth. *Acta Univérsitatis Carolinae, 33*, 5-16.
Nilsson, A., Ekelund, U, Yngve, A. & Sjostrom, M. (2002). Assessing physical activity
    among children with accelerometers using different time sampling intervals and
    placements. *Pediatric Exercise Science, 14*, 87-96.
O'Sullivan, S. O. (2002). The physical activity of children: A study of 1,603 Irish
    schoolchildren aged 11-12 years. *Irish Medical Journal, 95*, 78-81.
Przeweda, R. & Dobosz, J. (2003). Growth and physical fitness of Polish youths in two
    successive decades. *Journal of Sports Medicine and Physical Fitness, 43*, 465-474.
Raudsepp, L. & Jurimae, T. (1996). Physical activity, fitness and somatic characteristics of
    prepubertal girls. *Biology of Sport, 13*, 55-60.
Raudsepp, L., Liblik, R. & Hannus, A. (2002). Children's and adolescents' physical self-
    perception as related to moderate to vigorous physical activity and physical fitness.
    Pediatric Exercise Science, 14, 97-106.
Raudsepp, L. & Pall, P. (1998). Reproducibility and stability of physical activity in children.
    Pediatric Exercise Science, 10, 320-326.
Ribeiro, J., Guerra, S., Pinto, A., Oliveira, J., Duarte, J. & Mota, J. (2003). Overweight and
    obesity in children and adolescents: Relationship with blood pressure and physical
    activity. *Annals of Human Biology, 30*, 203-213.
Riddoch, C. (1990). *Northern Ireland health and fitness survey*. Belfast: Sports Council for
    Northern Ireland and Department of Health and Social Services.
Riddoch, C. J., Andersen, L. B., Wedderkopp, N., Harro, M., Klannson-Heggebø, Sardinha,
    L. B., Cooper, A. R. & Ekelund, U. (2004). Physical activity levels and patterns of 9-

and 15-yr-old European children. *Medicine and Science in Sports and Exercise, 36,* 86-92.

Rowland, T. W. (2000a). Pulmonary function. In N. Armstrong & W. Van Mechelen (Eds.), *Paediatric exercise science and medicine* (pp. 153-161). Oxford: Oxford University Press.

Rowland, T. W. (2000b). Cardiovascular function. In N. Armstrong & W. Van Mechelen (Eds.), *Paediatric exercise science and medicine* (pp. 163-171). Oxford: Oxford University Press.

Rowland, T. W. & Lisowski, R. (2001). Hemodynamic responses to increasing cycle cadence in 11-year-old boys: Role of the skeletal muscle pump. *International Journal of Sports Medicine, 22,* 405-409.

Rowland, T. W., Popowski, B. & Ferrone, L. (1997). Cardiac responses to maximal upright cycle exercise in healthy boys and men. *Medicine and Science in Sports and Exercise, 29,* 1146-1151.

Rutenfranz, J., Andersen, K. L., Seliger, V., Klimmer, F., Berndt, I. & Ruppel, M. (1981). Maximum aerobic power and body composition during the puberty growth period: Similarities and differences between children of two European countries. *European Journal of Pediatrics, 136,* 123-133.

Rutenfranz, J., Berndt, I. & Knauth, P. (1974). Daily physical activity investigated by time budget studies and physical performance capacity of schoolboys. *Acta Paediatrica Belgica, 28,* 79-86.

Rychtecky, A., Naul, R. & Neuhaus, W. (1996). Physical activity and motor performance of Prague and Essen school youngsters. *Acta Universitati Carolinae, 32,* 5-22.

Sainz, R. M. (1996). *La batería eurofit en euskadi.* Vitoria-Gasteig, Spain: Instituto Vasca de Educación Fisica.

Sallis, J. F. & Patrick, K. (1994). Physical activity guidelines for adolescents: A consensus statement. *Pediatric Exercise Science, 6,* 302-314.

Sallis, J. F., Patrick, K. & Long, B. J. (1994). Overview of the international consensus conference on physical activity guidelines for adolescents. *Pediatric Exercise Science, 6,* 299-302.

Sallo, M. & Silla, R. (1997). Physical activity with moderate to vigorous intensity in preschool and first grade schoolchildren. *Pediatric Exercise Science, 9,* 44-54.

Sallo, M. & Viru, A. (1996). Aerobic capacity and physical activity in 4 to 10-year-old children. *Biology of Sport, 13,* 211-219.

Saris, W. H. M. (1982). *Aerobic power and daily physical activity in children.* Meppel, Netherlands: Kripps Repro.

Saris, W. H. M., Noordeloos, A. M., Ringnalda, B. E. M., Van't Hof, M. A. & Binkhorst, R. A. (1985). Reference values for aerobic power of healthy 4 to 18 year old Dutch children: Preliminary results. In R. A. Binkhorst, H. C. G. Kemper & W. H. M. Saris (Eds.), *Children and exercise xi* (pp. 151-160). Champaign, Illinois: Human Kinetics.

Seliger, V., Cermak, V., Hendzo, S., Horak, J., Jirka, Z., Macek, M., Pribil, M., Rous, J., Skranc, O., Ulbrich, J. & Urbanek, J. (1971). Physical fitness of the Czechoslovak 12 and 15 year old population. *Acta Paediatrica Scandinavica, 217,* 37-41.

Seliger, V. S., Trefny, S., Bartenkova, S. & Pauer, M. (1974). The habitual physical activity and fitness of 12 year old boys. *Acta Paediatrica Belgica, 28,* 54-59.

Sirard, J. R. & Pate, R. R. (2001). Physical activity assessment in children and adolescents. *Sports Medicine, 31,* 439-454.

Skalik, K., Frömel, K., Sigmund, E., Vašendová, J. & Wirdheim, E. (2001). Weekly physical activity in secondary school students (a comparative probe into Czech, Polish and Swedish conditions). *Gymnica, 31*, 21-26.

Sleap, M. & Warburton, P. (1996). Physical activity levels of 5-11-year-old children in England: Cumulative evidence from three direct observation studies. *International Journal of Sports Medicine, 17*, 248-253.

Sprynarova, S., Parizkova, J. & Bunc, V. (1987). Relationships between body dimensions and resting and working oxygen consumption in boys aged 11 to 18 years. *European Journal of Applied Physiology, 56*, 725-736.

Strel, J., Kovaĉ, M. & Jurak, G. (2004). *Study on young people's lifestyle and sedentariness and the role of sport in the context of education and as a means of restoring the balance* (pp. 3-38). Ljubljana, Slovenia: University of Ljubljana.

Sundberg, S. & Elovainio, R. (1982). Cardiorespiratory function in competitive endurance runners aged 12-16 years compared with ordinary boys. *Acta Paediatrica Scandinavica, 71*, 987-992.

Sunnegardh, J. & Bratteby, L. E. (1987). Maximal oxygen uptake, anthropometry and physical activity in a randomly selected sample of 8 and 13 year old children in Sweden. *European Journal of Applied Physiology, 56*, 266-272.

Sunnegardh, J., Bratteby, L. E., Sjolin, S., Hagman, U. & Hoffstedt, A. (1985). The relation between physical activity and energy intake of 8 and 13 year old children in Sweden. In R. A. Binkhorst, H. C. G. Kemper & W. H. M. Saris (Eds.), *Children and exercise xi* (pp. 183-193). Champaign Illinois: Human Kinetics.

Szabó, T. & Pápai, J. (1997). Physical and motor structure characteristics of 11 to 17-year-olds. In N. Armstrong, B. J. Kirby & J. R. Welsman (Eds.), *Children and exercise xix* (pp. 99-104). London: Spon.

Telema, R., Naul, R., Nupponen, H., Rychtecky, A. & Vualle, P. (2002). *Physical fitness, sporting lifestyles and Olympic ideals: Cross-cultural studies on youth sport in Europe*. Schorndorf, Germany: Verlag Karl Hofmann.

Tomkinson, G. R., Leger, L. A., Olds, T. S. & Cazonla. (2003). Secular trends in the performance of children and adolescents (1980-2000). *Sports Medicine, 33*, 285-300.

Trost, S. G. (2001). Objective measurement of physical activity in youth: Current issues, future directions. *Exercise and Sport Sciences Reviews, 29*, 32-36.

Van Gerven, D. & Vanden Eynde, B. (1987). Aerobic capacity and ventilatory threshold of Belgian teenage boys. In H. Ruskin & A. Simkin (Eds.), *Physical fitness and the ages of man* (pp. 113-128). Jerusalem: Academan Press.

Van Mechelen, W. & Kemper, H. C. G. (1995). Body growth, body composition, and physical fitness. In H. C. G. Kemper (Ed.), *The Amsterdam growth study* (pp. 52-85). Champaign, Illinois: Human Kinetics.

Vermorel, M., Vernet, J., Bitar, A., Fellman, N. & Coudert, J. (2002). Daily energy expenditure, activity patterns, and energy costs of the various activities in French 12-16-y-old adolescents in free living conditions. *European Journal of Clinical Nutrition, 56*, 819-829.

Vinet, A., Mandigout, S., Nottin, S., Nguyen, L. D., Lecoq, A. M., Couteix, D. & Obert, P. (2003). Influence of body composition, haemoglobin concentration, and cardiac size and function of gender differences in maximal oxygen uptake in prepubertal children. *Chest, 124*, 1494-1499.

Watson, A. W. S. & O'Donovan, D. J. (1976). The physical working capacity of male adolescents in Ireland. *Irish Journal of Medical Science, 145*, 383-391.

Wedderkopp, N., Frobert, K., Hansen, H. S. & Andersen, L. B. (2004). Secular trends in physical fitness and obesity in Dutch 9-year-old girls and boys: Odense school child study and Danish substudy of the European youth heart study. *Scandinavian Journal of Medicine and Science in Sports, 14*, 1-6.

Welsman, J., Armstrong, N. & Kirby, B. (1994). Serum testosterone is not related to peak VO_2 and submaximal blood lactate responses in 12-16 year old males. *Pediatric Exercise Science, 6*, 120-127.

Welsman, J. R. & Armstrong, N. (2000a). Interpreting growth-related data. In N. Armstrong & W. Van Mechelen (Eds.), *Paediatric exercise science and medicine* (pp. 3-9). Oxford: Oxford University Press.

Welsman, J. R. & Armstrong, N. (2000b). Statistical techniques for interpreting body size-related exercise performance during growth. *Pediatric Exercise Science, 12*, 112-127.

Welsman, J. R. & Armstrong, N. (2000c). Physical activity patterns in secondary school children. *European Journal of Physical Education, 5*, 147-157.

Welsman, J. R., Armstrong, N., Kirby, B. J., Nevill, A. M. & Winter, E. M. (1996). Scaling peak VO_2 for differences in body size. *Medicine and Science in Sports and Exercise, 28*, 259-265.

Welsman, J. R., Bywater, K., Farr, C., Welford, D. & Armstrong, N. (2005). Reliability of peak VO_2 and maximal cardiac output assessed using thoracic bioimpedance in children. *European Journal of Applied Physiology, 94*, 228-234.

Westerstahl, M., Barnekow-Bergkvist, M., Hedberg, G. & Jansson, E. (2003). Secular trends in body dimensions and physical fitness among adolescents in Sweden from 1974 to 1995. *Scandanavian Journal of Medicine and Science in Sports, 13*, 128-137.

Weymans, M. L., Reybrouck, T. M., Stijns, H. J. & Knops, J. (1986). Influence of habitual levels of physical activity on the cardiorespiratory endurance capacity of children. In J. Rutenfranz, R. Mocellin & F. Klimt (Eds.), *Children and exercise xii* (pp. 149-156). Champaign Illinois: Human Kinetics.

Wilczewski, A., Sklad, M., Krawczyk, B., Saask, J. & Majle, B. (1996). Physical development of fitness of children from urban and rural areas as determined by Eurofit test battery. *Biology of Sport, 13*, 113-126.

Williams, J., Armstrong, N., Winter, E. & Crichton, N. (1992). Changes in peak oxygen uptake with age and sexual maturation in boys: Physiological fact or statistical anomaly? In J. Coudert & E. Van Praagh (Eds.), *Children and exercise xvi* (pp. 35-37). Paris: Masson.

Yamaji, K. & Miyashita, M. (1977). Oxygen transport system during exhaustive exercise in Japanese boys. *European Journal of Applied Physiology, 36*, 93-99.

Chapter 3:
Physical activity and physical fitness in relation to cardiovascular disease in children

Lars Bo Andersen, Karsten Froberg, Peter Lund Kristensen & Niels Christian Møller

Abstract

This chapter reviews the newest literature linking physical inactivity and low fitness to metabolic disorders and cardiovascular disease risk factors including obesity. There is a rationale for early prevention of CVD if a) children have a risk factor profile, which are known to increase risk for future disease in adults, b) physical activity and CVD risk factors track into adulthood, c) increased physical activity can improve the risk factor profile. There is convincing evidence for a progressive evolution of atherosclerosis which starts in childhood, and also that physical activity decreases the rate of the process through several mechanisms.

Among the central mechanisms mediating the effect of physical activity are a) increased insulin sensitivity, b) a non-insulin dependent glucose uptake, which causes lower insulin release, c) an improved ratio between HDL and LDL cholesterol because of increased activity of lipoprotein lipase, d) improved function of other metabolic hormones and enzymes for fat metabolism.

The association between CVD risk factors and physical activity/fitness is weak, when risk factors are analysed isolated. In the normal population of children, studies have shown that risk factors cluster and this clustering is strongly related to low physical activity and fitness. In European children it has been found that as many as 15 % of 9-year-old children has clustered risk. Most of the overweight and obese children have clustered risk, but clustering of risk factors is also observed in many lean and inactive children, who might become overweight at a later point because of insulin resistance.

Obesity is increasing in Europe, but large geographical and social differences exist. The Northern and eastern European countries have less obese children than the Southern part of Europe, and obesity is more prevalent among the lower socio-economical classes.

It can be concluded that there is a large potential for primary prevention of CVD and obesity in European children, and lifestyle changes including increased physical activity as one of the key actions should be initiated.

Introduction

A sedentary lifestyle is common among adults and is associated with a higher mortality rate and rates of common diseases such as cardiovascular disease (CVD), diabetes and some cancers in adults (Vuori, Fentem, Andersen et al., 1995). These diseases are not manifest in children, but it may be anticipated that it becomes increasingly difficult to change to a more physically active lifestyle with higher age. Therefore, it might be a good idea to promote a healthy lifestyle in early life. Primary prevention as early as possible should always be preferred instead of prevention at a time where irreversible pathological changes have occurred. The latter may especially be related to metabolic diseases such as cardiovascular disease and type 2 diabetes.

There is a rationale for primary prevention in relation to CVD and health promotion in children if the following hypotheses are true:

1) A sedentary lifestyle causes increased levels in disease risk factors (cardiovascular), which is known to increase risk of premature death

2) A large percentage of children have a lifestyle sedentary to a degree that may increase the risk of developing atherosclerosis or other diseases prematurely

3) Risk factors or sedentary behaviour track during childhood and into adulthood

4) Interventions including increased physical activity in children at risk are efficient to decrease risk factor levels and change behaviour to a more physically active lifestyle.

In this review we will argue that the above hypotheses in fact are true.

In the following chapter we will focus on 1) a description of the atherosclerotic process, 2) key mechanisms which link physical activity to the biological CVD risk factors, 3) CVD risk factor levels in European children, 4) associations between physical activity/fitness and CVD risk factors, 5) tracking of physical activity, fitness and CVD risk factors, 6) overweight and obesity in children, 7) final conclusions.

Physical activity levels (primary risk factor) are described elsewhere, but the secondary risk factors, which are the biological markers such as blood pressure, blood lipids and serum insulin, are negatively associated to physical fitness/activity, and will be described here. These risk factors are thought to be part of the causal pathway linking physical inactivity to atherosclerosis. Overweight/obesity, which is recognised as a CVD risk factor, will be described in a separate chapter, because of the importance of this risk factor.

Atherosclerosis

Atherosclerosis is degenerative changes in the arterial wall which decreases the elasticity and narrows the lumen, and eventually may result in coronary heart disease, stroke or peripheral artery disease depending on the site of the atherosclerosis. Atherosclerosis develops over decades from the first microscopic changes in the wall until clinical symptoms may occur later in life. The causes of atherosclerosis are multi-factorial and especially the initial steps in the development of atherosclerosis are only partly elucidated. The arterial wall consists of different layers and atherosclerosis is probably caused by a dysfunction in the inner layer, the endothelial layer. From the endothelium LDL cholesterol intrudes the intima, which is just inside the endothelium. LDL is oxidised and attracks microphags, which thickens the wall. This condition is called a fatty streak. Fatty streaks does not give symptoms and they are reversible. The macrophags with their content of LDL cholesterol are called foam cells and they are thought of as the early stages of atherosclerosis.

The content of cholesterol in the macrophags and later in the smooth muscle cells of the arterial wall gradually increases, and this process is most pronounced where the arteries split or where the transmural pressure is great. A layer of collagen tissue covers the lesion and it develops into an atherosclerotic plaque or raised lesion. An atherosclerotic plaque is not entirely reversible, but it can decrease in size. However, the usual process is that it increases in size and eventually it will decrease the blood flow in the artery and symptoms will appear; e.g. angina pectoris. This stage is common in middle aged persons. If the plaque bursts and come in contact with the blood, a thrombosis develops and the artery can be completely blocked.

The whole process of atherosclerosis starts in early childhood and progresses throughout life. There is no proof that fatty streaks develops into atherosclerotic plaques in children, but the site of fatty streaks in children are similar to where plaques are found in the coronary arteries and aorta in adults, which could speak against fatty streaks as an early stage of atherosclerosis. Further, morphological studies have found a progression of the early fatty streaks and plaques with increasing age and depending on the level in the CVD risk factors (McGill, McMahan, Zieske et al., 2000). Plaques and thrombosis are rare in children, but morphological studies at necropsy of coronary arteries in children have shown an increasing number of fatty streaks from the age of 3 years until adulthood (Berenson, Wattigney, Tracy et al., 1992). The PDAY study (Pathological Determinants of Atherosclerosis in Youth study) found visible changes in the coronary artery walls in 60 % of adolescents 15-19 years of age with an increase in the prevalence to 80-90 % among men and women at the age of 30-34 years (Strong, Malcom, McMahan et al., 1999). The changes in the coronary artery walls are primarily fatty streaks at younger age, and more progressed lesions start after puberty and are apparent in 25 % at the age of 30 years (Strong et al., 1999).

The degree of atherosclerosis is related to the level of biological CVD risk factors. The coronary arteries and aorta were studied in almost 3000 subjects, who died from other causes than disease (accidents, murder and suicide), in the PDAY study. Atherosclerotic changes were related to the level of total cholesterol, HDL, LDL, blood pressure, fatness and insulin resistance (McGill, Herderick, McMahan et al., 2002). The risk of atherosclerotic lesions and the severity of the lesions were related to the number of risk factors over the whole age range from 15 to 34 years of age. The association between risk factors and the level of atherosclerosis is apparent even in younger age groups. The Bogalusa Heart study included 204 subjects who were 2-39 years of age at death, and among these 93 subjects had their CVD risk factor profile assessed while they were alive (Berenson, Srinivasan, Bao et al. 1998). The amount of fatty streaks and atherosclerotic plaque were associated with fatness, blood pressure, total cholesterol, HDL, LDL, triglyceride and smoking. Physical activity and fitness were not measured. Further, subjects having more risk factors had more widespread atherosclerosis, and subjects with 0, 1, 2 and 4 risk factors had 1.3 %, 2.5 %, 7.9 % and 11 %, respectively, of the arterial wall covered with fatty streaks.

During the last years ultrasound technique has made it possible to measure the thickness of the layers intima and media of the arterial wall of arteria carotis. Davis et al. and Li et al. found that children with more risk factors had greater thickness of the carotis wall as adults (Li, Chen, Srinivasan et al., 2003). The Cardiovascular in Young Finns Study studied CVD risk factors in children 12-18 years of age and found that levels in LDL, systolic blood pressure, BMI and smoking were associated to arterial wall thickness at the age of 24-39 years even after adjustment for risk factor level in adulthood (Raitakari, Juonala, Kähönen et al., 2003). The Amsterdam Growth and Health Study measured risk factors several times from childhood (age 12 years) through adolescence and into adulthood, and boys with a low fitness level in childhood had greater arterial wall thicknesses at the age of 36 years, and in those where fitness increased, the walls of the artery was less stiff (Ferreira, Twisk, Stehouwer et al., 2003). Other studies have shown that obesity, a low level of HDL and an increased blood pressure during childhood are associated with increased atherosclerosis of the coronary arteries 15-20 years later (Mahoney, Burns, Stanford et al., 1996). Finally, children with hypertension and especially obese children with hypertension have developed an increased wall thickness of the heart, a condition which in adults is associated with increased risk of heart disease (Hansen, Nielsen, Froberg et al., 1992).

In conclusion, atherosclerosis develops over decades starting in early childhood with the development of fatty streaks. Fatty streaks may develop into plaques which can be seen in some adolescents. Plaques may later result in infarctions in the heart, the brain or in the legs. Morphological studies of coronary arteries have shown a gradually increase in fatty streaks from the age of 3 years and plaques from puberty, and the degree of atherosclerosis is related to the level in CVD risk factors.

Physiological mechanisms behind the benefit of physical activity

The most convincing evidence, which is normally used when causal conclusions shall be drawn between an exposure and a disease, comes from randomised controlled trials. This type of study has not been performed with respect to any of the major life style risk factors where hard endpoints are considered. Knowledge of biological mechanisms is therefore important in our evaluation of possible causal relationships between physical activity and CVD risk factors, and in our understanding of type, frequency and intensity of the physical activity beneficial for health. Benefits of physical activity can be separated into acute changes caused by the activity itself and more long term physiological changes caused by the training effects of physical activity on the muscle-, and fat tissues, the heart, and the action of enzymes and hormones. Most of the biological CVD risk factors are linked to the metabolism, which are regulated by enzymes and hormones, mainly the oxidative enzymes, insulin and noradrenalin/adrenalin. Clustering of CVD risk factors are closely linked to high levels of fasting insulin (Andersen, Boreham, Young et al., 2006a). It is therefore important to understand the relationship between physical activity and insulin, and how insulin affects CVD levels, but it is also important to understand that physical activity have beneficial effects through different independent mechanisms, which all change risk factor levels in a positive direction.

Substrates (glucose, fat, and amino acids) are transported via the bloodstream for storage or utilisation in the muscle tissue as shown in figure 1. Insulin binds to its receptor in the cell membrane to start the cascade of signalling steps that eventually lead to the allocation of glucose transport protein (GLUTs, mainly GLUT4) to the cell membrane to allow glucose transport. A failure in any of the steps in this cascade could result in insulin resistance. Physical activity is believed to alter this mechanism. Further, acute muscle contraction primarily allocates Glut4 to the cell membrane through an insulin-independent mechanism (Ploug & Ralston, 2002). This mechanism is very important, because it works whenever a contraction occurs even if the physical activity is not sufficient to create a training effect. The amount of glucose up-take by this mechanism can be as large as the insulin mediated glucose uptake. Further, the insulin mediated

Fig. 1:   Overview of substrate routes. GLUT=Glucose Transporter protein, FFA=Free Fatty
          Acid (~NEFA), FABPPM=Fatty Acid Binding Protein Plasma Membrane isoform,
          FAT=Fatty Acid Transporter (CD36), FATP=Fatty Acid Transporting Protein.
          (Adapted from Franch, 2002)

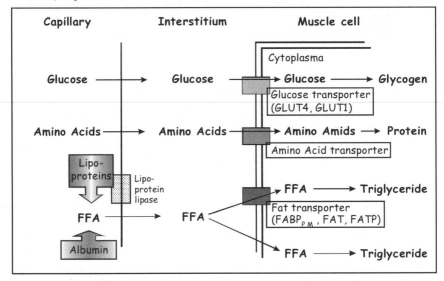

glucose uptake decrease when adrenalin increases in the blood, which can be the
case in stressful situations, but the contraction mediated uptake is not negatively
influenced by adrenalin (Franch, Aslesen, Jensen et al., 1999). Therefore, in
periods with much stress the hormonal regulation of blood glucose demands
more insulin, because the action of insulin is partly blocked by adrenalin, but
exercise can diminish this tension on the regulation (Franch et al. 1999). This
mechanism may be one explanation for the benefit of low intensity physical
activity, such as walking or cycling (Andersen, Schnohr, Schroll, Hein et al.,
2000), which has been found in prospective studies.

The positive chronic effect of physical activity may be linked to the
accumulation of activity bouts, in particular. However, it is likely that physical
activity stimulates insulin action and glucaemic control by more than one
mechanism. One simple hypothesis is that physical activity leads to an up-
regulation of the enzymes Hexokinase (HK), Citrate Synthase (CS), and
Glycogen Synthase (GS), which are the rate-limiting enzymes in glycolysis, in
Krebs' cycle, and in glycogen synthesis, respectively. This would ensure
maintenance of the concentration gradient during the time when the GluT4s are
incorporated in the membrane, because glucose is more rapidly being either
metabolised or stored as glycogen. Another mechanism is that exercise have

been shown to induce hyperexpression of GluT protein and mRNA (Richter, Derave, Wojtaszewski et al., 2001), making more GluTs available for translocation. Another pathway by which frequent exercise influence insulin sensitivity could be revealed by the fact, that physically active people have lower triglycerides (TG) and non-esterified fatty acids (NEFA or free fatty acids, FFA) levels in the blood and muscle. These lipids could impair the function of the proteins in the insulin cascade (Boden, 2003). Also suggested is a change in membrane fluidity, due to a preferential incorporation of saturated fatty acids into the plasma membrane when fat utilisation is low.

It can be concluded that insulin sensitivity is increased after acute exercise and that training induces more persistent changes in insulin sensitivity.

As fat metabolism is such an integrated part of the insulin resistance syndrome, it is appropriate to review mechanisms, by which this is regulated by physical activity and what effect this will have on lipid levels.

Fatty acids, in the form of TG or NEFA, are ingested in the diet or synthesized by the liver. In the bloodstream, NEFA is bound to albumin and TG is bound to cholesterol. TG is the most significant source of fatty acids, because this is the form in which dietary lipids are assembled by the gut and liver. TG made up of long chain fatty acids, in the form of chylomicrons (from intestinal absorption) or lipoproteins (from hepatic synthesis), is hydrolyzed to glycerol and free fatty acids by the enzymes lipoprotein lipase (LPL) and monoacylglycerol lipase, which is incorporated into endothelial cells, once it is synthesized. LPL is located on the inside of the capillary wall and training increase the number of capillaries. The rate of this synthesis is increased by physical activity and decreases with age (Hamilton, Areiqat, Hamilton et al. 2001). Exercise training increase HDL cholesterol levels via LPL and other enzymes. Increased lipoprotein lipase-mediated TG clearance and reduced hepatic TG secretion are both likely to contribute to the exercise-induced TG reductions (Gill & Hardman, 2003). LPL is also activated by apoprotein, which is associated with higher levels of physical activity. Insulin plays an important role in the lipogenic process, the net effect being enhancement of storage and blocking of mobilization and oxidation of fatty acids. Insulin exerts its effect by enhancing hepatic VLDL synthesis, stimulating LPL formation (so that circulating TG is hydrolyzed and free fatty acids can enter muscle or adipose tissue) and reduces mobilization of fatty acids from adipose tissue by inhibiting TG lipases. Exercise improves the anti-lipolytic response of insulin (Hickner, Racette, Binder et al., 1999). Insulin is also required for the transport of glucose via GluT into the adipocytes, which is needed for re-esterification of the NEFA inside the adipocytes.

In other words, insulin resistance is not a phenomenon that is isolated to skeletal muscle, thus high circulating insulin levels may result from reduced insulin sensitivity in other tissues, but muscle tissue is by far the most metabolic active tissue and is responsible for 90 % of the substrate utilisation. Reduced insulin sensitivity results in increased insulin levels and therefore increased fat storage.

Regular physical activity also has an effect on resting blood pressure, possibly linked with insulin and also the renin-angiotension-aldosterone system (DeFronzo & Ferrannini, 1991). Blood pressure is influenced by the diameter of the blood vessels, which is acutely controlled by vaso-dilatation / vaso-constriction, but also influenced by the elastic compliance of the vessel wall (and thus also mediated by factors that influence cell membrane fluidity (Ferrara, Guida, Iannuzzi et al., 2002)). Dilatation / constriction is determined by stimulation of either the α-adrenoceptors (more frequently found in greater arteries) or the β-adrenoceptors (more frequently found in smaller blood vessels) by adrenaline during sympathetic activity. The density ratio between α- and β-adrenoceptors is important in determining blood pressure, and β-adrenoceptors is upregulated by physical activity (Maki, Naveri, Leinonen et al., 1990). Moreover, training results in a more efficient recruitment of the motor units in the muscle, thus requiring less sympathetic activity for the same amount of work. Insulin has vasodilatory effects but this is uneffective if the muscles are not well capillarised (Krotkiewski, Lithell, Shono et al., 1998). Additionally, insulin stimulates the sympathetic nervous system, inhibits the parasympathetic, and enhance renal sodium reabsorption, but decrease uric acid clearance, which are all important factors in blood pressure regulation (Ferrannini, 1999). However, changes in sympathetic activity after training is also related to changes in mean arterial blood pressure, independently of changes in insulin sensitivity, body fat, and VO$_2$max (Brown, Dengel, Hogikyan et al., 2002).

Potassium ion (K$^+$) release, increased plasma osmolality, increase in blood pH and CO$_2$, hypoxemia, histamine release occur during exercise and cause vasodilatation to increase blood flow to exercising muscles, whereas blood vessels of other tissues are constricted. Interestingly, these factors also stimulate endothelial release of nitric oxide (NO), which is believed to have a stimulatory effect on glucose transport. The release of NO is chronically increased with regular exercise. Indeed, aerobic training increases the large-artery compliance, contributing to a reduction in systolic blood pressure and an attenuation of the cardiac afterload, which may be explained by the NO pathway (Kingwell & Jennings, 1997).

In conclusion, among the acute effects of physical activity are changes in blood lipids caused by the metabolism of triglycerides during exercise, and acute effects on HDL cholesterol (Hicks, MacDougall & Muckle, 1987), but important is also the insulin independent glucose uptake in the muscle cell when it contracts (Franch et al., 1999), because it decreases the insulin response after a meal. Most of the acute changes are reversed after 2-3 days, but they are very important in the prevention of CVD, obesity and diabetes type 2. Exercise should be frequent, preferably every day, because the acute changes gradually disappear. When a muscle contracts, it metabolites sugar and fat. The substrates for this process may come from stores in the cell, but the blood will supply the muscle cell with substrate afterwards. Triglyceride will enter the cell and be removed from the blood during and after an exercise bout, and this will cause a transient decrease in triglyceride in the blood, which lowers the risk of CVD if it happens often. Some of the triglyceride will come from LDL or VLDL cholesterol, and the remaining part of the molecule (HDL cholesterol) will be able to absorb new triglyceride. Lipoprotein lipase (LPL) is responsible for the brake down of LDL and VLDL. This enzyme is attached to the inside of the capillary in the muscle, and one of the long term training effects is an increase in capillaries and therefore LPL. However, even without an increase in LPL there will still be an acute effect of exercise on triglyceride in the blood.

Effects of physical training beneficial for health include an increase in the number of capillaries in the muscles and the heart, increased insulin sensitivity, adrenalin sensitivity, oxidative enzymes, improved blood lipid profile, and decreased blood pressure. It can be difficult to separate changes caused by acute exercise and chronic training effects, because an aerobic training program includes two to several sessions a week. However, some changes caused by training do not occur after one bout of exercise and they do not disappear from day to day. Capillaries, VO$_2$max and oxidative enzymes increase gradually over months of training and decrease at almost the same rate during detraining (Klausen, Andersen & Pelle, 1981). During the first two weeks of training oxidative enzymes and VO$_2$max increase at the same rate, but after two month of training oxidative enzymes had increased about 40 % whereas VO$_2$max only increased 20 %. After cessation of training, oxidative enzymes decreased at a much faster rate than VO$_2$max. Changes in fitness are therefore not identical with changes in health parameters, but there is of cause a quite close relationship. Insulin sensitivity may be increased after one bout of exercise and drop again after a few days, but the amount of GLUT4 increases gradually with training and stays elevated for longer time (Dela, Plough, Handberg et al., 1994). Other long term effects of training are a decrease in peripheral resistance in the arterioles and a lower resting heart rate (Clausen, 1977). These changes reduce the work of the heart both during rest and at a certain absolute work load.

Many of the changes are localised to the trained muscle, but are important for the whole body, when a large muscle mass is trained. In one leg training models, capillaries, GLUT4 and oxidative enzymes only increase in the trained muscles (Dela et al., 1994; Klausen et al., 1981). The improvements are therefore local, but the effect is global, because insulin sensitivity improves, and the blood lipid profile improves caused by the local changes.

CVD risk factor levels in European children

A negative association between physical activity and CVD was found as early as in 1953 (Morris, Heady, Raffle et al., 1953), and the association between CVD risk factors and both physical activity and fitness, respectively, received increasing attention in the prospective studies initiated during the 1970's. In a comparison of age-standardised CVD mortality in the age group of 35-64 years between Sweden and Finland in the mid 1970's a much higher rate was found in Finland, and in 1982 rates were 72 % higher in men and 41 % higher in women according to official cause-of-death statistics (Åkerblom, Viikari, Kouvalainen et al., 1985). As a consequence of the results found in the 1970's, the Cardiovascular Risk of Young Finns study was started in 1980, and pilot studies were conducted in the late 1970's. The study included a large representative sample of 3,596 Finnish children 3-18 years of age (Åkerblom, Uhari, Pesonen et al., 1991). In 1983 and in 1986 the cohort studied in 1980 was followed up, and tracking of serum lipids was measured (Åkerblom, Porkka, Viikari et al., 1991). At the 6-year follow-up, population data on serum lipids and physical activity were extended to young adults (Porkka, Viikari, Rönnemaa et al., 1994). This increased interest in CVD risk factors in children took place in many countries simultaneously, and the Amsterdam Growth and Health Study was started almost at the same time (Kemper & Vanthof, 1978). The Leuven Longitudinal Study started a little earlier, but this study focused more on growth and motor performance than CVD risk factors during the first years (Beunen, Claessens, Lefevre et al., 1988). In the early 1980's data on CVD risk factors and physical activity and fitness were collected in many other European countries as well.

In Denmark, three population studies in children were initiated: The Danish Youth and Sport Study (Andersen, 1996), the First Year of Gymnasium Study (Andersen, 1994), and the Odense Schoolchild Study (Hansen, Hyldebrandt, Froberg et al., 1990). The Danish Youth and Sport Study assessed risk factor levels and direct measurement of aerobic fitness in a representative cohort of adolescents (Andersen, Henckel, Saltin et al., 1987, 1989), and this cohort was followed up after two and eight years, respectively. A widening of the distribution of VO_2max and other CVD risk factors was found from adolescence to young adulthood, especially in men, most likely caused by a change to a more sedentary lifestyle in 25 % of the men. Former trade and vocational school children had more unfavourable changes in risk factors compared to former gymnasium students.

As a part of the Odense Schoolchild Study a controlled intervention trial studying the effect of 8 months of physical training on blood pressure in hypertensive and normotensive children (Hansen, Hyldebrandt, Froberg et al., 1990; Hansen, Froberg, Hyldebrandt, et al., 1991). Systolic and diastolic blood pressure was reduced and fitness was increased significantly after 8 months of training, in both the hypertensive and the normotensive group.

Among the early studies of CVD risk factors in children was the "Know Your Body" program, which included several European countries (Wynder, Williams, Laakso et al., 1981). Participating European countries were Finland, France, West Germany, Greece, Italy, Holland, Norway and Yugoslavia. Quite large differences were found in cholesterol and blood pressure levels in 13-year-olds between countries resulting in different prevalences of these risk factors. In boys, the prevalence of children having a cholesterol level above 180 mg/dl varied between 10 % in Greece and Italy and 69 % in Finland. Similar differences were found in girls, where 9 % of Greek girls and 70 % of Finnish girls, respectively, were found to be above this level. The prevalence of children having a systolic blood pressure above 130 mmHg varied between none and 21 % between countries, but large differences were found between genders. In some countries girls had higher blood pressure compared to boys but in other countries boys had the highest blood pressure. However, within each country differences between boys and girls were persistent from study to study, and the differences may therefore be attributed to environmental or lifestyle factors.

Later in the 1980's other large European studies including CVD risk factors were initiated in children. Armstrong and Simons-Morton studied CVD risk factors in English adolescents (Armstrong & Simons-Morton, 1994). The Northern Ireland Young Hearts Study was started in the late 1980's, and this study has been extended to a mixed longitudinal study, where the cohort is still being followed (Boreham, Twisk, Murray et al., 2001). Recently, Twisk et al. analysed clustering of CVD risk factors in this cohort. They found that risk factors clustered, but lifestyle parameters was not significantly related to this clustering (Twisk, Boreham, Cran et al., 1999). Clustering of CVD risk factors have also been analysed in the European Youth Heart Study (EYHS) (Andersen, Harro, Sardinha et al., 2006b). The EYHS is a European multi-centre study, where data including physical activity, other CVD risk factors and determinants of these variables have been collected in Denmark, Norway, Portugal and Estonia using identical protocols. Using identical protocols makes it possible to compare results between countries and to make pooled analyses. Data collection has been finished in Iceland and started in Spain in 2004. A planned six year follow-up of the cohorts will extend the EYHS-project into a mixed longitudinal study, and in Denmark the follow-up data collection was completed in 2004. In the first part of the Danish EYHS, fitness was a strong predictor of clustering of biological CVD risk factors at baseline (Wedderkopp, Froberg, Hansen et al., 2003). The risk of having three or more risk factors was eleven times higher in the children belonging to least fit quartile compared to the children belonging to the most fit quartile, and the risk of having four or more

CVD risk factors was elevated 24 times. These results are supported by results from the Danish Youth and Sport Study, and further, those who had clustered risk had a six times increased risk of having clustered risk after eight years compared to subjects without clustered risk at baseline (Andersen, Hasselstrøm, Grønfeldt et al., 2004).

CVD risk factor levels have recently been assessed in other European countries, but mostly in single factors.

In conclusion, risk factor levels have been assessed in most European countries, but clustered risk, which is a more severe health problem, is only calculated in very few studies. Interventions should focus on eliminating the causes of clustered risk, which include lack of physical activity and obesity potentially leading to insulin resistance.

Association between physical activity/fitness and CVD risk factors in the population

The causal chain leading from physical inactivity to CVD is multi-factorial, and a description of associations between physical activity/fitness and CVD risk factors is therefore a superficial way to describe the problem of inactivity. Aerobic exercise exerts a direct effect on the circulatory system including the heart. It changes the sensitivity of insulin and adrenalin, and it changes the concentration of the oxidative enzymes in the metabolism of fat and carbohydrates (see chapter 2). Insulin and adrenalin are metabolic hormones responsible for changes in fat and carbohydrate metabolism. They are influenced by physical training and they are related to most of the biological CVD risk factors. Therefore, physical activity causes changes in CVD risk factors such as cholesterol fractions, triglyceride, blood pressure, and abdominal fat simultaneously, and part of the benefit from physical activity is caused by changes in these risk factors. Analysis of the association between physical activity/fitness and the combined effect on risk factors gives a much stronger picture of the real benefit, than when only single risk factors are considered. Only few controlled intervention studies have been conducted in children and our main knowledge is coming from cross-sectional studies and longitudinal observational studies.

The cross-sectional association between physical activity and single CVD risk factors in adolescents is weak and only statistical significant in large studies. This is also the case in adults, but in children the relationship is somewhat weaker, partly explained by the fact that there are less entirely sedentary children than adults. Armstrong and Simons-Morton reported that data showing a beneficial association between activity and lipids and lipoproteins were minimal, but there was some evidence that HDL might be enhanced (Armstrong

& Simons-Morton, 1994). A great number of recent studies have found no associations between physical activity and blood lipids, but almost the same number of studies have found a weak association. Regarding blood pressure most studies have found a relation to physical fitness and some to physical activity. The relationship between physical activity and blood pressure in children is confounded by body weight, because body weight increases with increasing physical activity in normal weight children, and body weight is an independent predictor of blood pressure. Shear et al. found a positive relationship between blood pressure and body fat in adolescents (Shear, Freedman, Burke et al., 1987), but Stallones, Mueller & Christensen (1982) found that the weight to blood pressure association was due to components of body weight other than body fat. Furthermore, because body weight is included in the measure of aerobic fitness, some of the effect of fitness disappears when the association is adjusted for weight, but there is still a beneficial effect of a high fitness level left (Nielsen & Andersen, 2003).

The main reason for the weak relationship is a large variation in both CVD risk factors and in physical activity variables. Most children are quite physically active and negative effects of inactivity may mainly be apparent when the activity level becomes very low. Also, some of the effects may develop gradually over many years and are not yet manifest in children. When extremely sedentary groups are analysed, relationships become stronger. Relationships between physical fitness and CVD risk factors are also stronger, because the error variation in fitness is smaller compared to physical activity, and the relationship between fitness and clustered risk is very strong.

The association between blood pressure, BMI and physical fitness was analysed in a cross-sectional study of 13,000 Danish adolescents (Nielsen & Andersen, 2003). Physical fitness and BMI were independent predictors of hypertension with an increased risk of being hypertensive of almost five times in the obese compared to normal weight adolescents. A similar increase was found in adolescents with a low fitness level and the relative risk between groups of different BMI of hypertension increased with lower fitness. In the study of Nielsen and Andersen it was not possible to separate abdominal fatness, but in other studies especially abdominal fatness has been shown to be associated with higher risk (Lenthe, van Mechelen, Kemper et al., 1998).

Risk factor levels are lower in children than in adults, but conditions similar to the metabolic syndrome in adults are seen in children. The risk factors included in the metabolic syndrome, i.e. fatness, blood pressure, blood lipids and insulin levels, cluster in children already at the age of 9 years (Andersen, Wedderkopp, Hansen et al., 2003). Andersen et al. found an eight times higher risk of having a high number of risk factors compared to the number of children expected to have this number of risk factors if risk factors had been randomly distributed in the population. Clustered risk was found in 15 % of the children, who may already be partly resistant to insulin. The clustering of risk factors is found both in children and adolescents and it is associated with low level of fitness (Wedderkopp, Froberg, Hansen et al., 2003). In the European Youth Heart Study, odds ratio for having clustered risk was calculated between quartiles of fitness. When clustered risk was defined as being in the upper quartile of three of five possible risk factors, the risk was 11.4 (95 % CI: 5.7-22.9) for the lower quartile of fitness compared to the upper quartile, and the risk was 24 (95 % CI: 5.7-101.1) times higher for the low fit if clustered risk was defined as having four or more risk factors (Wedderkopp et al., 2003). Therefore, the observed decline in physical fitness in Danish 8 to 10-years-old girls between 1997-98 and 2003-04 gives rise to concern regarding future generations with unfavourable CVD risk status. Physical inactivity is recognised as a strong risk factor for CVD in adults, where inactivity can be analysed against hard endpoints (US Department of Health and Human Services, 1997). Myocardial infarction is usual a result of high levels in many risk factors simultaneously for many years, and therefore, in an analytical sense, it can be compared to clustered risk. It is difficult to define at which level in a CVD risk factor that risk is elevated and children are at risk, but there is little doubt that clustered risk will increase the rate of atherosclerosis.

Few randomised controlled trials exist where the effect of physical training on CVD risk factors have been studied in children. Hansen et al. found an increase in aerobic fitness and a decrease in blood pressure after eight months of training in hypertensive children (Hansen et al., 1991). Longitudinal observational studies support this finding. In these studies, changes are observed and the associations between changes in physical activity or fitness can be analysed against changes in risk factors. Also, childhood levels of physical activity or fitness can be analysed as predictors of adulthood risk. The European studies include the Young Finns Study (Åkerblom et al., 1985), the Danish Youth and Sport Study (Andersen et al., 1989), the Amsterdam growth and Health Study (Kemper & Vanthof, 1978), the Leuven Longitudinal Growth Study (Beunen et al., 1988) and the Young Hearts Study from Northern Ireland (Boreham, Savage, Primrose et al. 1993). The Danish Youth and Sport Study followed a cohort initially 15-19 years of age for eight years (Hasselstrøm, Hansen, Froberg et al., 2002). Blood pressure, skinfold, blood lipids, waist to hip ratio, physical activity and physical fitness were assessed. No association was found between physical activity or fitness during adolescence and CVD risk factors as young adult, but changes in fitness were related to risk in adulthood and to changes in risk from adolescence to adulthood. The Amsterdam Growth and Health Study observed a cohort through their teenage years and found that physical fitness during these years predicted adult levels after 20 years of follow-up in fatness and serum cholesterol (Twisk, Kemper & van Mechelen, 2002).

Tab. 1:   Magnitude of changes in cardiovascular risk factors due to exercise. Studies are mainly in adults, but may indicate the magnitude of expected changes in risk factors by increased physical activity levels.

Risk factor	Males and females	95% CL/ P-values	High risk individuals	95% CL/ P-values
Systolic blood pressure	−3 [1]	(p <0.01)	−10 [2]	(p <0.001)
Diastolic blood ressure	−3 [1]	(p <0.01)	−8 [2]	(p <0.001)
Triglycerides (mmol/l)	−0.18[3]	(p <0.01)	−0.41 [4] −0.13 [5]	p <0.05 NS
HDL-cholesterol mol/l)	+0.03 [3]	(NS)	+0.03 [4] +0.04 [5]	(NS) (NS)
LDL-cholesterol mol/l)	−0.13 [3]	(p <0.05)	−0.13 [4] −0.17 [5]	(NS) (NS)
Total cholesterol mol/l)	−0.26 [3]	(p <0.01)	−0.04 [4] −0.17 [5]	(NS) (NS)
Insulin sensitivity (%)	27 [6]		61-65 [7]	(P<0.05)

[1](Hansen et al., 1991); [2](Powell, Thompson, Caspersen et al., 1987); [3](Anderssen, Haaland, Hjermann et al., 1995); [4](Wood, Haskell, Blair et al., 1983); [5](Leon, Conrad, Hunninghake et al., 1979); [6](Bray, 1990); [7](Heath & Kendrick, 1989)

In conclusion, associations between physical activity or fitness and each of the CVD risk factors do exist, but they are weak. Controlled trials with physical activity have shown a positive effect on risk factors. Strong relationships are found when clustered risk is related to physical fitness or activity.

Tracking of physical activity, physical fitness and CVD risk factors

Tracking is a measure of how well subjects keep rank order within a variable. It can be expressed as a correlation calculated over the whole distribution or as an odds ratio of staying at risk from one point of time to another. The former is a good way to express stability in a variable if risk increases linearly, which it does in many CVD risk factors, and there is no well defined cut off point in the different risk factors for children above which risk increases. Odds ratio of staying at risk or staying above a defined level in a risk factor may be a better way to analyse relationships if they are not linear or to analyse clustered risk. It may be of less importance if a subject changes from the lower part of the distribution to the middle than a change from the middle to the top. However, many CVD risk factors are linearly associated to CVD. A high tracking coefficient gives a high predictive value of the risk factor measured later in life, but a low value doesn't necessarily mean the opposite, because it may be caused by measurement error or short time fluctuations, i.e. total cholesterol is very precisely measured in a particular blood sample, but day to day fluctuations are great. A tracking coefficient can never be better than the error variation in the risk factor, and it is therefore difficult to compare tracking coefficient between risk factors. Assessment of physical activity is difficult and both accelerometer measurements and self-reported activity have a low reproducibility, so tracking coefficients are always low, which does not necessarily mean that the activity level in childhood is not a determinant of adult activity. Fitness is more stable and changes gradually if physical activity is changed, and a precise assessment is possible. The tracking coefficient normally decreases with increasing time span between the measurements.

Tracking of physical activity

Low tracking coefficients are found in studies where self-reported physical activity has been analysed. Part of the explanation may be assessment problems related to self-reported activity, but some studies have found that childhood participation in sports, educational level, other life experiences and fitness level predicts adult physical activity level (Telema, Laakso & Yang, 1994). To our knowledge, only one large population study has reported tracking of physical activity measured with accelerometers (Kristensen, Wedderkopp, Moller et al., 2006).

The Danish Youth and Sport Study followed subjects for eight years from adolescence to young adulthood and found correlations of 0.31 for men (p <0.01) and 0.20 for women (n.s.) (Andersen & Haraldsdóttir, 1993). The risk for a sedentary man to stay inactive was 2.2 times higher than expected, but for women more sedentary women than expected from a random distribution became active. Similar results were found in the Young Finns Study and in the Amsterdam Growth and Health Study (Raitakari, Porkka, Taimela et al., 1994; Twisk, Kemper & van Mechelen, 2000).

Tracking of physical fitness

Physical fitness is assessed as aerobic fitness or as different measures of strength, flexibility, and motor coordination often assessed by field test batteries. When tracking of aerobic fitness is analysed, the results depend on the assessment method, because indirect methods include measurement error. Only few studies have used direct measurements of VO_2max. Aerobic fitness tracks moderately with correlation coefficient around 0.5 (Andersen, 1995; Twisk et al., 2000). Somewhat higher coefficients are found when isometric strength is assessed ($r = 0.7$), but if strength is expressed relative to body size values similar to aerobic fitness are found. Even higher coefficients were found in the Leuven Longitudinal study (Maia, Beunen, Lefevre et al., 2003).

Tracking of CVD risk factors

Only a few studies have measured tracking of CVD risk factors from adolescence to young adulthood, and they found similar results (Andersen, 1996). Both blood lipids and blood pressure (BP) track in children, but higher correlation coefficients are usually found in cholesterol fractions (0.5-0.7) compared to BP and to triglyceride (0.3-0.4). Tracking of BP was assessed in an American study, which followed 211 subjects from childhood (3-11 years) to adulthood (30 years and 50 years of age) (Nelson, Ragland & Syme, 1992). Correlations between juvenile blood pressure and adult blood pressure were low, but lower for measurements at age 50 years compared to measurements at age 30 years. Tracking in systolic blood pressure was higher than in diastolic blood pressure. However, more hypertensive subjects dropped out, which could influence tracking coefficients. Also, many subjects at age 50 years use drugs for hypertension, which is an additional bias. Correlations for blood pressure vary between 0.2 and 0.5. Associations between blood pressures measured with years interval are weakened by large intra-subjects variability from day to day and even within minutes. Part of this variation could be diminished by more measurements before the follow-up and after the follow-up, but such data are not available.

Blood lipids and lipoproteins are more stable than physical activity and blood pressure from childhood to adulthood except for triglyceride (Twisk, Kemper, van Mechelen et al., 1997). Most correlation are between 0.5 and 0.7 for total cholesterol and LDL cholesterol, and somewhat lower for triglyceride and other lipoproteins. This is quite high because big fluctuations occur from day to day in total cholesterol. Subjects in the highest quintile of total cholesterol as children have a 2-3 fold increased risk of being in the highest quintile after 8 years of follow-up (Andersen & Haraldsdóttir, 1993) and a doubled risk after 15 years of follow-up (Bao, Srinivasan, Wattigney et al., 1996).

Tracking of clustered risk

In the Danish Youth and Sport Study a total risk score was calculated as the sum of scores in the single risk factors (ranked into 1 to 6) (Andersen, 1996). A high correlation coefficient was found from adolescence to adulthood in men (r = 0.67, p <0.001) but not in women (r = 0.33, p <0.01). Recently, a report analysing tracking of clustered risk was published from this cohort, and those who had clustered risk as teenagers had a six fold increased risk of having clustered risk as young adults (Andersen et al., 2004).

In conclusion, CVD risk factors and physical fitness tracks. Blood pressure, triglyceride and physical activity only show weak tracking which in part could be due difficulties in assessing these variables, but clustered risk tracks strongly.

Overweight and obesity in children

Overweight and obesity are now at epidemic proportions in most countries. About 15 percent of the European school-aged children are carrying excess body fat (Table 2), with an increased risk of developing chronic disease. Of these overweight children, a quarter are obese, with a strong likelihood of some having multiple risk factors for type 2 diabetes, heart disease and a variety of other co-morbidities before or during early adulthood. The prevalence of overweight is dramatically higher in economically developed regions, but is rising significantly in most parts of the world. Prof. Philips James, Chairman of International Obesity Task Force (IOTF) says: *"Obesity constitutes one of the most important medical and public health problems of our time"*.

Tab. 2:   Prevalence of overweight and obesity among school-age children in global regions. Overweight and obesity defined by IOTF criteria. Children aged 5–17 years. Based on surveys in different years after 1990.

Prevalence (%)	Overweight	Obese
Worldwide	8	2
the Americas	26	8
Europe	15	4
Near/Middle East	11	6
Asia-Pacific	4	1
Sub-Sahara Afrika	2	0

Data from individual countries indicates that in Europe 10-20 % of men and 10-25 % of women are obese (Body Mass Index >30) (2004).The prevalence of obesity has increased by 10-40 % in European countries since 1990. Between 2-8 % of the total sick care costs of western countries is estimated to be attributable to obesity. But the full burden upon the health services cannot yet be estimated. Although childhood obesity brings a number of additional problems – hyper-insulineamia, a raised risk of type 2 diabetes, hypertension, sleep apnoea, social exclusion and depression – the greatest health problems will be seen in the next generation of adults as the present childhood obesity epidemic passes through to adulthood. Greatly increased rates of heart disease, diabetes, certain cancers, gall bladder disease, osteoarthritis, endocrine disorders and other obesity related conditions will be found in young adult populations, and their need for medical treatment may last for their remaining life-time, and their could be forced to early retirement and disability pension. Also indirect costs are attributable to obesity such as psychological stress and social dysfunction. The costs to the health services, the losses to society and the burdens carried by the individuals involved will be great.

The aetiology of obesity is likely to exist in the interactive effects of genotype and critical environmental influences such as physical activity levels and food intake. A range of additional psychosocial and demographic influences can modify these relationships. We have only limited data that address these complex relationships. Many studies have investigated linear relationships between individual – or a limited range of antecedent factors and obesity, but this approach disregards the complex nature of the relationships between the aetiological factors, the disease itself and its co-morbidities.

Obesity in childhood

Childhood obesity is becoming an increasingly important issue. There are clear indications that overweight and obesity in children are increasing, and there is substantial evidence that obesity during childhood lays the metabolic groundwork for adult cardiovascular disease (Gidding, Leibel, Daniels et al., 1996). Obesity is related to blood pressure, serum cholesterol, LDL cholesterol, triglycerides, serum glucose and serum insulin, even in childhood, and it is therefore likely to be a major contributor to morbidity and mortality from adult coronary heart disease in later years (Jebb, 1997). US data show that between 5 and 14 years of age, the prevalence of overweight increased from 15 % to 24 %. Compared with non-obese peers, children who were obese at ages 6-9 have been shown to be 8.8 times as likely to be obese in their 20s (Whitaker, Wright, Pepe et al., 1997). It has been reported, that overweight in adolescence predicts a broad range of adverse health effects in adulthood that are independent of adult weight (Whitaker et al., 1997). Adolescence is one of the most vulnerable periods for the development overweight/obesity and overweight during adolescence is therefore concluded to be a more significant predictor of a range of future diseases than overweight as an adult (Must, Jacques, Dallal et al., 1992).

The three principal causes of overweight and obesity are likely to be low energy expenditure, high energy intake and genetic predisposition. The dramatic secular increase in the prevalence of obesity over recent years is unlikely to be explained by genetic factors, as the gene pool is largely unchanged. However, it is important to assess whether some children are genetically predisposed to be more susceptible to the adverse effects of an environment that is toxic to physical activity and healthy eating.

The changing nature of the environment towards greater inducement of obesity has been described in WHO Technical Report on chronic disease as follows:

'Changes in the world food economy have contributed to shifting dietary patterns, for example, increased consumption of energy-dense diets high in fat, particularly saturated fat, and low in unrefined carbohydrates. These patterns are combined with a decline in energy expenditure that is associated with a sedentary lifestyle-motorized transport, labour-saving devices at home, the phasing out of physically demanding manual tasks in the workplace, and leisure time that is preponderantly devoted to physically undemanding pastimes.'

This emphasis on the environmental causes of obesity leads to certain conclusions: firstly, the treatment of obesity is unlikely to succeed if we deal only with the child and not with the child's prevailing environment, and secondly that the prevention of obesity will require a broad-based, public health program.

Since genetic predisposition is likely to be an important determinant of the risk of developing obesity, it will be important to assess variations in genotype/ phenotype, as well as examining factors that influence gene expression. Such evidence will be critical in the design of future obesity prevention programs.

Genetic evidence

Twin studies suggest a strong genetic component to obesity. Comparing the combined skinfold thicknesses of monozygotic twins gives a correlation co-efficient of 0.81, compared with 0.49 for dizygotic twins (Hawk & Brook, 1979). Studies of twins brought up in separate environments have shown that a genetic predisposition to gain weight could account for 60–85 % of the variation in obesity (Allison, Matz, Pietrobelli et al., 1999). For most of these children the genes for overweight are expressed where the environment allows and encourages their expression (obesogenic' environment). A genetic predisposition to accumulate weight is a significant element in the development of obesity, but the genetic components are complex, therefore the amount and rate of weight gain are unlikely to be related to a single gene in the majority of obesity.

In children, we can assess the unmodified effect of genetic variations on many health risk factors – including obesity. The young age enables us to disregard some of the risk factors, which may either modify the genetic variation or be more important than the genetic variation in an adult population. In this way, we are able to estimate the importance of interaction between genotype and environmental factors on obesity and its co-morbidities.

Children at risk - life factors

Given the high level of genetic predetermination of obesity risk it is clear that large numbers of children are likely to develop excess body weight wherever the situation permits it. However, there appear to be certain physical and social environments that particularly encourage weight gain and certain groups of children that might be at special risk, including children with physical disability, adolescents with type 1 diabetes, children with psychological problems and children with eating disorders. But also ethnicity, parental obesity, and low birth weight and not least social deprivation linked to family and school function are essential and influencing factors (Lobstein, Baur, & Uauy, 2004).

For some children, foetal growth is related to obesity. Significant correlations have been observed between maternal skinfold thickness and the skinfold thickness of the baby suggesting that either nutritional deprivation of the mother early in pregnancy affected the regulation of food intake and growth, or nutritional deprivation affected a critical period of development for adipose tissue cellularity (Whitelaw, 1976). Also the influence of breast-feeding have been suggested to have a protective influence on subsequent childhood obesity (Armstrong & Reilly, 2002). The evidence in this field is still tentative, so the accumulating evidence suggesting foetal and infant origins of many diseases that are co-morbidities of obesity make this an important field of investigation.

Diet and physical activity

The two main environmental influences on obesity are likely to be low physical activity and high energy intake. There appears to have been a modest decline in the energy intake in adults over the past 2-3 decades (Hill & Melanson, 1999). It has therefore been argued that low levels of physical activity are the main cause of the rise in obesity. Obesity is rising in the face of unchanged or slightly declining energy intake in adults, whereas indices of physical inactivity (car ownership, TV viewing, computer games) are increasing. Similar trends have been reported in children (Prentice & Jebb, 1995). Mean energy intakes of 14-year-old girls have declined from 2,600 kcal./day to 1,800 kcal./day over the last 50 years, and the decline in 14-year-old boys over the same period is 3,100 kcal./day to 2,400 kcal./day. Again, it appears that fatness is increasing in the face of declining energy intakes, and an important issue in this context is sedentary behaviour. Multivariate studies have found that television viewing and playing video games for longer periods of time, or not participating in sports outside of school, promotes obesity, whilst physical activity shows protective effects (Berkey, Rockett, Field et al., 2000; Wedderkopp, Andersen, Hansen et al., 2001). There is little evidence that obese children consume more calories than non-obese children (Rolland-Cachera, Deheeger, Pequignot et al., 1988). However, the possibility of higher levels of under-reporting by obese children cannot be discounted, and the precision of the methodology is questionable. It is therefore critical that studies of childhood obesity use sophisticated methods of measurement, as it will be important to detect subtle differences in the critical measures.

Measures of body fatness

An ideal measure of body fat should be accurate in its estimate of body fat; precise, with small measurement error; accessible, in terms of simplicity, cost and ease of use; acceptable to the subject; and well documented, with published reference values. No existing measure satisfies all these criteria at the moment. Measurement of adiposity in children and adolescents occurs in a range of settings, using a range of methods.

Body fat: direct measures and derived estimates.

Direct measures of body composition provide an estimation of total body fat mass and various components of fat free mass. Such techniques include underwater weighing, magnetic resonance imaging (MRI), computerized axial tomography (CT or CAT) and dual energy X-ray absorptiometry (DEXA). The methods are used predominantly for research and in tertiary care settings, but may be used as a 'gold standard' to validate anthropometric measures of body fatness (Goran, 1998).

Anthropometric measures of relative fatness.

Among the anthropometric measures of relative adiposity or fatness are waist and hip, skinfold thickness and indices derived from measured height and weight such as Quetelet's index (BMI or W H-2), the ponderal index (W H-3) and similar formulae. All anthropometric measurements rely to some extent on the skill of the measurer, and their relative accuracy as a measure of adiposity must be validated against a 'gold standard' measure of adiposity.

Definitions of 'overweight' and 'obesity' in young people.

The primary purposes for defining overweight and obesity are to predict health risks and to provide comparisons between populations. Faced with a continuous distribution, criteria need to be set which defines cut-off points that best fulfil these purposes. For practical reasons, the definitions have usually been based on anthropometry, with waist circumference and BMI being the most widely used.

Waist circumference

In a large-scale epidemiological study of young people aged 5-17 years, Freedman et al. showed that central fat distribution (particularly as assessed by waist circumference) was associated with an adverse lipid profile and hyperinsulinaemia (Freedman, Dietz, Srinivasan et al., 1999). A high waist circumference has also been shown to track well into adulthood (Goran, Gower, Treuth et al., 1998). Although waist circumference percentile charts have been described, appropriate cut-off points for defining high or low health risks have not been identified.

Waist circumference may be useful in clinical practice as a means of determining a child or adolescent's response to weight control measures. In epidemiological studies, it may be used to characterize a population in terms of abdominal fat distribution and to determine the prevalence of risk factors. Abdominal fat is a metabolic active tissue and secrete substances that decrease insulin sensitivity, and is therefore the most important fat storage in relation to health. At present, however, waist circumference cannot be used to categorize a child as being at a high or low risk because there is no consensus of cut points for risk.

Body mass index (BMI).

BMI is significantly associated with relative fatness in childhood and adolescence, and is the most convenient way of measuring relative adiposity.

BMI for age reference charts and BMI for age percentiles

BMI varies with age and gender. It typically rises during the first months after birth, falls after the first year and rises again around the sixth year of life: this second rise is sometimes referred to as 'the adiposity rebound'. A given value of BMI therefore needs to be evaluated against age- and gender-specific reference values. Several countries, including France, the UK, Singapore, Sweden, Denmark and the Netherlands, have developed their own BMI-for-age gender-specific reference charts using local data. In the USA, reference values (Must, Dallal, & Dietz, 1991) derived from US survey data in the early 1970s, have been widely used and were recommended for older children (aged 9 years or more) by a WHO expert committee in 1995. More recently, the US National Center for Health Statistics (NCHS) has produced reference charts based on data from five national health examinations from 1963–1994 (Kuczmarski, Ogden, Grummer-Strawn et al., 2000).

The advantage of using BMI-for-age charts is that a child can be described as being above or below certain centile lines (for example the 85th or 90th centile), which can be useful in a clinical setting. Data, however, are usually derived from a single reference population, and classifying an individual as overweight or obese assumes that the individual is comparable to that reference population. Furthermore, clinicians may wrongly interpret the centiles as representing an ideal population, when the figures may in fact come from a reference population with a high prevalence of obesity, such as the USA NCHS data.

The NCHS documentation recommends that those children with a BMI greater than or equal to the 95th percentile are classified as 'overweight' and those children with a BMI between the 85th and 95th percentile are classified as 'at risk of overweight' (Kuczmarski et al., 2000).

Tab. 3:   International cut-off points for body mass index for overweight and obesity by sex
          between 2 and 18 years (Cole et al, 2000)

Age (years)	Body mass index 25 kg m-2		Body mass index 30 kg m-2	
	Males	Females	Males	Females
2	18,41	18,02	20,09	19,81
2,5	18,13	17,76	19,80	19,55
3	17,89	17,56	19,57	19,36
3,5	17,69	17,40	19,39	19,23
4	17,55	17,28	19,29	19,15
4,5	17,47	17,19	19,26	19,12
5	17,42	17,15	19,30	19,17
5,5	17,45	17,20	19,47	19,34
6	17,55	17,34	19,78	19,65
6,5	17,71	17,53	20,23	20,08
7	17,92	17,75	20,63	20,51
7,5	18,16	18,03	21,09	21,01
8	18,44	18,35	21,60	21,57
8,5	18,76	18,69	22,17	22,18
9	19,10	19,07	22,77	22,81
9,5	19,46	19,45	23,39	23,46
10	19,84	19,86	24,00	24,11
10,5	20,20	20,29	24,57	24,77
11	20,55	20,47	25,10	25,42
11,5	20,89	21,20	25,58	26,05
12	21,22	21,68	26,02	26,67
12,5	21,56	22,14	26,43	27,24
13	21,91	22,58	26,84	27,76
13,5	22,27	22,98	27,25	28,20
14	22,62	23,34	27,63	28,57
14,5	22,96	23,66	27,98	28,87
15	23,29	23,94	28,30	29,11
15,5	23,60	24,17	28,60	29,29
16	23,90	24,37	28,88	29,43
16,5	24,19	24,54	29,14	29,56
17	24,46	24,70	29,41	29,69
17,5	24,73	24,85	29,70	29,84
18	25,00	25,00	30,00	30,00

BMI for age Z-scores.

BMI can be compared with a reference data set and reported as Z-scores. A BMI Z-score is calculated as follows:

(observed value) – (mean reference value of a population)

standard deviation of reference population

A Z-score of 0 is equivalent to the median or 50th centile value, a Z-score of +1.00 is approximately equivalent to the 84th centile, a Z-score of +2.00 is approximately equivalent to the 98th centile and a Z-score of +2.85 is >99th centile. As with other measures, BMI Z-scores can be used to compare an individual or specified population against a reference population. BMI for age Z-scores, however, require suitable statistical skills or software programs and furthermore, it is difficult to choose an appropriate reference population, and there are only arbitrary cut-off points for categorizing into non-overweight, overweight and obese.

BMI based on adult cut-off points.

An expert committee convened by the International Obesity Task Force in 1999 determined that although BMI was not ideal as a measure of adiposity, it had been validated against other, more direct measures of body fatness and may therefore be used to define overweight and obesity in children and adolescents. As it is not clear at which BMI level adverse health risk factors increase in children, the group recommended cut offs based on age specific values that project to the adult cut offs of 25 kg m-2 for overweight and 30 kg m-2 for obesity. Using data from six different reference populations (Great Britain, Brazil, the Netherlands, Hong Kong, Singapore and the USA) Cole et al. derived centile curves that passed through the points of 25 kg m-2 and 30 kg m-2 at age 18 years, provide age and gender specific BMI cut offs to define overweight and obesity, corresponding to the adult cut off points for overweight and obesity (Cole, Bellizzi, Flegal et al., 2000).

The tables developed by Cole et al. (reproduced in Table 3) are useful for epidemiological research in that children and adolescents can be categorized as non-overweight, overweight or obese using a single standard tool. The cut off points were developed using several data sets. Therefore they represent an international reference that can be used to compare populations world-wide.

Since BMI is proportional to the height of the subject (wt/ht^2) and increases with sexual maturation in children, it is questionable to use this measure in the evaluation of secular trends over many decades within an age group, since children to day have become taller and more mature compared to earlier decades.

But the reference cut-offs from Cole et al. are suitable for research use and for monitoring and evaluating changes in populations, because the cut-offs provide a standard benchmark against which all population groups can be compared and trends assessed. In terms of defining groups at special risk of health problems due to excess weight, the cut-off points may need to be adjusted to account for local factors.

In clinical practice, the variations found in body fat mass and non-fat mass for a given bodyweight may make any judgement based on weight (adjusted for height and/or for age) unreliable as an estimate of an individual's actual body fat. At higher levels, BMI and the BMI cut-offs may be helpful in informing a clinical judgement, but at levels near the norm additional criteria may be needed. For clinical assessment, more direct measures, such as bio-impedance, as well as indirect measures such as waist circumference, are sometimes used.

Weight for height relations

Various alternatives to the weight-to height ratio have been developed examining different powers of N in the formula weight/heightN, such as the ponderal index (w/h3). 'N' is sometimes referred to as the Benn index.

The power of the height value has been studied according to the Benn index (Franklin, 1999).

Adjusted weight = weight/height^p where p is a value between 1 and 3. In the special case that $p = 2.0$ it is called BMI. If different sized individuals are considered geometrically similar with the same shape and body density the p value would be 3.0, meaning that weight would be adjusted simply for volume.

As shown in Figure 2 studies have estimated the p value for boys in 4 countries. The studies shows that the estimated p value change according to the age of the boys. P lay just below 3.0 for children aged 6 years, rising to 3.5 for children aged around 10 and fell to around 2.0 just before the age of 18. Thus BMI is not optimal as an indicator of obesity in children. According to figure 4 different powers for the height should be used with different ages. However, attaining worldwide unanimity on standardized p-values seems unlikely and would require innumerable verifying studies. Basically Franklins study show how difficult it is to agree on a final set of measuring weight for height on children.

Recommendations for the definition of 'overweight' and 'obesity' (Lobstein Baur, & Uauy, 2004).

• Body mass index should be used as the main measure of overweight and obesity in childhood and adolescence for survey purposes.

• Research studies involving epidemiological or clinical data should ensure that BMI for age is expressed as a mean and standard deviation for each gender;

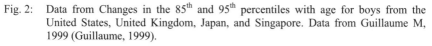

Fig. 2:   Data from Changes in the 85th and 95th percentiles with age for boys from the United States, United Kingdom, Japan, and Singapore. Data from Guillaume M, 1999 (Guillaume, 1999).

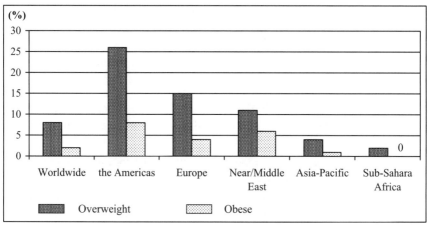

and prevalence is estimated by using cut-off points from a clearly established reference. This will allow international comparison of data.

- Researchers should be encouraged to collect data on waist circumference in childhood and adolescence when performing epidemiological or clinical studies.

- Further research is needed to validate the BMI-for age or waist-for-age cut-off points associated with health risks in childhood and adolescence.

- Further research is needed into the effect of ethnicity on the interpretation of the definitions of 'overweight' and 'obesity'.

- Further work is needed in establishing clinical definitions of 'overweight' and 'obesity' that are congruent with research definitions.

Prevalence and trends in childhood obesity

As mentioned before, our understanding of the circumstances surrounding obesity in children and adolescents is limited due to the lack of comparable representative data from different countries and, in particular, due to the use of varying criteria for defining obesity among different countries and researchers.

This methodological problem of consistency between classifications of childhood obesity is the major obstacle in studying global secular trends for younger age groups. The data reviewed on 7 to 10-year-old children are the published data and some additional unpublished data collected by the International Obesity Task Force in collaboration with regional task forces and members of the International

Association for the Study of Obesity (Lobstein et al., 2004). The data on 13 and 15-year-old children is data from the WHO survey: Young people's health in context – Health behaviour in school aged children (HBSC) study: International report from the 2001/2002 survey. This report divides subjects in boys and girls and in two age groups and into pre-obese and obese groups, which correspond to the adult BMI values of 25.0-29.9 and >30.0 and over.

The method used in the HBSC study is self reported questionnaire, asking:

- How much do you weigh without clothes?

- How tall are you without shoes?

Age- and gender-specific BMI international cut-off points were used to calculate the prevalence of overweight (Cole et al., 2000).

There are several constraints on the use of survey data for interpreting trends in obesity in children and adolescents.

- Sampling issues. Some of the results presented are based on national representative surveys, while others are based on smaller surveys that do not represent national populations.

- Sexual maturation influences body fatness: fat gain occurs in both boys and girls early in adolescence, then ceases and may even temporarily reverse in boys but continues throughout adolescence in girls. There are large intra- and inter-population variations in the patterns of sexual maturation.

- Secular trends in growth and development. Over recent decades, children world-wide have become taller, they mature earlier, and in some cases, become heavier for a given age. These trends have affected some populations more than others, and at different rates of change. Comparisons between populations should take these secular trends into account.

- Measurement errors and missing data. Data collected in different studies and countries and over time may not have the same quality.

The potential influence of measurement errors should not be ignored. All these factors may influence the observed trends. Nonetheless, survey material is an invaluable source of data for understanding the rising epidemic of childhood obesity and the continued collection of such data is essential.

In European countries a number of studies have examined the trends in childhood obesity, including material collected by IOTF in collaboration with the European Childhood Obesity Group (International Obesity task Force with the European Childhood Obesity Group, 2002) and Lobstein TJ and Frelut M-L. (Lobstein et al., 2004). The data suggest that childhood obesity has increased steadily in this region over the past two to three decades, although there are complex patterns in the prevalence and trends, which vary with time, age, sex and geographical region. The highest prevalence levels are observed in southern European countries, as table 4 show. Children in northern Europe generally have overweight prevalence rates of 10-20 %, while in southern Europe the prevalence rates are 20-35 %.

Tab. 4:   Prevalence (percentage) of overweight children in various European countries. Overweight defined by IOTF criteria (includes obese). Children aged around 7-10 years. Based on surveys in different years after 1990 (Lobstein et al., 2004)

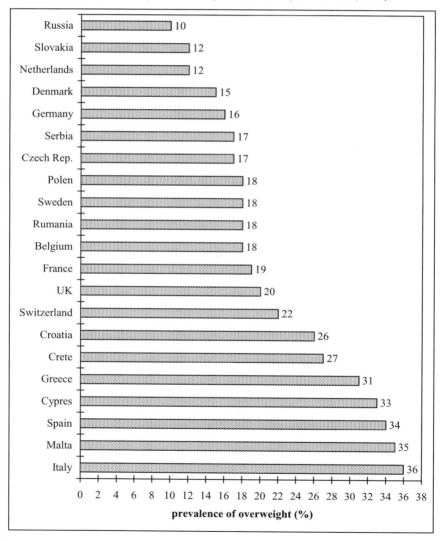

The reasons for a north-south gradient are not clear. Genetic factors are unlikely, because the gradient can be shown even within a single country, such as Italy. The child's household or family income may be a relevant variable, possibly mediated through income-related dietary factors such as maternal nutrition during pregnancy, or breast or bottle-feeding in infancy. Several studies have reported an inverse association between socio-economic status and body fatness in children, and recently heterogeneous trends in BMI and the prevalence of overweight across socio-economic gradients has been observed in Danish third grade school children between 1997-98 and 2003-04, with results in general showing less favourable trends in children coming from families with low socio-economic status (Kristensen, Wedderkopp, Moller et al., 2006).

Economic recession may affect the rate of increase in obesity levels. Some countries in the region have reported a fall in obesity rates; in Russia the prevalence of overweight and obesity declined from 15.6 % to 9.0 % between 1992 and 1998, a period when the country suffered severe socio-economic difficulties (Wang, Monteiro & Popkin, 2002). In Poland in 1994, during a period of economic crisis, a survey of over two million young people found 8 % to be overweight compared with the national reference figure of 10 % (Oblaciska Wrocawska & Woynarowska, 1997). In Croatia, which experienced less economic recession, the Croatian Health Service Year Book 1998 documented little change in excess weight levels in schoolchildren between the early and later 1990, while in the Czech Republic, also less economically damaged than Russia, overweight (above 90th centile 1991 reference) rose modestly from 10 % to 12.5 % in the period 1991-1999 (Bláha & Vignerová, 2002).

The data in table 5 and 6 show a clear relationship between the prevalence of overweight and the development of obesity: countries with higher percentages of overweight also report a higher prevalence of obesity.

In both 13 and 15-year-olds, overweight appears to show a geographical pattern confirming the mentioned north–south gradient with the UK countries as an exception. Prevalence is highest in England, Scotland and Wales and some southern European countries: Greece, Italy, Malta, Portugal and Spain.

The Scandinavian countries and the central European countries have a lower proportion of overweight young people, and prevalence is lowest in the eastern half of the WHO European Region.

Among 13-year-olds, boys have higher rates than girls in a number of countries, with the highest gender differences found in Malta and Spain. Among 15-year-olds, again boys have higher rates than girls in 10 countries with the highest gender differences in Croatia, Greece, Italy, Malta and Slovenia.

Tab. 5:   Young people who are overweight/obese according to BMI, (%) (Data from World Health Organization 2004).

Country	13-year-olds (%)			
	owerweight boys	owerweight girls	obese boys	obese girls
Malta	24,7	18,1	9,1	5,4
Wales	17,8	15,1	4,4	1,7
Spain	21,5	11,1	3,2	0,6
England	13,4	12,9	4,4	1,3
Italy	17,9	10,9	3,1	1,5
Portugal	16,1	11,6	4,3	1,3
Greece	17,5	10,4	2,8	1,7
Scotland	13,4	10,6	2,4	2,4
Slovenia	12,4	11,0	3,3	1,4
Finland	12,8	9,8	3,1	1,2
Austria	13,3	10,1	1,7	0,9
Hungary	13,0	9,5	2,5	1,4
Ireland	10,5	8,4	3,9	2,1
Belgium (Fr)	11,2	9,7	1,9	1,1
Norway	11,7	6,6	3,6	1,3
Macedonia	13,3	5,8	3,2	1,0
Germany	11,9	7,2	2,6	1,1
France	11,8	7,9	2,0	0,8
Sweden	10,5	7,0	0,7	1,5
Belgium (Fl)	10,2	7,0	1,5	1,1
Croatia	11,1	5,4	1,9	0,7
Czech Rep.	10,3	6,4	1,4	0,7
Denmark	7,5	8,3	0,9	0,9
Poland	9,7	3,9	1,2	0,4
Switzerland	7,8	5,6	1,9	0,6
Estonia	9,0	4,1	1,1	0,3
Netherlands	7,4	4,2	0,7	0,3
Latvia	6,9	3,0	0,6	0,6
Russia	6,3	3,6	0,5	0,1
Lithuania	5,3	3,6	0,4	0,1
Ukraine	5,0	2,9	0,0	0,2
HBSC mean	12,0	7,9	2,4	1,2

Tab. 6:   Young people who are overweight/obese according to BMI, (%) (Data from World
          Health Organization 2004).

Country	15-year-olds (%)			
	owerweight boys	owerweight girls	obese boys	obese girls
Malta	18,6	11,9	9,3	4,8
Wales	16,6	14,4	5,6	3,0
Greece	20,3	7,5	2,7	1,1
Spain	17,7	10,0	2,9	0,7
England	11,8	10,1	4,5	2,8
Finland	14,3	7,9	2,8	1,4
Italy	17,1	6,6	2,5	1,1
Slovenia	16,6	6,2	1,9	0,8
Scotland	12,6	8,1	1,7	2,3
Norway	12,6	8,4	2,0	1,1
Ireland	9,6	10,8	1,4	1,8
Denmark	12,8	8,6	1,4	0,9
Portugal	15,1	6,4	1,7	0,8
Hungary	11,7	7,5	3,7	1,8
Germany	13,7	5,5	2,1	1,1
France	10,3	7,6	1,8	2,4
Austria	10,0	7,5	3,3	0,7
Belgium (Fl)	10,7	7,2	2,0	1,0
Sweden	12,7	6,0	1,9	1,1
Croatia	14,7	5,6	1,5	0,5
Belgium (Fr)	10,3	7,9	1,3	1,6
Macedonia	13,0	4,6	1,8	1,2
Czech Rep.	11,5	5,0	1,6	0,5
Switzerland	10,2	5,5	1,2	1,2
Netherlands	8,8	7,1	1,0	0,8
Estonia	8,1	3,8	1,2	0,8
Poland	7,0	4,2	0,8	1,1
Latvia	7,9	3,5	0,7	0,7
Ukraine	6,1	4,3	0,4	0,3
Russia	6,4	2,8	0,6	0,3
Lithuania	4,4	3,0	0,6	0,3
HBSC mean	12,2	7,1	2,3	1,4

A comparison of the age groups does not reveal a relationship between the levels of overweight at 13 and 15 years. Except in Denmark, Sweden, Latvia and Ukraine, the prevalence of obesity is much higher in boys: up to five times the levels in girls and the results are similar among 15-year-olds. The gender difference is not as large, however; levels for boys are on average two or three times higher. Again, similar to the findings for overweight, there does not appear to be a relationship between levels of obesity at 13 and 15 years. In all countries and regions, prevalence does not increase or decrease greatly between the two ages.

In table 7 the IOTF data on 7-10 years is compared with the WHO data on 13 and 15 years. There is a clear difference in the gradients of overweight, showing

Tab. 7: Comparison of young people who are overweight/obese (ow/ob) according to BMI, (%) between WHO data and IOTF data.

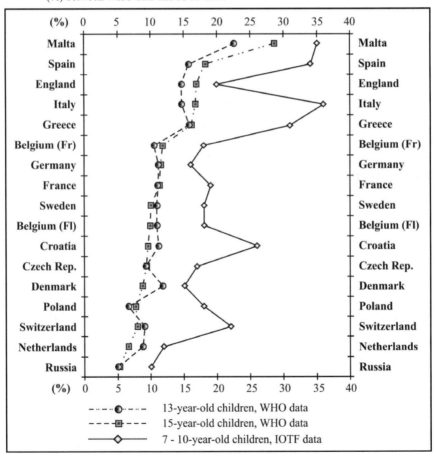

much lower percentage of overweight children in the WHO data. The reason for this is not clear. But the proportion of missing BMI data in the WHO data was high, and analysis of the characteristics of the young people who did not report their height and weight, compared with those who did, revealed that the youngsters who did not report their height and weight were: less likely to come from higher socioeconomic groups; less likely to be physically active; more likely to be dieting or feel the need to lose weight; more likely to consume less fruit and vegetables. These findings suggest that young people who do not report their height and weight are more likely to be overweight or obese, and dissatisfied with the size and weight of their bodies. These concerns may have influenced them in responding to the questionnaire. Another possibility is a shift in overweight and obesity from child to adolescent, but this has not been seen in longitudinal studies following children from childhood into adolescents.

Conclusion

In order to take our understanding of obesity to a higher level, large-scale studies are needed that can identify the subtle relationships and interactions that influence fat deposition. A comprehensive range of influencing factors and co-morbidities must be measured to allow meaningful models of obesity to be generated. Precise and detailed measurement of critical factors such as physical activity and eating behaviour are needed that allow intuitive investigation of the complex and differing dimensions of these behaviours. For example, the timing, quality and patterning of meals, and the frequency, intensity and mode of physical activity are important dimensions to investigate in relation to obesity. The level of sedentary behaviour – rather than physical activity – can be a key factor in the development of obesity.

The use of objective motion sensors is a very important technological advancement in the measurement of physical activity and sedentary living in studies relating to the development of obesity, but this has only recently become feasible. An additional requirement is that measures of body composition include determination of the distribution of fat – or 'fat patterning' – as there are indications that central obesity is a particularly undesirable form of obesity and that sexual dimorphism in fat patterning exists (Goran & Gower, 1999; Taylor Jones, Williams et al., 2000).

Obesity interventions with adults have achieved minimal success, and prevention of obesity during childhood is therefore a key public health strategy, especially in view of the fact that the prevalence of childhood obesity is also rising. In order to intervene successfully with children there is a need to identify with some precision the main factors that influence the development of overweight and obesity at this stage of life. At another level, it may also be important to identify additional factors related to the influencing factors themselves – in particular the determinants of physical activity and diet. In this way, a more sophisticated model of the development of obesity in children can be generated. Much previous research in this field relies heavily on self-report methodologies and these normally carry unacceptable levels of measurement error, especially in children. It is unsurprising that the existing data relating diet, physical activity and overweight in children is equivocal , as until very recently we have been unable to detect the subtle differences in behaviour that – over time – cause excess fat deposition.

Prevention is the only realistic solution.

Many questions regarding what constitutes the best treatment remain unanswered: there have been few sufficiently large multicentre clinical trials initiated in order to test the efficacy and safety of well-defined obesity treatment programs. Such trials may reveal which non-pharmacological and non-surgical interventions can help manage obesity over the long term. Losing weight over the short term, and then experiencing a rebound gain in weight, remains the usual experience for the majority of obese children and adolescents. The importance of further research cannot be over stated.

The most logical settings for preventive interventions are school settings and home-based settings. A number of interventions have been tried at these levels. A Cochrane review of those trials of sufficient duration to detect the effects of intervention concluded that there was little evidence of success (Campbell, Waters, O'Meara et al., 2002). It suggested that a more reliable evidence base is needed in order to determine the most cost-effective and health promoting strategies that have sustainable results and can be generalized to other situations and prevention strategies will require a co-ordinated effort between the medical community, health administrators, teachers, parents, food producers and processors, retailers and caterers, advertisers and the media, recreation and sport planners, urban architects, city planners, politicians and legislators.

Trends in cardio-respiratory fitness

Despite several anecdotal reports suggesting that there has been a decline in physical fitness in children in recent years, rather few studies have examined secular trends in cardio-respiratory fitness (CF) in children using a CF-test to exhaustion. However, secular trends in CF measured objectively to exhaustion have recently been examined twice in Danish school children participating in the European Youth Heart Study. Declining CF was demonstrated in Danish boys between 1985-86 and 1997-98, whereas no overall difference in CF was found in girls overall during that period of time (Wedderkopp, Froberg, Hansen et al., 2004). In the same study, however, a polarization in CF over time was found in both boys and girls since an increased difference between the least fit and the most fit boys and girls, respectively, was observed. When examining secular trends in CF including a comparable sample of Danish children six years later, results showed a significant 2.8 % decline in CF in girls whereas no further change was found in boys in the period between 1997-98 and 2003-04. When examining the secular trends in CF across socio-economic gradients in the Danish school children between 1997-98 and 2003-04, results in general showed a tendency towards more favourable trends in boys coming from families with high socio-economic position (Moller, Andersen, Wedderkopp et al., 2006).

Other studies have reported a secular decline in physical fitness, but they used different and less reliable tests such as running distance covered in 9 minutes, the 1 mile run/walk test, the 50m sprint test, and the 20m shuttle run test as fitness variables. Disadvantages of aerobic field tests which potentially could complicate secular comparison include parameters like practice, motivation, strategy, and environmental conditions. However, when examining secular changes in directly measured peak VO_2 in US boys and girls, by comparing available data from the 20th century (1930s-1990s), Eisenmann et al. found no changes in absolute or weight-relative peak VO_2 in boys aged 6-18 years since 1938, and no changes in young girls since 1960. However, a decrease in CF was observed in adolescent girls since 1980 (Eisenmann, 2003).

Final Conclusion

Atherosclerosis develops over decades from the first microscopic changes in the arterial walls until clinical symptoms such as thrombosis in heart, brain or legs. Atherosclerotic lesions are seen in teenagers and at the age of 25-35 years they are apparent in 25 % of the population. There is a clear relationship between CVD risk factor levels and development of atherosclerosis, and low physical fitness is a strong predictor of clustered risk. Physiological changes caused by training give plausible explanations for the positive relationship between physical activity and improved risk factor profile. Clustering of CVD risk factors and physical fitness track from childhood into adulthood and there is therefore a strong rationale for early prevention of cardiovascular risk.

The international reference charts for making international comparisons and for monitoring the secular trends in childhood obesity need to be continually refined and evaluated.

Collection of longitudinal data, which can be used to track the development of obesity and evaluate interventions, needs to be encouraged. Longitudinal studies may prove particularly valuable for examining the social, environmental, behavioural and biological factors that may contribute to the secular trends in childhood obesity.

It can be concluded that there is a large potential for primary prevention of CVD and obesity in European children, and lifestyle changes including increased physical activity as one of the key actions should be initiated.

References

Åkerblom, H. K., Uhari, M., Pesonen, E., Dahl, M., Kaprio, E. A., Nuutinen, E. M., Pyörälä K. & Viikari, J. (1991). Cardiovascular risk in young Finns. *Annales de Médecine Interne, 23*, 35-39.

Åkerblom, H. K., Viikari, J. & Kouvalainen, K. (1985). Cardiovascular risk factors in Finnish children and adolescents. *Acta Paediatrica Scandinavica, 318 (Suppl.)*, 5-6.

Allison, D, B., Matz, P. E., Pietrobelli, A., Zanolli, R. & Faith, M. S. (1999). Genetic and environmental influences on obesity. In A. Bendich & R. J. Deckelbaum (Eds.), *Primary and secondary preventive nutrition* (pp. 147-164). Totawa, New Jersey: Humana Press.

Andersen, L. B. (1994). Blood pressure, physical fitness and physical activity in 17-year-old Danish adolescents. *Journal of International Medical Research, 236*, 323-330.

Andersen, L. B. (1995). Tracking of VO2max, strength and physical activity from teenage to adulthood. *Journal of Pediatrics, Exercise and Science, 6*, 315-329. .

Andersen, L. B. (1996). Tracking of risk factors for coronary heart disease from adolescence to young adulthood with special emphasis on physical activity and fitness. *Danish Medical Bulletin, 43*, 407-418.

Andersen, L. B., Boreham, C. A., Young, I. S., Davey, S. G., Gallagher, A. M., Murray, L. & McCarron, P. (2006a). Insulin sensitivity and clustering of coronary heart disease risk factors in young adults. The Northern Ireland Young Hearts Study. *Preventive Medicine, 42*, 73-77.

Andersen, L. B. & Haraldsdóttir, J. (1993). Tracking of cardiovascular disease risk factors including maximal oxygen uptake and physical activity from late teenage to adulthood. An 8-year follow-up study. *Journal of International Medical Research, 234*, 309-315.

Andersen, L. B., Harro, M., Sardinha, L. B., Froberg, K., Ekelund, U., Brage, S. & Anderssen, S. A. (2006b). Physical activity and clustered cardiovascular risk in children: a cross-sectional study (The European Youth Heart Study). *Lancet 368*, 299-304.

Andersen, L. B., Hasselstrøm, H., Grønfeldt, V., Hansen, S. E. & Froberg, K. (2004). The relationship between physical fitness and clustered risk, and tracking of clustered risk from adolescence to young adulthood: eight years follow-up in the Danish Youth and Sport Study. *International Journal of Behavioral Nutrition and Physical Activity, 1*, 6.

Andersen, L. B., Henckel, P., Saltin, B. (1987). Maximal oxygen uptake in Danish adolescents 16-19 years of age. *European Journal of Applied Physiology and Occupational Physiology, 56*, 74-82.

Andersen, L. B., Henckel, P., Saltin, B. (1989). Risk factors for cardiovascular disease in 16-19-year-old teenagers. *Journal of International Medical Research, 225*, 157-163.

Andersen, L. B., Schnohr, P., Schroll, M. & Hein, H. O. (2000). All-cause mortality associated with physical activity during leisure time, work, sports, and cycling to work. *Archives of Internal Medicine, 160*, 1621-1628.

Andersen, L. B., Wedderkopp, N., Hansen, H. S., Cooper, A. R., Froberg, K. (2003). Biological cardiovascular risk factors cluster in Danish children and adolescents. Danish part of the European Heart Study. *Preventive Medicine, 37*, 363-367.

Anderssen, S. A., Haaland, A. , Hjermann, I., Urdal, P., Gjesdal, K. & Holme, I. (1995). Oslo Diet and Exercise Study: a one year randomized intervention trial; effect on hemostatic variables and other risk factors. *Nutrition, Metabolism and Cardiovascular Diseases, 5,* 189-200.

Armstrong, J. & Reilly, J. J. (2002). Breastfeeding and lowering the risk of childhood obesity. *Journal Lancet, 359,* 2003-2004.

Armstrong, N. & Simons-Morton, B. (1994). Physical activity and blood lipids in adolescents. *Journal of Pediatrics, Exercise and Science,* 6, 381-405.

Bao, W., Srinivasan, R. S., Wattigney, W. A. & Berenson, G. S. (1996). Usefulness of childhood low-density lipoprotein cholesterol level in predicting adult dyslipidemia and other cardiovascular risks. *Archives of Internal Medicine, 156,* 1315-1320.

Berenson, G. S., Srinivasan, R. S., Bao, W., Newman, W. P., Tracy, R. E., Wattigney, W. A., (1998). Association between multiple cardiovascular risk factors and atherosclerosis in children and young adults. *New England Journal of Medicine, 338,* 1650-1656.

Berenson, G. S., Wattigney, W. A., Tracy, R. E., Newman, W. P., Srinivasan, S. R., Webber, L. S., Dalferes, E. R. & Strong, J. P. (1992). Atherosclerosis of the Aorta and Coronary-Arteries and Cardiovascular Risk-Factors in Persons Aged 6 to 30 Years and Studied at Necropsy (the Bogalusa Heart-Study). *American Journal of Cardiology, 70,* 851-858.

Berkey, C. S., Rockett, H. R., Field, A. E., Gillman, M. W., Frazier, A. L., Camargo, C. A & Colditz, G. A. (2000). Activity, dietary intake, and weight changes in a longitudinal study of preadolescent and adolescent boys and girls. *Pediatrics, 105,* E56.

Beunen, G. P., Claessens, A. L., Lefevre, J., Ostyn, M., Renson, R., Simons, J. & Gerven, D. G. (1988). Simple body fatness indices in youths 12-20 year of age. *American Journal of human Biology, 18,* 25-30.

Bláha, P. & Vignerová, J. (2002). Investigation of the growth of Czech children and adolescents. Prague, Czech Republic: National Institute of Public Health.

Boden, G. (2003). Effects of free fatty acids (FFA) on glucose metabolism: Significance for insulin resistance and type 2 diabetes. *Experimental and Clinical Endocrinology & Diabetes, 111,* 121-124.

Boreham, C., Savage, J. M., Primrose, D., Cran, G. & Strain, J. (1993). Coronary risk factors in schoolchildren. *Archives of Disease in Childhood, 68,* 182-186.

Boreham, C., Twisk, J. W. R., Murray, L., Savage, M., Strain, J. J. & Cran, G. (2001). Fitness, fatness, and coronary heart disease risk in adolescents: the Northern Ireland Young Hearts Project. *Medicine and Science in Sports and Exercise, 33,* 270-274.

Brown, M. D., Dengel, D. R., Hogikyan, R. V. & Supiano, M. A. (2002). Sympathetic activity and the heterogenous blood pressure response to exercise training in hypertensives. *Canadian Journal of Applied Physiology, 92,* 1434-1442.

Campbell, K., Waters, E., O'Meara, S., Kelly, S. & Summerbell, C. (2002). Interventions for preventing obesity in children. Cochrane database of systematic reviews, CD001871.

Clausen, J. P. (1977). Effect of physical training on cardiovascular adjustments to exercise in man. *Physiological Reviews, 57,* 779-815.

Cole, T. J., Bellizzi, M. C., Flegal, K. M. & Dietz, W. H. (2000). Establishing a standard definition for child overweight and obesity worldwide: international survey. British Medical Journal, 320, 1240-1243.

DeFronzo, R. A. & Ferrannini, E. (1991). Insulin resistance. A multifaceted syndrome responsible for NIDDM, obesity, hyperten sion, dyslipidemia, and atherosclerotic cardiovascular disease. *Diabetes Care, 14,* 173-194.

Dela, F., Plough, T, Handberg, A., Petersen, L. N., Larsen, J. J., Mikines, K. J., Galbo, H. (1994). Physical training increases muscle GLUT4 protein and mRNA in patients with NIDDM. *Diabetes, 43*, 862-865.

Eisenmann, J. C. (2003). Secular trends in variables associated with the metabolic syndrome of North American children and adolescents: a review and synthesis. *American Journal of human Biology, 15*, 786-794.

Ferrannini, E. (1999). Insulin resistance and blood pressure. In G. M. Reaven & A. Laws (Eds.), Insulin resistance. The metabolic syndrome X (pp. 281-308). Totowa, New Jersey: Humana Press.

Ferrara, L. A., Guida, L., Iannuzzi, R., Celentano, A., Lionello, F. (2002). Serum cholesterol affects blood pressure regulation. *Journal of Human Hypertension, 16*, 337-343.

Ferreira, I., Twisk, J. W. R., Stehouwer, C. D. A., van Mechelen, W., Kemper, H. C. G. (2003). Longitudinal changes in VO2max: associations with carotid IMT and arterial stiffness. *Medicine and Science in Sports and Exercise, 35*, 1670-1678.

Franch, J. (2002). *Regulation of fat and carbohydrate metabolism in skeletal muscle.* Denmark: Institute of Sports Science and Biomechanics, University of Southern Denmark.

Franch, J., Aslesen, R., Jensen, J. (1999). Regulation of glycogen synthesis in rat skeletal muscle after glycogen-depleting contractile activity: effects of adrenaline on glycogen synthesis and activation of glycogen synthase and glycogen phosphorylase. *Biochemical Journal, 344*, 231-235.

Franklin, M. F. (1999). Comparison of weight and height relations in boys from 4 countries. *American Journal of Clinical Nutrition, 70*, 157-162.

Freedman, D. S., Dietz, W. H., Srinivasan, R. S. & Berenson, G. S. (1999). The relation of overweigth to cardiovascular risk factors among children and adolescents:The Bogalusa heart study. *Pediatrics, 103*, 1175-1182.

Gidding, S. S., Leibel, R. L., Daniels, S., Rosenbaum, M., Van Horn, L. & Marx, G. R. (1996). Understanding obesity in youth. A statement for healthcare professionals from the Committee on Atherosclerosis and Hypertension in the Young of the Council on Cardiovascular Disease in the Young and the Nutrition Committee, American Heart Association. Writing Group. *Circulation, 94*, 3383-3387.

Gill, J. M. & Hardman, A. E. (2003). Exercise and postprandial lipid metabolism: an update on potential mechanisms and interactions with high-carbohydrate diets (review). *Journal of Nutritional Biochemistry, 14*, 122-132.

Goran, M. I. (1998). Measurement issues related to studies of childhood obesity: assessment of body composition, body fat distribution, physical activity, and food intake. *Pediatrics, 101*, 505-518.

Goran, M. I. & Gower, B. A. (1999). Relation between visceral fat and disease risk in children and adolescents. *American Journal of Clinical Nutrition, 70*, 149-156.

Goran, M. I., Gower, B. A., Treuth, M. & Nagy, T. R. (1998). Prediction of intra-abdominal and subcutaneous abdominal adipose tissue in healthy pre-pubertal children. *International Journal of Obesity and Related Metabolic Disorders, 22*, 549-558.

Guillaume, M. (1999). Defining obesity in childhood: current practice. *American Journal of Clinical Nutrition, 70*, 126-130.

Hamilton, M. T., Areiqat, E., Hamilton, D. G. & Bey, L. (2001). Plasma triglyceride metabolism in humans and rats during aging and physical inactivity. *International Journal of Sport Nutrition & exercise metabolism, 11*, (Suppl), 97-104.

Hansen, H. S., Froberg, K., Hyldebrandt, N. & Nielsen, J. R. (1991). A controlled study of eight months of physical training and reduction of blood pressure in children: the Odense schoolchild study. *BMJ, 303*, 682-685.

Hansen, H. S., Hyldebrandt, N., Froberg, K.& Nielsen, J. R. (1990). Blood pressure and physical fitness in a population of children - the Odense Schoolchild Study. *Journal of Human Hypertension, 4,* 615-620.

Hansen, H. S., Nielsen, J. R., Froberg, K., Hyldebrandt, N. (1992). Left ventricular hypertrophy in children from the upper five percent of the blood pressure distribution - the Odense Schoolchild Study. *Journal of Human Hypertension, 6,* 41-45.

Hasselstrøm, H., Hansen, S. E., Froberg, K., Andersen, L. B. (2002). Physical fitness and physical activity during adolescence as predictors of cardiovascular disease risk in young adulthood. *International Journal of Sports Medicine, 23,* 27-31.

Hawk, L. J. & Brook, C. G. (1979). Family resemblances of height, weight, and body fatness. *Archives of Disease in Childhood, 54,* 877-879.

Heath, G. W. & Kendrick, J. S. (1989). Outrunning the risks: a behavioral risk profile of runners. *Preventive Medicine, 5,* 347-352.

Hickner, R. C., Racette, S B., Binder, E. F., Fisher, J. S. & Kohrt, W. M. (1999). Suppression of whole body and regional lipolysis by insulin: Effects of obesity and exercise. *Journal of Clinical Endocrinology and Metabolis, 84,* 3886-3895.

Hicks, A. L., MacDougall, J. D. & Muckle, T. J. (1987). Acute changes in high-density lipoprotein cholesterol with exercise of different intensities. *Journal of Applied Psychology, 63,* 1956-1960.

Hill, J. O., Melanson, E. L. (1999). Overview of the determinants of overweight and obesity: current evidence and research issues. *Medicine and Science in Sports and Exercise, 31,* 515-521.

International Obesity task Force with the European Childhood Obesity Group (2002). Obesity in Europe. Copenhagen, Denmark.

Jebb, S. A. (1997). Aetiology of obesity. *British Medical Bulletin, 53,* 264-285.

Kemper, H. C. G. & Vanthof, M. A. (1978). Design of A Multiple Longitudinal-Study of Growth and Health in Teenagers. *European Journal of Pediatrics, 129,* 147-155.

Kingwell, B. A.& Jennings, G. L. (1997). The exercise prescription: focus on vascular mechanisms. *Blood Pressure Monitoring, 2,* 139-145.

Klausen, K., Andersen, L. B & Pelle, I. (1981). Adaptive changes in work capacity, skeletal muscle capillarization and enzyme levels during training and detraining. *Acta Physiologica Scandinavica, 113,* 9-16.

Kristensen, P. L., Wedderkopp, N., Moller, N. C, Andersen, L. B., Bai, C. N. & Froberg, K. (2006). Tracking and prevalence of cardiovascular disease risk factors across socio-economic classes: a longitudinal substudy of the European Youth Heart Study. *Bmc Public Health, 6,* 20.

Krotkiewski, M., Lithell, H., Shono, N., Wysocki, M. & Holm, G. (1998). High blood pressure and muscle morphology/metabolism--causal relationship or only associated factors? *Clinical Physiology, 18,* 203-213.

Kuczmarski, R. J., Ogden, C. L., Grummer-Strawn, L. M., Flegal, K. M., Guo, S. S., Wei, R., Mei, Z., Curtin, L. R., Roche, A. F.& Johnson, C. L. (2000). *Growth Charts: United States Advance Data from Vital and Health Statistics.* Atlanta: National Center for Health Statistics.

Lenthe, F. J. v, Mechelen W. v, Kemper, H. C. G. & Twisk, J. W. R. (1998). Association of a central pattern of body fat with blood pressure and lipoproteins from adolescence into adulthood. The Amsterdam Growth and health study. *American Journal of Epidemiology, 147,* 686-693.

Leon, A. S., Conrad, J., Hunninghake, D. B. & Serfass, R. (1979). Effects of a vigorous walking program on body composition, and carbohydrate and lipid metabolism of obese young men. *American Journal of Clinical Nutrition, 33,* 1776-1787.

Li, S., Chen, W., Srinivasan, R. S., Bond, M. G., Tang, R., Urbina, E. M.& Berenson, G. S. (2003). Childhood risk factors and carotid vascular changes in adulthood. The Bogalusa Heart study. *JAMA, 290,* 2271-2276.

Lobstein, T., Baur, L. & Uauy, R. (2004). Obesity in children and young people: a crisis in public health. *Obesity Review, 5 (Suppl 1),* 4-85.

Mahoney, L. T., Burns, T. L., Stanford, W., Thompson, B. H., Witt, J. D. & Rost, C. A. (1996). Coronary risk factors measured in childhood and young adult life are associated with coronary artery calcification in young adults: the Muscatine Study. *Journal of the American College of Cardiology, 27,* 277-284.

Maia, J. A., Beunen, G., Lefevre, J., Claessens, A. L., Renson, R. & Vanreusel, B. (2003). Modelling stability and change in strength development: a study in adolescent boys. *American Journal of Human Biology, 15,* 579-591.

Maki, T., Naveri, H., Leinonen, H., Sovijarvi, A., Lewko, B., Harkonen, M.& Kontula, K. (1990). Effect of propranolol and pindolol on the up-regulation of lymphocytic beta adrenoceptors during acute submaximal physical exercise. A placebo- controlled double-blind study. *Journal of Cardiovascular Pharmacology, 15,* 544-551.

McGill, H. C., Herderick, E. E., McMahan, C. A., Zieske, A. W., Malcom, G. T., Tracy, R. E. & Strong, J. P. (2002). Atherosclerosis in youth. *Minerva Pediatrica, 54,* 437-447.

McGill, H. C., McMahan, A., Zieske, A. W., Sloop, G. D., Walcott, J. V., Troxclair, D. A., Malcolm, G. T., Tracy, R. E., Oalmann, M. C. & Strong, J. P. (2000). Associations of coronary heart disease risk factors with the intermediate lesion of atherosclerosis in youth. *Atherosclerosis, Thrombosis and Vascular Biology, 20,* 1998-2004.

Møller, N. C., Andersen, L. B., Wedderkopp, N. & Froberg, K. (2006). Secular trends in cardiovascular fitness and overweight in Danish third grade school children. Danish substudy of the European Youth Heart Study. Scandinavian Journal of Medicine and Science in Sports, 16 (4).

Morris, J. N., Heady, J. A., Raffle, P. A. B., Roberts, C. G. & Parks, J. W. (1953). Coronary heart-disease and physical activity of work. *Lancet,* 262 (6800),1053-1057.

Must, A., Dallal, G. E. & Dietz, W. H. (1991). Reference data for obesity: 85th and 95th percentiles of body mass index (wt/ht2) and triceps skinfold thickness. *American Journal of Clinical Nutrition, 53,* 839-846.

Must, A., Jacques, P. F., Dallal, G. E., Bajema, C. J. & Dietz, W. H. (1992). Long-term morbidity and mortality of overweight adolescents. A follow-up of the Harvard Growth Study of 1922 to 1935. *New England Journal of Medicine, 327,* 1350-1355.

Nelson, M. J., Ragland, D. R. & Syme, S. L. (1992). Longitudinal prediction of adult blood pressure from juvenile blood pressure levels. *American Journal of Epidemiology, 136,* 633-645.

Nielsen, G. A. & Andersen, L. B. (2003). The association between high blood pressure, physical fitness and body mass index in adolescents. *Preventive Medicine, 36,* 229-234.

Oblaciska, A., Wrocawska, M. & Woynarowska, B. (1997). Frequency of overweight and obesity in the school-age population in Poland and health care for pupils with these disorders. *Pediatria Polska, 72,* 241-245.

Ploug, T., & Ralston, E. (2002). Exploring the whereabouts of GLUT4 in skeletal muscle (Review). *Molecular Membrane Biology, 19,* 39-49.

Porkka, K. V. K., Viikari, J. S. A. & Åkerblom, H. K. (1991). Tracking of serum HDL-cholesterol and other lipids in children and adolescents: The cardiovascular risk in young Finns study. *Preventive Medicine, 20,* 713-724.

Porkka, K. V. K., Viikari, J. S. A., Rönnemaa, T., Marniemi, J. & Åkerblom, H. K. (1994). Age and gender specific serum lipid and apolipoprotein fractiles of Finnins children and young adults. The Cardiovascular Risk in Young Finns Study. *Acta Paediatrica, 83,* 838-848.

Powell, K. E., Thompson, P. D., Caspersen, C. J. & Kendrick, C. S. (1987). Physical activity and the incidence of coronary heart disease. *Annual Review of Public Health, 8,* 253-287.

Prentice, A. M. & Jebb, S. A. (1995). Obesity in Britain: gluttony or sloth? *BMJ, 311,* 437-439.

Raitakari, O. T., Juonala, M., Kähönen, M., Taittonen, L., Laitinen, T., Mäki-Torkko, N., Järvisalo, M. J., Uhari, M., Jokinen, E., Rönnemaa, T., Åkerblom, H. K. & Viikari, J. S. A. (2003). Cardiovascular risk factors in childhood and carotid artery intima-media thickness in adulthood. *JAMA, 290,* 2277-2283.

Raitakari, O. T., Porkka, K. V. K., Taimela, S., Telema, R., Räsänen, L. & Viikari, S. A. (1994). Effects of persistent physical activity and inactivity on coronary risk factors in children and young adults. *American Journal of Epidemiology, 140,* 195-205.

Richter, E. A., Derave, W. & Wojtaszewski, J. F. (2001). Glucose, exercise and insulin: emerging concepts. *Journal of Physiology, 535,* 313-322.

Rolland-Cachera, M. F., Deheeger, M., Pequignot, F., Guilloud-Bataille, M., Vinit, F. & Bellisle, F. (1988). Adiposity and food intake in young children: the environmental challenge to individual susceptibility. *British Medical Journal (Clinical Research Ed.), 296,* 1037-1038.

Shear, C. L., Freedman, D. S., Burke, G. L., Harsha, D. W. & Berenson, G. S. (1987). Body fat patterning and blood pressure in children and young adults. The Bogalusa Heart Study. *Hypertension, 9,* 236-244.

Stallones, L., Mueller, W. H. & Christensen, B. L. (1982). Blood pressure, fatness, and fat patterning among USA adolescents from two ethnic groups. *Hypertension, 4,* 483-486.

Strong, J. P., Malcom, G. T., McMahan, C. A., Tracy, R. E., Newman, W. P., Herderick, E. E. & Cornhill, J. F. (1999). Prevalence and extent of atherosclerosis in adolescents and young adults: implications for prevention from the Pathobiological Determinants of Atherosclerosis in Youth Study. *JAMA, 281,* 727-735.

Taylor, R. W., Jones, I. E., Williams, S. M., Goulding, A. (2000). Evaluation of waist circumference, waist-to-hip ratio, and the conicity index as screening tools for high trunk fat mass, as measured by dual-energy X-ray absorptiometry, in children aged 3-19 y. *American Journal of Clinical Nutrition, 72,* 490-495.

Telema, T. R., Laakso, L. & Yang, X. (1994). Physical activity and participation in sports of young people in Finland. *Scandinavian Journal of Medicine and Science in Sports, 4,* 65-74.

Twisk, J. W. R., Boreham, C., Cran, G., Savage, J. M., Strain, J. & Mechelen W. v. (1999). Clustering of biological risk factors for cardiovascular disease and longitudinal relationship with lifestyle of an adolescent population: the Northern Ireland Young Hearts Project. *Journal of Cardiovascular Risk, 6,* 355-362.

Twisk, J. W. R., Kemper, H. C. G. & Mechelen, W. v. (2002). The relationship between physical fitness and physical activity during adolescence and cardiovascular disease risk factors at adult age. The Amsterdam Growth and Health Study. *International Journal of Sports Medicine, 23,* 8-14.

Twisk, J. W. R., Kemper, H. C. G., Mechelen, W. v. & Post, G. B. (1997). Tracking of risk factors for coronary heart disease over a 14-year period: a comparison between lifestyle and biologic risk factors with data from the Amsterdam Growth and Health Study. *American Journal of Epidemiology, 145,* 888-898.

Twisk, J. W. R., Kemper, H. C. G. & Mechelen, W. v. (2000). Tracking of activity and fitness and the relationship with cardiovascular disease risk factors. *Medicine and Science in Sports and Exercise, 32,* 1455-1461.

US Department of Health and Human Services (1997). Physical activity and health: a report of the Surgeon General. Atlanta: U.S.Department of Health and Human Services. Centers for Disease Control and Prevention, National Center for Chronic Disease Prevention and Health Promotion.

Vuori, I., Fentem, P., Andersen, L. B., Felten, R. W., Rubana, M., Strömme, S. B., Haulicá, J. & Ekblom, B. (1995). The significance of sport for society (pp. 19-87). Strasbourg: Council of Europe Press.

Wang, Y., Monteiro, C. & Popkin, B. M. (2002). Trends of obesity and underweight in older children and adolescents in the United States, Brazil, China, and Russia. *American Journal of Clinical Nutrition, 75,* 971-977.

Wedderkopp, N., Andersen, L. B., Hansen, H. S. & Froberg, K. (2001). Fedme blandt børn - med særlig vægt på danske forhold. *Ugeskrift for Laeger, 163,* 2907-2912.

Wedderkopp, N, Froberg, K., Hansen, H. S. & Andersen, L. B. (2004). Secular trends in physical fitness and fatness in Danish 9-year old girls and boys. Odense School child Study and Danish substudy of The European Youth Heart Study. *Scandinavian Journal of Medicine and Science in Sports, 14,* 1-6.

Wedderkopp, N., Froberg, K., Hansen, H. S., Riddoch, C. & Andersen, L. B. (2003). Cardiovascular risk factors cluster in children and adolescents with low physical fitness. *Pediatric Exercise Science, 15,* 419-422.

Whitaker, R. C., Wright, J. A., Pepe, M. S., Seidel, K. D. & Dietz, W. H. (1997). Predicting obesity in young adulthood from childhood and parental obesity. *New England Journal of Medicine, 337,* 869-873.

Whitelaw, A. G. L. (1976). Influence of maternal obesity on subcutaneous fat in the newborn. *British Medical Journal, 2,* 985-986.

Wood, P.D., Haskell, W. L., Blair, S. N., Williams, P. T., Krauss, R. M., Lindgren, F. T., Albers, J. J., Ho, P. H. & Farquhar, W. (1983). Increased exercise level and plasma lipoprotein concentrations: a one year, randomized, controlled study in sedentary middle-aged men. *Metabolism, 32,* 31-39.

Wynder, E. L., Williams, C. L., Laakso, K. & Levenstein, M. (1981). Screening of risk factors for scronic disease in children from fifteen countries. *Preventive Medicine, 10,* 19-120.

Chapter 4:
Health, Development and Education in an Integral Perspective

Paolo Parisi

This presentation is meant to approach our theme in broad terms, and offer some general considerations attempting to look at the relation of health and lifestyle in the context of an integral perspective on human development, as a possible theoretical fundament in shaping future action plans in health and education, which is in fact what is implied by the EU declaration of 2004 as the *European Year of Education through Sport.*

As the EU declaration highlights, we are living a time when society, culture and science have become increasingly aware of the great importance of sport, broadly understood, for individual and social health and wellbeing. If we look at the EYES motto, *"Move Your Body, Stretch Your Mind"*, we can say much is known on its first part, which is actually the focus of current research. We know that "moving our body" has a fundamental role in promoting health: an overwhelming evidence points to the positive correlates of physical activity in countering risk factors, delaying the aging process, etc. We know that lack of exercise increases the risk of at least 20 diseases, and we all share the emphasis on the high individual and social costs of sedentariness and unhealthy lifestyles, and the need of effective strategies to counter their harmful effects.

So, as the editors implied suggesting a title reversing the EYES Motto's into *"Stretch Your Body, Move your Mind"*, here we will mainly refer to the second part of the Motto, *the mind,* and consider "moving our mind" in two interconnected perspectives – behavioral, and psychosocial, attempting to somewhat put the action of biological factors in a wider context.

We will shortly address a number of intricate issues, as listed in Table 1, trying to link them together in an intellectual path, to suggest that our ordinary categories in the study of human development, health and disorder, fundamental to empirical studies as they are, may at times prove excessively fragmented and simplistic, and that a more integral perspective might contribute to a wider understanding.

In this context, sport appears to play a central role – and the point we wish to make is that this is not just because it helps spending calories and keeping up with certain parameters, but for its fundamental value in promoting homeostasis, hence physical and mental health and wellbeing, as is in fact true of any form of activity stimulating the body's physical and emotional expressions.

The obesity epidemic

Overweight, nutrition, and exercise

As we focus on the epidemic of overweight and obesity, we obviously consider healthy diet and active lifestyle to provide the answer to it: their value has been recognised for a long time, and there is no question about this. Yet, things are not as clearcut as one might wish.

To start with, the obesity epidemic is actually part of a wider epidemic of chronic diseases, that a 2003 WHO/FAO Consultation (WHO, 2003a) has estimated at 46 % of the current global burden of disease, with a projected 57 % by 2020. Obesity is particularly worrying because it increasingly involves children and adolescents. And there is evidence suggesting that risks for chronic disease in general may already begin in fetal life (WHO, 2002). So, as the WHO/FAO panel recognised, a new platform is appearing, going beyond the simple energy intake/expenditure balance, and encompassing a wider concept of the human organism's subtle and complex relationship to its environment.

As I said, we can look at the issue in two interconnected perspectives, behavioral and psychosocial, and I will start with the former.

For now three decades, we have been literally deluged with all kinds of dietary and lifestyle recommendations, adapted in any possible way to help consumers understand and make wise choices. So, after so many campaigns, after so much talking about nutrition, sedentariness, risk factors, and what is healthy and what not, one would assume everyone to be reasonably informed, and there should be little question about that.

Yet, what we see is a widespread epidemic of overweight and obesity. Are the guidelines not so effective after all? Or is it that consumers just don't follow them? Perhaps because healthy eating is not as pleasurable as unhealthy one, and exercise is boring? Or because people find the guidelines uneasy to follow, contradictory with their periodical changes, or possibly ineffective?

All of these, and still other factors may well play a role. But anyway, the fact is that today the percentage of people complying with dietary guidelines appears to be discouraging: in the UK, for instance, just about 2-4 % of the population are reported to be currently consuming the recommended level of saturated fat. (WHO, 2003b). Surveys in the US have now shown for decades that Americans do have the basic knowledge needed to make wise choices, but that there is a widening gap between what consumers know and what they actually do – though frequently out of being "tired with deprivation" and with "feelings of guilt".

One just wonders, in the end, *is our behavior rational?* Why don't we just do what we know to be good for us, and frequently harm ourselves, as we do with eating, drinking, smoking, etc.?

Tobacco smoking has long been identified as the leading cause of premature illness and death in developed countries. Yet, reports from quite a few countries show that, over the past 10 years and after all our massive campaigns, the percentage of smokers has only decreased to a relatively minor degree. In Italy, for instance, it just passed from 25.1 % in 1994 to 23.8 % in 2002, and recent polls indicate that it may be even increasing among women. Increases are also found in adolescents: in Italy, again, in the 18-19-year-olds smoking passed in some polls from 20.7 % in 2001 to 23.1 % in 2002 (ISTAT, 2004).

According to a recent WHO survey (WHO 2004) on school-aged children in 35 countries, "most young people can recite the dangers associated with smoking", and yet many "view smoking as agreeable, adult and fashionable". And in fact, over 60 % of all 15-year-olds (and up to 80 % or more in some countries) report ever having smoked.

Clearly, although we pretend our behavior to be rational, that is frequently not so. Whether we like it or not, whether consciously or unconsciously, at basic levels our behavior is largely led by personal drives and emotions: pleasure and fear, and then the need to be accepted, frustration, anger, discomfort, and so on. We may ignore or rationalise this, but that makes it no less true.

If we want our strategies toward a healthy society really meet with some success, we must get to the roots of human behavior and address the basic, emotional levels that are behind it, and the personal and social factors that affect their intricate relations.

On the other hand, and coming now to the psychosocial perspective, one may note that whereas overweight and obesity have been going dramatically up for decades, the evidence we have on energy intake/expenditure is somewhat conflicting.

The FAO National Food Balance Sheets clearly show that, in all countries, there is more *food available*. Yet, this does not necessarily translate into *food intake*, since these data fail to account for such factors as unequal distribution, waste, etc. In fact, direct studies on actual food intake tend to indicate that in developed countries there has been a steady decrease in calories, and especially fat calories intake, while a variety of food substitutes have been introduced.

As it happens, people today may well be tired of deprivation and forget about the guidelines (though not systematically, and feeling guilty, as the reports tell us). But over the past decades, periodic surveys in the US indicated that the guidelines had been taken to heart, and in fact half Americans were reported to be on diet at any given time, with record sales of low-fat cookies, fake fats, etc. In the late 1980s, the Third National Health and Nutrition Examination Study (NHANES III) indicated that in the previous two decades total fat intake had been reduced from 40 % to 34 %. In the UK, food intake dropped from 3000 to 2000 calories. The US consumption of saturated fat dropped from 17 % of total calories in the 1960s to 12 % in the early 1990s, reaching about the same level as one century ago (Encyclopedia Britannica, Medical & Health Annual, 1992). The picture was already clear over ten years ago, when the contradiction with the still increasing obesity rate was stressed and summarised in a graph (Figure 1), calling instead for the importance of decreasing levels of physical activity (Prentice & Jebb, 1995).

Fig. 1:   Secular trends in diet and activity in relation to obesity (modified after Prentice & Webb, 1995)

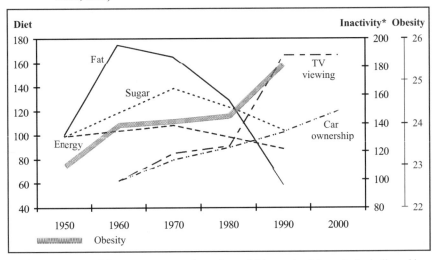

* Indirect measures. Direct measures tend to show childen and adolescents basically achieve recommended activity. (Riddoch et al. 2004)

That physical activity levels have dramatically decreased is an unquestionable fact, and the role this may have on individual and public health has now been stressed for several years. Yet, the claim that young people fail to meet activity recommendations, reasonable as it appears, does not seem to be confirmed by direct measurement. Recent reports from the European Youth Heart Study, based on objective quantitative measurements, indicate that all 9-year-olds (97.5 %) and over 70 % of 15-year-olds appear to achieve activity recommendations (Riddoch, Andersen, Wedderkopp et al., 2004). Also, the accumulated amount of time spent at moderate and rigorous physical activity was found to explain less than 1 % of the variance in body fatness (Ekelund, Sardinha, Anderssen et al., 2004).

Moreover, great increases in obesity have occurred also in developing countries, where average food intake and sedentary lifestyle are clearly not those of our societies. Prevalence increases of up to 40-65 % have been reported for some countries, with accompanying increases of up to 4.5 % in the prevalence of diabetes. The WHO recognises that the condition is "becoming a serious problem throughout Asia, Latin America and parts of Africa", and that in children "a disturbing increase has taken place over the past 20 years in developing countries as diverse as India, Mexico, Nigeria and Tunisia" (WHO, 2003c).

As a final, passing note, it may be observed that the current epidemic actually falls in line with other epidemics, and specifically disorders such as anorexia or bulimia, that involve aspects that are related and increasingly thought to have a strong psychosocial component.

All this is to say that perhaps the equation, *Obesity = too much food and/or too little exercise,* correct as it is in general terms, may fail to tell us all the story.

Other factors may play a role, such as genetic regulatory effects and the variability of individual response and adaptability, along with psychosocially induced variations in the metabolic handling of energy intake, in thermogenesis, etc. A deeper understanding is needed of the complex forces and interactions at work and much research is being conducted along these lines.

Clearly, health and disorder cannot be just mechanically explained, but need to also consider behavioral components, the sociocultural and individual context, and at a more subtle level, the related psychological mediators and interactions that characterise personal experience, and express themselves through those psychoendocrine, neuroimmunological networks that are now seen to play a fundamental, and previously unsuspected role in human health and wellbeing.

Psychosocial factors in human growth – Emotion, stimulation, and stress

An old story, which is particularly instructive, will help introduce the issue, which was more extensively reviewed elsewhere (Parisi & De Martino, 1980; Parisi, 1998).

In a 13th century chronicle attributed to the Franciscan Salimbene of Parma, the Holy Roman Emperor Frederick II, at the time King of Sicily, an enlightened sovereign known for his interest in culture and the study of languages, is reported to have performed an experiment,

"... to find out what kind of speech...children would have when they grew up, if they spoke to no one beforehand. So, he bade foster mothers and nurses to suckle the children, to bathe and to wash them, but in no way to prattle with them or to speak to them... But he laboured in vain, because the children all died. For they could not live without the petting and the joyful faces and loving words of their foster mothers."

Whatever its historical value, this account speaks for an early concern for the interactional needs of the infant. In the scientific literature, the consequences of a lack of stimulation and play activity on child growth and survival have also been known for a long time.

The high mortality of institutionalised infants was extensively discussed at meetings of the American Paediatric Society, early last century, substantiating a concept that, as Spitz was to report later, had already been highlighted by an 18th century bishop in Spain, as a sheer matter of observation:

"En la casa de niños expositos, el niño se pone triste y muchos de ellos mueren de tristeza"

("In the foundling home, children become sad and many of them die of sorrow").

It was in the 1940s when Bakwin pointed to the failure to thrive observed in children confined in hospitals and attributed it to emotional deprivation. And it was in the same years that a classic long-term investigation by Spitz on institutionalised infants showed that, irrespective of good nutritional and medical care, this could lead to physical and mental growth impairment, along with high susceptibility to infections and mortality rate (Parisi & De Martino 1980; Parisi, 1998).

Many cases were since reported, involving even children reared with their own families, described as showing a failure to thrive that could not be explained by inadequate nutrition, nursing or other organic cause, and seemed to be rather due to insufficient psychosocial stimulation. Mothering was frequently found to be emotionally inadequate, and this crossed all social classes. Many of these children exhibited the same symptoms we know today to characterise anorexia and bulimia, thereby confirming the strong emotional component underlying nutritional troubles. Endocrine alterations were described, but also seen to disappear under better emotional conditions, suggesting that biological correlates might rather be *an effect* of the trouble than a cause of it. Classical experiments meanwhile indicated contact comfort to be of critical importance also in non-human primates, with insufficient interaction leading even infant monkeys to develop depression or other behavioral troubles (Parisi & De Martino, 1980; Parisi, 1998).

The emergence of psychosomatics has considerably influenced later research trends, so that emotions, previously hardly a subject for scientific inquiry, have gradually become a prominent area of research, with increases in the number of scientific publications of up to 1000 % in the past three decades. Their metabolic effects have started to be described, and the clinical claims of an emotionally induced immunological depression have found support in much animal and clinical research (Steptoe, 1998; Chrousos, 2000; Yirmiya, Pollak, Morag et al., 2000; Kiank, Holtfreter, Starke et al., 2006) with such findings as, e.g., decreases in lymphocytes and resistance to infections associated to psychological feelings of self-devaluation, shame and guilt, and related findings. All this lends itself to some considerations.

Body and mind, however we define it, can no longer be held separate. As clinical observation has indicated for a long time and current research has confirmed, they interact in subtle ways in personal experience, so that emotional life influences body's health, and extreme troubles and suffering can reach a point where they translate into overt physical effects and disease.

Some amount of emotional stimulation and challenge is needed to maintain and stimulate homeostasis, hence the capability, increasingly developed throughout evolution, to respond and adjust to circumstances, and express optimal functioning. Stress represents a fundamental tuning mechanism in the maintenance of response capabilities, hence in fostering integral health and personal development. If stress levels are too low, or too high, the organism's homeostasis is affected.

The epidemic we are currently interested in, falls in line with a sequence of similar conditions, largely related to nutritional troubles and forms of addiction, all in various ways expressing, at increasing levels, emotional suffering and a loss of homeostasis, hence of self-regulation and response capabilities.

Play, hence games, sport and all kinds of activity and exercise, have a fundamental importance as primary sources of emotional stimulation and interaction, particularly in the more critical stages of development, as well as in the elderly and more generally across the lifespan.

This all speaks for the need to go beyond categorical deterministic approaches, and look at the complexity of things and their interactional nature.

Emergenesis and complexity – The integrative view

There is a growing tendency in biology, as more generally in science and epistemology, to shift the emphasis from determinism to complexity. However prevalent the classic mechanistic views may still be, emerging views are centered on the concept of increasing levels of interaction, self-organisation and complexity. The shift from a mechanistic, deterministic view to a more problematic, interactional view linked to complexity will be shortly discussed in the following and illustrated with some classic examples of well-known dualities.

Interaction and self-organisation: Reductionism versus Holism

Particularly in biology, things are increasingly seen to interact at the various levels and organise themselves in dynamic relation with the environment, so that increasingly complex open systems emerge and evolve. At all levels, novel properties emerge that were not present: a molecule of water has properties that could not be predicted by those of its components, the Hydrogen and Oxygen atoms, and have emerged as a result of their interactions. And that is increasingly so the higher the level of organisation. That is why the usual reductionistic approach, needed as it obviously is to conduct research, finds its limit and must at some point be integrated with a holistic view.

Though obviously guided by general principles, the process is not totally predetermined and has some degree of freedom which increases with increasing complexity and interaction. And this is where determinism and mechanistic views find their limit.

We have seen how easily natural phenomena can be affected in their delicate interconnections in the ecosystem, and how problematic reductionistic approaches can be when they are applied to higher levels of complexity. And human beings are by far the most complex systems in nature.

Nature and Nurture

The nature-nurture controversy is an old one, that modern genetic understanding has largely overcome, but that is culturally and ideologically loaded, so that it continuously reappears in one form or another.

How much is genetically determined and what is the role of environment? When we look at obesity, or other phenotypes in health and disease, we frequently find that clearcut explanations are unable to account for the complexity of things.

Is obesity genetic?

Yes, of course. It runs in families, is concordant in twins, resists treatment, and molecular studies show tens of genes to be involved in some way. But then why is it increasing year after year? Is it because of genetic changes? Not really: mutations take thousands of years to establish themselves, and our genes do not substantially differ from those of our cave men ancestors.

Is then obesity environmentally induced? Is it due to wrong nutrition and increasingly sedentary lifestyle?

Yes, of course. We all know it is. But then, again, why is it that there are people who eat a lot, do not exercise, and yet keep lean? And why is it that overweight and obesity continue to increase while food consumption does not accordingly? Why is it that in developing countries, where physical work is still widespread and the Westernised lifestyle has only reached a minority of the population, obesity can affect 40 % or more of the population?

Things are complicated and simple linear relations can be misleading. Obesity – we have come to realise – is neither genetically nor environmentally produced, but is rather the effect of complex interactions, as is true of many conditions. The old contrast viewing nature and nurture as alternative forces is in fact overcome today by an interactional view where they integrate (Figure 2).

Fig. 2: The changing view of obesity

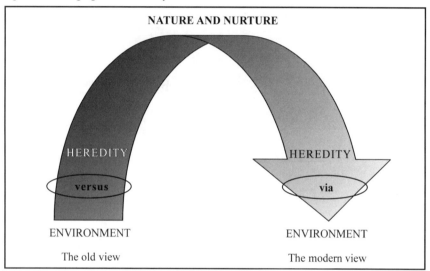

Gene-environment interactions

Gene-environment interactions represent today the core issue of the latest chapter in modern biology, the post-genomics or proteinomics, which in fact deals with gene expression in the course of development and throughout life events.

Genes do not operate in a vacuum, but in a physical context represented by the rest of their DNA and by cell environment, and can be influenced in their expression by other genes and by intracellular and extracellular events. Many phenotypes (particularly those related to continuous variables, as are in general anthropometric, physiological, or behavioural traits) are multifactorial in nature, and result from the actions, and interactions, of several genes and environmental factors (Figure 3).

Fig. 3: Gen-environment interactions

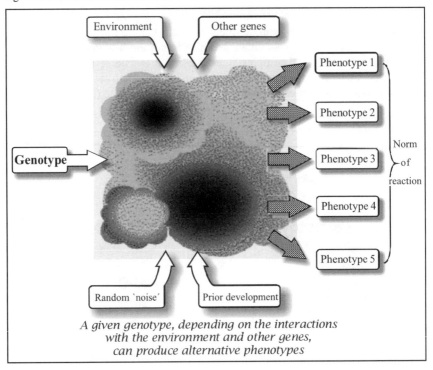

*A given genotype, depending on the interactions
with the environment and other genes,
can produce alternative phenotypes*

The expression of a gene in the course of ontogenesis was illustrated by Waddington (1975) with the evocative image of a stone rolling down the cragged slopes of a mountain: the general direction is given, but the path of development and its ending point are influenced by the epigenetic landscape (Figure 4). Conceived by the great evolutionary biologist half a century ago, the image still conveys a sense of how genes actually work in their given space-time context.

All this exemplifies the issue of the relative unpredictability implicit in the development of complex systems, and speaks for the great importance of environmental influences, and specifically of education (which in fact, from the Latin *e-ducere*, literally means to *lead out*, to *make to express*). Of course, the environment cannot do anything but develop or depress potentialities that, good or bad, must already be there, but we know that there is a great amount of information in the DNA and that complex gene regulation mechanisms allow a great plasticity in gene expression and development.

Fig. 4: Genes and development: The epigenetic landscape (from Waddington, 1975)

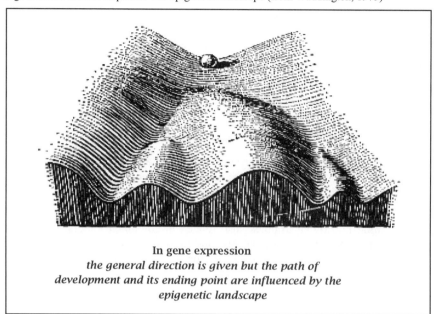

In gene expression
the general direction is given but the path of
development and its ending point are influenced by the
epigenetic landscape

So, in the end, possibly the best answer to this question was suggested several decades ago by the famous playwrighter George Bernard Shaw (1911):

"Take the utmost care to get born well, and well brought up."

Body and Mind

The Body/Mind issue is probably the best example of a classic duality based on strict mechanistic views, which current research now sees instead as a most complex, interactive, plastic system, likely to also greatly affect gene expression mechanisms, maximising or depressing genetic potentialities.

For example, as shown by research at the UCLA Psychoneuroimmunology Center, a simple feeling of shame can induce troubles in the cytokines, an immunologically controlled network of molecules. The levels of cortisol increase when stressful events are faced fighting and involve such emotions as anger or despise, directed outwards. When the reaction is directed inwards, instead, and emotions such as shame, sense of guilt and low self-esteem prevail, cortisol levels do not seem to increase, but lymphocytes decrease, thereby accelerating the progression of infectious conditions. Which might explain the frequent observation of decreased immune defenses in mentally depressed patients, and the high rates of infections and mortality in emotionally deprived children.

Bodily and mental structures coexist in human nature, and closely interact in what should be a harmonious totality, and is frequently not, one part of the self overriding the other. But unresolved emotional conflicts and needs, removed or confounded as they may be, unconsciously influence behaviour, as well as physical structures and functions alike, in health and disorder.

The loss of homeostasis – A sequence of epidemics

Four decades ago, psychosocial growth retardation appeared as an epidemic, to the point that a Presidential Address at the American Pediatric Academy was provocatively entitled, *"Has the failure to thrive taken the place of rickets in modern society?"*(Parisi & De Martino, 1980; Parisi, 1998).

Then, similar nutritional troubles, also related to emotional factors, made their appearance. In a matter of few years, conditions such as anorexia and bulimia became increasingly prevalent, and a new social and medical challenge.

Anorexia nervosa existed in the past, but was brought to public attention when celebrities, such as the singer Karen Carpenter or the gymnast Christy Henrich, died from it. It is estimated that in developed countries about 1 % of young adult females are affected, but this is probably an underestimate and the prevalence of the condition, which is almost exclusive of the female population, is increasing.

Bulimia is a symmetric condition to anorexia, involving overeating followed by vomiting and/or other compensatory behaviors, such as excessive amounts of physical exercise, drug intake, etc. About one-third of anorexics eventually turn to bulimia, and the two conditions may coexist or succeed one another. Here too, about 85 % of patients are female, and 2 % to 5 % of young adult females are estimated to be affected, with symptoms present in many more. A less serious form, *binge-eating*, affects an estimated 10 % of the student population.

Chronic disorders, frequently seen to also have a psychosocial component, are meanwhile increasing as well, with an impressive, steady progression, year after year (Figure 5).

So, what calls our attention today, the obesity epidemic, could actually be part of a wider, continuous epidemic involving a variety of conditions or behaviours and pointing to a homeostatic disruption, possibly psychosocially induced, eliciting gene effects in genetically predisposed individuals, particularly in the most sensitive layers of our society, children and adolescents in the first place.

To consider overweight only in terms of excess food and/or little exercise, may thus lead to simplify things too much. Eating disorders *are a symptom, not the disease*. Whether they stay within the limits of what we consider to be "normal", or reach the levels of overt clinical entities, they are always likely to be the expression of an underlying distress situation.

Fig. 5: The progression of chronic diseases

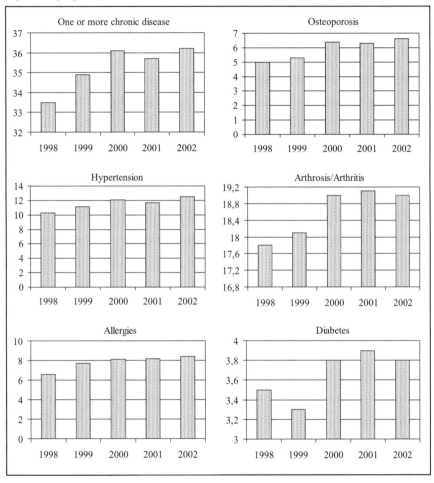

In terms of *behavior*, this may involve compensatory, compulsive habits – as is in fact overeating, to which people easily indulge because of its pleasurable aspect, and particularly so following the pressure against similar habits such as smoking or drinking. These habits are hard to overcome, because of their strong compensatory value. Being the expression of emotional needs, they cannot simply be matched by rational arguments; and because they are just a symptom and not the problem, when one of these habits is dismissed, some new compensatory habit is easily acquired.

At a *more subtle level,* then, involving the deep psychology of the individual, emotional troubles, if prolonged, may also eventually involve a loss of homeostasis, a loss of that fundamental capability of the organism to adjust to circumstances maintaining its health and equilibrium. Hence the instability of body weight and other physiological parameters, hence the possible modifications involving metabolism, and the endocrine and immune functions of the organism at various levels of manifestation.

As current research is increasingly showing, psychosocial stress might set forth a complex cascade of interconnected events eventually resulting in the clinical trouble. As shown in Figure 6, in the case of obesity, the stress may act through increased levels of a cytokine, Interleukin-6 (IL-6), increased sensitivity of the Hypothalamic-Hypophysis-Adrenal-Axis (HPAA), altered regulation of corticosteroids, possibly leading to increased accumulation of visceral fat, and eventually increased susceptibility to obesity and other metabolic disorders (Zhou, Kusnecov, Shurin et al., 1993, Bjorntorp, Holm & Rosmond, 1999; Bjorntorp, 2001; Ljung, Ottosson, Ahlberg et al., 2002). This is just an exemple, from current research in this area, and similar mechanisms may be involved in other conditions.

Fig. 6: Biological correlates of psychosocial stress – some likley mechanismus

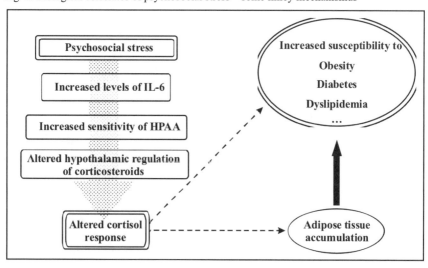

Many people do not diet, even eat what they want, and still have no overweight, hypertension or high cholesterol. Genetic factors play a role of course. But entire social groups exist where this is largely so.

The so-called *French Paradox,* the well-known association of high fat intake and low coronary heart disease in France, is then perhaps less of a paradox than it appears, considering that coronary heart disease is lowest in a region, that of Toulouse, which has the highest consumption of animal fat, but is also where eating has traditionally been a most central and pleasurable aspect of a generally enjoyable, easy lifestyle.

In a book appeared some ten years ago, and appropriately entitled, *The Hungry Soul,* the physician and humanist scholar, Leon Kass (1994), described eating disorders as a reflection of the increasing alienation of middle-class Americans from the emotional, cultural and spiritual values of food and life. An alienation that in fact seems generalised, and increasingly widespread and profound.

Perhaps, while still curing the symptoms as we can, we should start looking more seriously into our system of values and lifestyle – which implies more than just eating and exercise – and really pursue the goal of a healthy society getting to the roots of the problems, ensuring a wiser education, and a better development of the younger generations.

Homo Faber and Homo Ludens: Play, sport and lifestyle in health, development and education

Sport can in this context be extremely beneficial, and not just because it helps reset the calorie balance, but more generally.

The word, *sport,* originally signifies "that which diverts, amuses", and in fact it appears in King James' Bible in the sense of scenic play. That is of course the significance of play, which is the expression of fundamental emotional and spiritual needs, related to amusement, imagination, interaction, creativity, and is by definition "free from purpose" (as myth and religion tell us Creation is: in the Hindu cosmology, Creation is called *Lila,* the Game of Gods).

The fundamental aspect of spontaneity and pure play has long gone lost, as Johan Huizinga noted back in the 1930s, largely because of the increasing role of discipline and regulations, which characterised the transformation of traditional games into modern sport (Huizinga, 1950). The process, as noted by Norbert Elias, started with the Enlightenment and the project to transform pure performance into physical education and care of the body as a fundamental aspect of moral (later military) education (Elias, 1939).

The approach to the human condition that was then developed stressed the rational element and a social frame of reference, thereby generating the socially-oriented model of *Homo Faber,* focused on work, discipline, and endeavour toward continuous progress, health and welfare. The supposedly opposed *Homo Ludens* was reabsorbed, repressed or distorted. But spontaneity and will, just as Play and Work, Rationality and Emotionality, are not opposed categories but coexisting aspects of one and the same human being.

Real play is not much encouraged in our society. Parents tend frequently to project their expectations and frustrations upon their children, and want them to develop skills and abilities and achieve social success. They frequently don't see much value in play, unless it is purposeful, directed to some form of achievement. But then play loses its fundamental, imaginative function, and even becomes counterproductive in the perspective of a harmonious, integral development. Friedrich Froebel, the originator of Kindergarten, wrote that

> "Play is the highest development in childhood, for it alone is the free expression of what is in a child's soul." [reported in McDaniel, 1992]

Play has a high fitness value in mammals, and is essential for human development, as recognised long ago in the history of science and society. As highlighted by our initial story, children who have no opportunity to play are slow to develop, may end up mentally unbalanced or retarded, or even fail to survive. Play has obvious benefits for physical development and coordination, and for a healthy emotional functioning, as also recognised by Freud, for intellectual development and social adjustment. With play, children integrate all aspects of life and behavior, and unify mind, body, and spirit. Those who play in the consistent care of loving adults are considered to develop usually into healthy and mature adults, able to make maximum use of their intelligence and talents (McDaniel, 1992).

Play, as indeed sport and all forms of free activity and of physical and emotional expression, help to go beyond the outer level of superficial behaviors and symptoms, and allow the individual to express hidden energies and drives, reduce conflict and distress, and maintain mental and physical balance, and the effective functioning of homeostasis, without which the organism becomes defenceless and increasingly liable to environmental hazards and circumstances.

Sport, in its genuine sense, plays a most fundamental role in human health, development and education, in promoting a harmonious relation with one's body and emotional life, and its integration in personal growth and experience. Sport is a function of synthesis, allowing the irrepressible needs of the human person to creatively express themselves in a protected context. It fosters body awareness, and integrates with higher forms of self-analysis and meditation in reaching to the roots of one's profound needs and nature, and attain at that inner and outer harmony that is the fundamental aspiration of all human beings and the prerequisite of real health and wellbeing.

So, in the end, I think what I have to say comes to this. Let us do all we can to convince people, and particularly children, to eat less and better, and to exercise. That is for sure the best we can do in the short term.

But let us be aware that this is partly a symptomatic remedy, and so long as the roots of the problem remain untouched, we may continue to jump from one epidemic to the next.

References

Bjorntorp, P. (2001). Do stress reactions cause abdominal obesity comorbidities? *Obesity Review, 2,* 73-86.

Bjorntorp, P., Holm, G. & Rosmond, R. (1999). Hypothalamic arousal, insulin resistance and type 2 diabetes mellitus. *Diabetic Medicine, 16,* 373-383.

Chrousos, G. P. (2000). The stress response and immune function: clinical implications. *Annals of the New York Academy of Sciences, 91,* 738-767.

Ekelund, U., Sardinha, L. B., Anderssen, S. A., Harro, M., Franks, P. W., Brage, S., Cooper, A. R., Andersen, L. B., Riddoch, C. J. & Froberg, K. (2004). Associations between objectively assessed physical activity and indicators of body fatness in 9-to-10-yr-old European children: a population-based study from 4 distinct regions in Europe (the European Youth Heart Study). *American Journal of Clinical Nutrition, 80,* 584-590.

Elias, N. (1939). *Über den Prozess der Zivilisation.* Soziogenetische und Psychogenetische Untersuchungen. Bern: Haus zum Falken.

Huizinga, J. (1950): *Homo Ludens.* London: Routledge & Kegan Paul.

ISTAT -- Istituto Nazionale di Statistica (2004). *Indagine Multiscopo sulle Famiglie -- "Aspetti della vita quotidiana: Stili di vita e condizioni di salute" [Multipurpose Survey on the Families -- "Aspects of daily life: Lifestyle and health conditions"].* Rome: National Institute of Statistics.

Kiank, C., Holtfreter, B., Starke, A., Mundt, A., Wilke, C. & Schütt, C. (2006). Stress susceptibility predicts the severity of immune depression and the failure to combat bacterial infections in chronically stressed mice. *Brain, Behavior and Immunity, 20,* 359-368.

Leon Kass (1994): *The Hungry Soul.* Chicaog: University of Chicago Press.

Ljung, T., Ottosson, M., Ahlberg, A. C., Eden, S., Oden, B., Okred, S., Bronnegard, M., Stierna, P. & Bjorntorp, P. (2002). Central and peripheral GR function in abdominal obesity. *Journal of Endocrinological Investigation, 25,* 229-235.

McDaniel, C.-G. (1992). The serious business of child's play. *Encyclopedia Britannica's Medical and Health Annual (298-302).* Chicago: Encyclopedia Britannica.

McDaniel, C.- G. (1992)."Diet and Nutrition". *Encyclopedia Britannica's Medical and Health Annual (281-285).*Chicago: Encyclopedia Britannica.

Parisi, P. (1998). *Psychosocial development.* In S. J. Ulijaszek, F. E. Johnston, M. A. Preece (Eds.), *Cambridge Encyclopedia of Human Growth (253-255).* Cambridge: Cambridge University Press.

Parisi, P. & De Martino, V. (1980). Psychosocial factors in human growth – Deprivation and failure to thrive. In F. E. Johnston, A. F. Roche & Susanne Eds.), *Human Physical*

Growth and Maturation--Methodologies and Factors (pp-339-356). New York: Plenum Press.

Prentice, A. M. & Jebb, S. A. (1995). Obesity in Britain: gluttony or sloth? *British Medical Journal, 311,* 437-439.

Riddoch, C. J., Andersen, L. B., Wedderkopp, N., Harro, M., Klasson-Heggebo, L., Sardinha, L. B., Cooper, A. R. & Ekelund, U. (2004). Physical activity levels and patterns of 9- and 15-yr-old European children. *Medicine & Science in Sports and Exercise, 36,* 86-92.

Steptoe, A. (1998). Coping, control, and health risk. *Annals of the New York Academy of Sciences, 851,* 470-476.

Waddington, C. H. (1975). *The Evolution of an Evolutionist.* Edinburgh: University Press of Edinburgh.

World Health Organisation (2002). *Programming of chronic disease by impaired fetal nutrition: evidence and implications for policy and intervention strategies.* Geneva: Documents WHO/NHD/02.3 and WHO/NPH/02.1.

World Health Organisation (2003a). Diet, nutrition, and the prevention of chronic diseases. Report of a Joint WHO/FAO Expert Consultation. *WHO Technical Report Series, 916,* 4.

World Health Organisation (2003b): Diet, nutrition, and the prevention of chronic diseases. Report of a Joint WHO/FAO Expert Consultation. *WHO Technical Report Series, 916,* 45.

World Health Organisation (2003c). Diet, nutrition, and the prevention of chronic diseases. Report of a Joint WHO/FAO Expert Consultation. *WHO Technical Report Series, 916,* 5, 8.

World Health Organisation (2004). *Young people's health in context. Health Behavior in School-aged Children (HBSC) study.* Copenhagen: Health Policy for Children and Adolescent, No.4.

Yirmiya, R., Pollak, Y., Morag, M., Reichenberg, A., Barak, O., Avitsur, R., Shavit, Y., Ovadia, H., Weidenfeld, J., Morag, A., Newman, M. E. & Pollmächer, T. (2000). Illness, cytokines, and depression. *Annals of the New York Academy of Sciences, 917,* 478-487.

Zhou, D., Kusnecov, A. W., Shurin, M. R., DePaoli, M. & Rabin, B. S. (1993). Exposure to physical and psychological stressors elevates plasma interleukin-6: relationship to the activation of hypothalamic-pituitary-adrenal axis. *Endocrinology, 133,* 2523-2530.

Chapter 5:
Sedentary lifestyles and physical (in-)activity in youth, a social risk perspective

Bart Vanreusel & Bert Meulders

Introduction

Due to technological, economic, cultural, biomedical and social developments, European societies have reached a high level of comfortable living for a very large group of inhabitants. For large groups in society, the need to perform considerable physical activity in daily life no longer exists. This results in a growing number of people who develop a sedentary lifestyle. As Mandal (1981) has put it, we have created a new kind of human, homo sedens, a sedentary human being. Homo sedens emerged from intense work carried out throughout the 20th century by homo sapiens to create a society which does not need to move to meet most daily needs (Rutten et al, 2003). Although the increasing level of comfort in everyday life is a major achievement in European societies, this achievement at the same time causes some serious risks. In a conceptualization of the 'risk society', Beck & Ritter (1992) pointed out that developments in society, commonly considered as progress, often include risks or threats to the same society. Transferring the concept of risk society to the issue of diminishing physical activity in daily life, health risks are caused by a physically inactive and a sedentary lifestyle. The epidemic of inactivity in everyday life throughout western industrialized countries is the result of the effort put into producing these sedentary lifestyles (Rzewnicky, 2003). Today's young generation in Europe is the first generation to grow up in a society that at the same time produces the comfort leading to a sedentary lifestyle and the health related risks caused by such a lifestyle. At the same time extensive evidence about the importance of physical activity for health and well-being has been produced. Youngsters grow up in a society with a risk for the development of a sedentary lifestyle in youth, and with a risk to continue a sedentary lifestyle into adulthood. Recent reports in almost all European countries reveal alarming figures on the rise of sedentariness in youth and on the health related risks of this development.

It is the aim of this paper to look at the emergence of a sedentary lifestyle as a 'social risk' concept. This means that a sedentary lifestyle is not only an individual and biomedical issue to be studied from a medicalized perspective of the human body. A 'social risk' approach of sedentariness suggests that (1) the problem of sedentariness is generated by developments in society (2) a coordinated social policy is needed to cope with this problem. In this chapter we will address this 'socially generated risk' approach of sedentariness, with a special focus on the role of sport. In this chapter, a broad definition of sport is used, including recreational physical activity for young people. We are aware of significant lifestyle features such as nutrition in the context of sedentariness. Yet in this chapter the focus will be on physical (in-) activity.

The social paradox of sedentarines.

As an attempt to respond to the rise of a sedentary lifestyle, most European countries have developed population based sport for all programs. These programs offer recreational sport related physical activities for everyone. Easy access and democratic participation have been the guiding principles. Most evaluations of such programs point at increasing participation figures among youth, including different modes and styles of participation in sport activities. (Scheerder, Taks, Vanreusel et al., 2002)

But in strong contrast to these rising sport participation figures, studies on physical fitness and physical activity show decreasing numbers of young people meeting fitness norms, increasing levels of sedentariness and increasing prevalence of overweight and obesity among youngsters.

These contrasting tendencies are an intriguing paradox: increasing participation in sport and physical activity on the one hand, increasing sedentariness and related features on the other.

This paradox forces us to reconsider the position of sport and physical activities as a means to cope with sedentariness. First, participation in sport and physical activities may not, or not completely be valid indicators of successful coping with the risks related to sedentariness. Second, sedentariness must be caused and affected in more different ways by other lifestyle features than participation in sport and physical activity.

As a consequence of this paradox, a gradual shift of paradigm can be observed in the approaches of physical activity as a practice, as a policy tool and as an object of study (Figure 1).

Fig.1:   A changing paradigm in the approach of physical activity

A paradigm shift in physical activity practice, policy and research
• from performance related physical activity to…
• health deficit related physical (in-) activity to…
• health enhancing physical activity (HEPA)

The performance paradigm with its cultural connection to sport performance and elite sport has dominated the physical activity concept for a long time. A health deficit paradigm, culturally connected to a medicalized perspective on (the lack of) physical fitness gradually gained momentum in physical activity practices, policy and research. The focus was on the deficits of a lack of physical activity: the risk of disease, economic loss, decreasing quality of life etc. More recently a 'health enhancing physical activity' (HEPA) paradigm has entered the physical activity discourse. The focus is on the benefits related to physical activity: positive approaches of health, psychological benefits increasing quality of life etc.

This paradigm shift is taking place in different applied fields of physical activity. In research, the health enhancing physical activity (HEPA) concept is widely accepted and fostered (Beunen, De Bourdeaudhuij, Vanden Auweele et al., 2001) In public policies, HEPA programs are generating interest, both as large scale population based initiatives and as local initiatives for specific target groups with a high risk for sedentariness. The educational system is incorporating the HEPA concept in its pedagogical methods and models. Instead of isolated lessons in physical education, recent HEPA models promote a so-called 'enlarged school' concept. In this concept, the school environment needs to create a physical activity stimulating climate that stretches from the classroom to the entire school into daily life. Interesting and innovative try out-projects in this field guided by research, are carried out (De Bourdeaudhuij, Van Waes, De Martelaer et al., 2006).

But in contrast to the well established HEPA approach in research policy and education, the position of HEPA in the everyday lifestyles of youngsters remains unclear. This is a remarkable situation because a HEPA approach of coping with sedentariness can only be successful if it is integrated in the everyday life and lifestyle of youngsters.

Young people's lifestyle features, changes and determinants are crucial parameters of knowledge and practice in the physical activity – sedentariness debate. Therefore, lifestyle research in relation to sedentariness, such as developed in the European project by Brettschneider and Naul (2004), is a crucial step needed in research, policy and action on sedentariness.

Three working hypotheses on sedentariness as a social risk

We have argued that the development of a sedentary lifestyle is part of growing up in a 'risk society' and that lifestyle analysis is needed in order to get a more adequate grasp on the issue of sedentary youth. From a social science perspective, three working hypotheses can be elaborated and tested in future research. These three hypotheses are based on the assumption that sedentariness in youth is a 'social construction' caused by developments in society. An analysis of this social construction of sedentariness is needed in order to facilitate coping strategies.

Fig. 2:   Three working hypotheses on the social construction of a sedentary life style in youth.

Hypothesis 1. A sedentary life style in youth is culturally learned, confirmed and rewarded.

Hypothesis 2. The development of a sedentary life style is the result of a socialization process towards physical inactivity developed in youth and continued into adulthood.

Hypothesis 3. The development of a sedentary life style in youth is reinforced by social inequality.

Hypothesis 1: A sedentary lifestyle in youth is culturally learned, confirmed and rewarded.

It is often taken for granted that young people are educated towards a physically active lifestyle. This hypothesis suggests the opposite: many aspects of consumer culture, of educational institutions, of family life and leisure are directly enhancing the risk for a sedentary lifestyle. In the daily life of young people, impulses that foster sedentariness may be much more frequent and intensive than impulses for being active. Furthermore little is known about the relative impact of different lifestyle influencing variables. For example, what is the impact on the lifestyle of youngsters of traditional P E lessons, compared to the impact of consumer culture as it presents itself in shopping streets and supermarkets?

The hypothesis also suggests that youth subcultures may be confirmative to a non-active lifestyle. Learning processes from the 'hidden curriculum' type such as leisure experiences in subgroups, chatting on the internet and informal peer group interaction also may play a confirmatory and rewarding role with regard to a sedentary lifestyle much more than we like to think.

A study on young people's participation in sport clubs may illustrate the hypothesis (Kliksons, 2004). This study covers a representative sample (N = 35,542, age 10 to 18) in Flanders, Belgium. The youngsters in the sample expressed a number of positive claims on the role of sport clubs in their lifestyle:

- sport clubs provide stimulating environments for physical activity
- sport clubs provide social support by peers and significant others
- sport clubs are easy accessible and open minded organisations.

These statements confirm the common perception of sport clubs as outspoken child friendly and physical activity stimulating environments. But the same sample also expressed experiences of disappointment and failure in sport clubs, resulting in dropout from the club.

- 38 % lost their interest by negative experiences in the sport club
- 24 % were unsatisfied with trainers and coaches
- 20 % experienced negative group pressure
- 18 % disliked the competitive spirit
- 10 % perceived themselves as incompetent

  (non accumulative percentages) (Kliksons, 2004)

Such data show that sport clubs not just are positive stimulating environments for an active lifestyle. For a number of young people, sport clubs produce a 'hidden curriculum' of negative experiences which may cause the withdrawal from physical activities such as sport.

More general studies on social environment correlates of physical activity and sedentariness have been summarized by Rzewnicky (2003). Physically active and inactive groups of young people systematically differ from each other with regard to:

- feelings of competence in physical activities
- attitudes towards physical activity
- perceived social support from peers
- perceived family norms towards physical activity

In general, data confirm the social construction hypothesis on sedentariness. A complex set of social variables in the social climate of everyday life of young people will perform a determining role in the development of a sedentary lifestyle. Modern societies appear to create formal and informal learning processes which reinforce a sedentary lifestyle.

Hypothesis 2: The development of a sedentary lifestyle is the result of a socialization process towards physical inactivity developed in youth and continued into adulthood.

This hypothesis is dealing with the intriguing question of longitudinal socialization. It is based on the general assumption that youth experiences affect or even determine adult lifestyle patterns. In the context of sedentariness as a social risk, the question is wether a sedentary lifestyle in youth leads towards a sedentary lifestyle in adulthood?

In contrast to the tempting nature of this hypothesis, empirical data are scarce. From a rather limited set of studies, Rzewnicki (2003) concluded that tracking of psychosocial determinants of sedentariness between youth and adulthood is moderate to high. (Tracking refers to the relative position in a group over a period of time). Longitudinal data on involvement in sport and physical activity from youth to adulthood in Belgium (Vanreusel, Renson, Beunen et al., 1997) and Finland (Telama & Yang, 2000) seem to confirm similar trends: tracking of involvement in physical activities such as sport is but low to moderate, yet significant. But tracking of low activity or inactivity from youth to adulthood is moderate to high. Figure 3 and 4 show tracking profiles for men and women who are categorized as 'inactive' in youth.

Fig. 3:   Level of sports participation at age 30

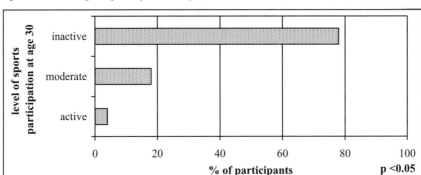

Fig. 4:   Level of sports participation at age between 35-41

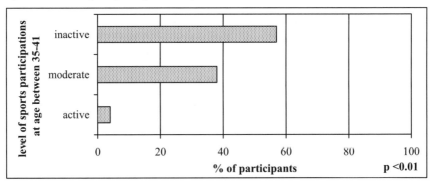

At age 30, 78 % of the males, inactive in youth, still are inactive. Only 4 % changed from inactive at 17 to active at 30 years of age. 57 % of inactive women at age 17, still are inactive at 30 years. Again, only 4 % of inactive women at age 15-18 changed to active sport involvement at age 35-41. These data suggest that an inactive lifestyle may be reinforced by a longitudinal socialization process from youth to adulthood. The hypothesis that a sedentary lifestyle is learned and acquired in youth and likely to be continued into adulthood is challenging. But more longitudinal research on representative samples is needed to test this hypothesis.

Limited and preliminary data certainly do not allow general conclusions. Yet, they suggest that a socialization process towards a sedentary lifestyle is taking place between youth and adulthood. Adequate research on the social risk for sedentariness needs to elaborate on this longitudinal socialization process as a key element.

Hypothesis 3: The development of a sedentary lifestyle is reinforced by social inequality.

Throughout all studies, social inequality appears as a constant and important determinant of involvement in physical activity among youngsters. Indices of social inequality, such as socio-economic status, educational status, financial status, degree of dependency on the service of others etc, all point in the same direction. Youngsters growing up in unfavourable conditions in average have a less physically active lifestyle than youngsters that live in a more advantaged environments. This general observation is confirmed in multivariate studies on determinants of physical activity (Scheerder, 2003) Table 1 dramatically illustrates how social inequality relates to children's chances to be active in leisure sport. Less than 5 % of children from parents with high status jobs are not participating in sports. In contrast, 1 out of 4 children from unemployed parents is a non-participant.

Tab. 1:   Social inequality and non-participation in leisure sport by children (Scheerder, 2003)

Children from:	% of non-participation in leisure sports
Unemployed parents	23.5
Lower education parents	23.4
Low-education of child	22.9
Labour class parents	19.5
Unsportive parents	16.2
Two-income class parents	11.0
Highschool education parents	6.9
Sportive parents	5.8
Higher education parents	5.1
Parents with high status jobs	4.4

The general observation that health problems occur more among children from lower socio-economic groups is complemented by the observation that more highly educated people meet the fit norm than lower educated people. Social inequality is the result of in low opportunities in education, living environment, access to wellbeing, economic living conditions etc. The lifestyle of young people is molded by equality issues. Underprivileged young people develop a higher risk for a sedentary lifestyle than the more privileged ones. Different opportunities to participate in physical activities between privileged and underprivileged youngsters are just one expression of the impact of social inequality on the risk of sedentariness.

The former three hypotheses on the 'social construction' of a sedentary lifestyle come together in the concept of social capital as developed by Bourdieu (1978). Social capital refers to the whole of practices, attitudes, tastes and styles acquired by combined interaction of formal and informal education, schooling, dwelling area, socio-economic situation, etc. Future research on the risk for sedentariness in youth will profit from a social capital perspective. Preliminary data suggest that a sedentary lifestyle is related to low social capital features in youth. A sedentary lifestyle may be part of a low social capital profile.

Interventions by state, market and civil society

We have argued that a sedentary lifestyle in youth is part of today's risk society and that it is related to one's social capital. Consequently, interventions to prevent sedentariness need a lifestyle encompassing approach, based on an integrated social policy.

Three major players in such an integrated intervention model can be distinguished:

(1)   the state, by developing a public policy

(2)   the market by providing services and goods and by using marketing methods

(3)   the civil society by taking initiatives by citizens and local communities.

As shown in the model by Ibsen (1998), state, market and civil society meet each other at various intersections of society (figure 5).

The public sector, the for profit sector and the civil sector together have an enormous potential to intervene in the problem of sedentariness in youth. Interactive and cooperative policy models between these different sections of society create a richness of strategies to decrease the risk of sedentariness. Again, it sounds ironical that state, market and civil society have created the social risk of sedentariness in the first place. The same institutions who contributed to the rise of sedentariness as a public health concern will be needed to fight it.

Fig. 5:   Different fields of society between state, market and civil society (Ibsen, 1998)

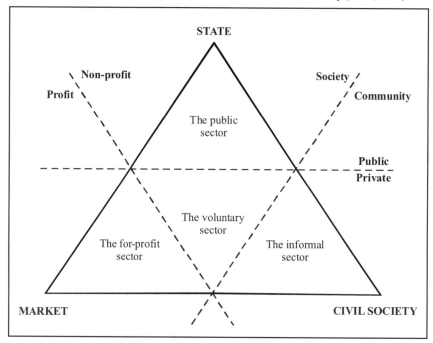

Although a combined effort of public policy, market impact and civil society initiatives is needed, each sector can act according to its specific capacities:

state initiatives and public policy:

• campaigns on awareness and attitudes of healthy lifestyles

• development and implementation of programs against sedentariness

• activating other institutions such as education, health system, public transport, families

• regulating measures such as laws, taxes, subsidies, reward systems, monitoring systems

market initiatives:

• providing services and goods that promote an active lifestyle and prevent sedentariness

• address specific target groups and underserved youth

• develop and promote active role models and images

- using marketing methods to decrease sedentariness and promote physical activity

civil society initiatives:

- facilitating self organisation and responsibility
- provide formal and informal support
- training of volunteers and 'activity coaches'
- family and peer group initiatives
- organised memberships

Summary and recommendations

It is argued in this chapter that a sedentary lifestyle is part of a 'risk society' and that different social institutions need to launch a cooperative effort for lifestyle changes to minimize this risk. All following policy recommendations are based on this perspective.

The recommendations in this document are inspired by the work of a HEPA working group of experts in Belgium (Beunen et al, 2001). The goal of the HEPA-group was to create an integrated framework that maximizes opportunities for health promoting physical activities and that minimizes the risk for sedentariness.

Recommendations for policy: between state, market and civil society.

Although research on youth lifestyles and sedentariness is incomplete and preliminary, there is sufficient evidence that sedentariness is a growing and serious health risk in the population and particularly in youth. Intervention strategies need to include major actors with an impact on youth lifestyles. Public policy measures, market strategies and civil society action together will have to address the growing sedentariness issue.

- Public policy measures need to facilitate, promote, implement and regulate health enhancing physical activity programs in all areas of youth culture, including daily life physical activity, mobility, play, physical education, formal and informal sport, exercise and nutrition.
- Market and media strategies need to emphasize health enhancing physical activity in the marketing of youth and lifestyle images, goods, services, attitudes and mentalities.
- The potential impact of civil society on youth lifestyle tends to be under-estimated. It is crucial to raise awareness and responsibility among young

citizens themselves. Responsibility for a healthy and active lifestyle, after all, lies in the hands of groups and individual youngsters themselves. Self organisation and action by parents, children play groups, youth movements, teenage clubs, neighbourhood initiatives, etc can be a most effective measure.

- Public policy, market and civil society need to act in a synergetic way towards the common objective of fighting sedentariness. Contradictory signals from the market will harm or eradicate HEPA initiatives by public policy and civil society.

- Policy makers need to create legal, fiscal and budgetary space to encourage physical activity. They need to create strategies to shift social values and norms towards a more physically active lifestyle and have to make these strategies a priority for public health.

- Policy makers have to take measures to create a more 'movement friendly environment', through the construction of safe, accessible and attractive footpaths and bicycle lanes. Active promotion of biking, walking, use of stairs and other examples of active transportation have to be incorporated in the local, regional and national policy.

Recommendations to the educational system

Major changes are needed to implement an effective HEPA strategy in the educational system.

- HEPA needs to be an integrated part of the educational system: home centered education of young children, child care institutions, preschool, junior school, highschool and higher education institutions. HEPA programs cannot be isolated to curricula of physical education only.

- The concept and content of physical education programs need to address HEPA in a more in depth way. New modules and concepts of physical activity in the school context need to be developed and implemented. Transfer of physical education classes to everyday life physical activity needs to be realized.

- Physical education programs at school need to monitor, advise, and guide physical activity of children and youth. Counselling and implementation of individual trajectories of physical activity need to be developed.

- The amount of time spent on HEPA needs to be increased at all levels of the educational system. Curricular and extra-curricular initiatives are needed.

- School HEPA programs need to raise the responsibility of every individual child and teenager for her or his physically active lifestyle.

- The socialization role of the educational environment is crucial. Young children have to be encouraged to be more physically active in the first place by their parents, who also have to be encouraged to be more active themselves. When children go to school, teachers (next to parents) have an initiating and supportive role. As children grow older the supportive role of friends, siblings, partners and colleagues becomes more important.

- Increase in knowledge is necessary but not sufficient to induce a behavioural change. Nevertheless it is necessary that the current norms for physical activity become common knowledge for educators. For example, a widely spread misconception exists that mainly intense sports generate beneficial effects. As a person is involved in 'more' and 'more intense' physical activities, this will, to a certain extent, have an additional and beneficial health effect. The (intrinsic) motivation for a lifelong active lifestyle will be stimulated by increasing the positive outcomes of physical activity such as fun, social contact and health.

- Perceived barriers to (more) physical activity have to be eliminated. 'Lack of time' can be taken care of by setting different priorities or by more effective time management. The common idea of 'I'm not the athletic type' can be mediated through the promotion of physical activities of mainly low and moderate intensity.

- More creativity is required in the provision of and / or tolerance towards 'free choice moments' of different physical activity types at school. Concrete, for these situations we consider transport to and from school and breaks as good opportunities to increase physical activity level.

- Physical activity has to be promoted as an efficient and cheap means to increase health and wellness. This can be done through promotion of daily physical activities, active transport to and from school, physical activities at school (breaks, organization of classes, ...), and an active lifestyle during leisure time.

- Policy can also have an important impact on physical activities at school, through the provision of sufficient (more) hours of Physical Education, which have to include physical activities oriented towards a lifelong active and healthy lifestyle. It is important to educate children and youngsters during those Physical Education classes about ways to maintain and increase physical fitness. It is also important that those classes are used to create a positive attitude towards a lifelong active lifestyle (by offering fun physical activity types) and to teach movement routines that can be executed at all ages. In other words, present school infrastructure in terms of classrooms, class schedules, curriculum, and qualified teachers have to be organized as efficient as possible to reach short- and long-term health objectives.

- It should be made clear to educators (teachers, youth coaches, parents) that the positive effects on health and wellness do not result automatically from physical activity, but through good planning and reflective effort, adjusted to each education level (with inclusion of special education). As such, guidelines have to be put in place to maximize the potential for beneficial outcomes.

- Guidelines (curricula, methodologies) have to be set in place to help parents, teachers and coaches maximize chances at school, at home and in sporting clubs for a lifelong fit and healthy lifestyle through their own unique approach.

Recommendations to sports organizations

The social network of sport clubs is a unique supporting structure for the systematic promotion of physical activities in youngsters. This network needs full support of local, regional and national public authorities.

- Sport clubs need to develop a membership strategy to include youngsters with an inactive or a sedentary lifestyle and to avoid drop-out by youngsters.

- Sport clubs need to target specific subgroups of participants. Whereas some sport clubs will focus on elite sport and competitive sport, others need to specialize in the recruitment of non-sport oriented or sedentary youth. This means that such sport clubs need to redefine their objectives, recruiting strategies, membership profiles, programs and coaches' profiles towards a HEPA approach.

- The social and pedagogical climate of sport clubs is a major source of drop-out. Sport clubs need to create an inclusive social and pedagogical climate.

- Sport clubs need to be managed as grass roots centres for involvement in physical activities for all youngsters.

- Voluntary and (semi-)professional staff in sport clubs need to develop knowledge, practical skills, methodologies and didactics related to HEPA.

Recommendations for further research

- Research on youth lifestyles and sedentariness is incomplete and suffering from conceptual and methodological shortcomings.

- A lack of transfer exists between research findings and policy development on youth and sedentariness.

- Levels of physical (in-) activity in youth need to be monitored by research in a systematic, reliable and valid way on representative samples of youth.

- Research needs to focus on causalities of a sedentary lifestyle in youth, rather than on correlations.

- Effects of intervention strategies (e.g. indirect intervention, media campaigns) have to be evaluated continuously in a scientific manner, in order to draw conclusions about the most effective strategies to promote physical activity. Determinant studies for children and youngsters are rare. In this age category, there exists a need in the first place for knowledge about determinants of daily physical activity and not so much for knowledge about factors that affect sports in sporting clubs. Further research is needed to identify determinants that intervene in the different behavioural stages of change. Knowledge about such determinants will allow applying specific interventions that are most relevant for an individual in a certain stage of change.

- It is clear that research studies about 'environmental determinants' are still in the embryonic stage. This subfield of research is seen as very promising for the future. Further research about the impact of objective and subjective environmental determinants for physical activity of individuals in different age categories is needed.

References

Beck., U. & Ritter, M. (1992). Risk society: towards a new modernity. London: Sage.

Beunen, G., De Bourdeaudhuij, I., Vanden Auweele, Y. & Borms, J. (Eds.) (2001). Fysieke activiteit, fitheid en gezondheid (Physical activity, Fitness and Health). *Vlaams tijdschrift voor sportgeneeskunde en sportwetenschappen, special edition,112 p.*

Bourdieu, P. (1978). Pratiques sportives et pratiques sociales. In HISPA (Ed.), 7ème Congrès international de l'Association de l'Histoire de l'Education Physique et du Sport (HISPA; Paris; 28 mars – 2 avril 1978) (17-37). Paris: Insep.

Brettschneider, W.- D. & Naul, R. (Eds.) (2004). Study on young people's lifestyles and sedentariness and the role of sport in the context of education and as a means of restoring the balance (final report). Paderborn, Essen: University of Paderborn, University of Duisburg Essen.

De Bourdeaudhuij, I., Van Waes, E., De Martelaer, K. & Vanreusel, B. (2006). Brede school met sportaanbod (the enlarged school concept and sport). Rapport steunpunt sport, beweging, gezondheid, (unpublished report of the policy research center for sport,movement and health). Gent: University of Gent.

Kliksons (2004). Online database on leisure time of Flemish children and teenagers (www.kliksons.be). Brussel: kinderrechtencommissariaat (Office for children's rights of the Flemish government).

Ibsen, B. (1998). Sport and the welfare society, the development of sport between state, market and community, paper presented at the conference of the international society for the sociology of sports. Montreal: unpublished paper.

Mandal, A. C. (1981). The seated man, homo sedens. *Applied Ergonomics, 12 (1),* 19-26.

Rzewnicky, R. (2003). Health Enhancing Physical Activity. Measurement and determinants of daily activity at home, work, travel, and leisure. Leuven: KU Leuven, Doctoral dissertation.

Scheerder, J., Taks, M., Vanreusel, B. & Renson, R. (2002). 30 jaar breedtesport in Vlaanderen, participatie en beleid, (30 years of sport for all in Flanders, participation and policy) (series on sport and society), Gent: BVLO publicatiefonds.

Scheerder, J. (2003). Gelijke Speelvelden? Sociale gelaagdheid van de vrijetijdssport vanuit een sociaal-cultureel veranderingsperspectief (Level Playing Fields, social stratification of leisure sport from a cultural change perspective). Leuven: KU Leuven, Doctoral dissertation.

Telama, R. & Yang, X. (2000). Decline of physical activity from youth to young adulthood in Finland. *Medicine & Science in Sport and Exercise, 32 (9)*, 1617-1622.

Vanreusel, B., Renson, R., Beunen, G., Claessens, A.L., Lefevre, J., Lysens, R. & Vanden Eynde, B. (1997). A longitudinal study of youth sport participation and adherence to sport in adulthood. *International Review for the Sociology of Sport, 32 (4)*, 373-387.

Chapter 6:
Obesity prevention in the homes, schools and neighbourhoods of Mexican-American children

Susan C. Duerksen, Nadia R. Campbell, Elva M. Arredondo, Guadalupe X. Ayala, Barbara Baquero, John Elder

In the southwestern corner of the United States, an urban interface between the U.S. and Mexico, a randomized community intervention trial known as *"Aventuras para Niños"* (Adventures for Children) tackled the environmental influences contributing to childhood obesity. Using a *promotora* (lay health advisor) model, the intervention sought to change the home, school and community environments of young Mexican-American children to improve their opportunities for both *physical* activity and healthy eating. The three-year intervention, implemented in two waves beginning in 2003 and 2004, was designed to achieve both behavioral and body weight outcomes. The study was funded to the San Diego State University Research Foundation through a National Institutes of Health initiative seeking environmental answers to childhood obesity.

The research focused on Mexican-American children of ages 5-7, because they represent a population disproportionately affected by the obesity epidemic and young enough to provide a prevention opportunity before the adiposity rebound of the preteen years. The rate of overweight among Mexican-American children is higher and growing faster than that of non-Hispanic white children or children overall (Hedley, Ogden, Johnsen et al., 2004; Flegal, Ogden & Caroll, 2004). In the 1999-2000 NHANES survey, which over-sampled Mexican-American children to improve the estimate, the prevalence of overweight at ages 6-11 was 23.7 % of Mexican-American children, 19.5 % of non-Hispanic black children and 11.8 % of non-Hispanic white children (Hedley et al., 2004; Ogden, Flegal, Caroll et al., 2002). For Latinos of all ages, a disproportionate prevalence of overweight and obesity leads to higher risk of diabetes and other health problems (Flegal, Caroll, Ogden et al., 2002; Cossrow & Falkner, 2004).

Study design

Aventuras para Niños participants were students at 13 public elementary schools in three school districts in southern San Diego County. The districts were chosen for high Latino enrollment. Schools within the districts were invited to participate if they had Latino enrollment of at least 70 %, had not had any other obesity-related programs or special physical education training within the past 4 years, and had defined attendance boundaries (as opposed to charter or magnet schools that draw students from a broad region). Children entering kindergarten, 1st or 2nd grades were eligible to participate in the study, regardless of ethnicity, if they lived within the school attendance boundaries and had no major health problems. Participating families (one child and one primary caregiver per household) were enrolled in two waves, the first five schools at the beginning of the 2003–04 school year and the rest in the fall of 2004, and were each followed for three years. The height and weight of each child and caregiver were measured each year, and the caregiver – usually the mother – completed a questionnaire on family history, behavior and demographics. A total of 812 children were enrolled, 86 percent of them Latino. The participating schools were randomly assigned to one of four intervention conditions: microenvironment only (home), macroenvironment only (school and community), both types of intervention ("micro + macro"), or a no-treatment control condition. This 2X2 factorial design allowed *Aventuras para Niños* to compare the effects of environmental changes in the home, in the school and larger community, and the interaction of both at once.

Intervention design

The intervention was based on the Social Ecological Theory, which holds that the conditions in which people live are important determinants of individual behavior (Stokols, 1996). The influence of environmental conditions has repeatedly been shown to be a major force behind the rapidly rising wave of overweight and obesity (Hill & Peters, 1998; French, Story & Jeffery, 2001; Jeffery & Utter, 2003). Cohen, Scribner & Farley (2000) identified four types of structural factors beyond individual control that influence behavior: 1) availability of protective or harmful products, 2) physical structures, 3) social structures and policies, and 4) media and cultural messages. The *Aventuras para Niños* intervention was designed to impact all three environmental levels – home, school and community – and to address all four of the categories of environmental influences as they relate to the promotion of physical activity and healthy eating among young children. Specifically, those influences included such things as: parenting practices and the types of foods and toys available at home; play facilities, equipment and physical activity opportunities at school; school policies and availability of foods and drinks; the types of food and recreation facilities accessible to families in the community, and culturally aligned messages to parents regarding all of the above factors.

The intervention was built on a *promotora* model, which has been identified as one of the most culturally appropriate and well-received intervention methods for Latinos (Navarro, Senn, Mc Nicholas et al., 1998; Elder, Ayala, Campbell et al., 2005; Candelaria, Lyons, Elder et al., 1998). The *promotora* model is based on the assumption that within every community there are formal and informal social networks through which health information is exchanged and predisposing interpersonal environments are created. Research shows that *promotoras* – women from the community trained in basic health promotion – have the capacity to create awareness, disseminate and tailor health information, and support behavior change (Navarro et al., 1998; Navarro, Senn, Kaplan et al., 1995; Elder, 2005). *Aventuras* staff recruited and trained two groups of *promotoras* for the micro and macro interventions, which involved very different kinds of work.

Home (micro) intervention

The home (micro) intervention involved structured one-on-one peer counseling for parents of participating children in the family's home. Home environments of young children are shaped almost entirely by adults in the home, so the parents were given health education and encouragement to create a home where children were able and likely to engage in physical activity and healthy eating. Each participating family was assigned a *promotora*, who visited the home monthly for seven months over the course of one school year, with a break for the winter holidays. At each visit, the *promotora* reviewed a 4-page project-generated newsletter with the parent (see below), provided other materials and guided the parent in setting incremental goals for the next month to improve eating and physical activity aspects of the family life. A major part of the *promotoras'* job was to tailor the information and goal-setting to each family.

The project hired eight *promotoras* for the home intervention; all were veterans of other health education projects and six were monolingual Spanish speakers. They underwent 22 hours of training, in 11 sessions, on basic knowledge of obesity, nutrition and physical activity, as well as the specific content of each monthly home visit and how to conduct the discussions with parents. A detailed *promotora* training manual was developed by *Aventuras* staff and consultants during the initial year of planning. Biweekly meetings with a *promotora* coordinator throughout the intervention period bolstered the training with feedback from the visits, group discussions and role-playing. Depending on their efficiency and other job commitments, each promotora was able to handle monthly visits with between 12 to 30 families. The promotoras were paid a flat fee per completed visit, based on an average of 1.5 hours per visit, plus a stipend for mileage.

Home intervention content

Aventuras staff created the seven newsletters, which were printed on glossy paper in full color. Each newsletter addressed both nutrition and physical activity issues, with a general theme for each month, in the following order:

- Welcome and introduction
- Access and availability (of healthy options)
- Parental modeling/Family time
- Setting limits and rules
- Rewards and punishment
- Media messages and fast food
- Review/Get ready for summer

Each newsletter included a front-page story and photos of a local family that fit that month's theme, with quotes from the family about how and why they had made healthy changes, and how their children had benefited. The newsletters also contained short segments of information, tips, ideas, quizzes, exercises and healthy child-friendly recipes, using lots of bright colors, graphics and photos. Health messages focused specifically on increasing fruit and vegetable consumption, increasing consumption of water in place of sodas and sweetened drinks, decreasing TV viewing and increasing active play. Targeted environmental changes included physical changes such as having cut-up veggies within child's reach and moving a TV out of a child's bedroom, as well as social/policy changes in the rules and boundaries set by parents, discipline methods and family recreation and eating habits.

In addition to the newsletters, parents received informational handouts and other materials, including diaries to record their child's eating and physical activity for 4 days and goal-setting sheets to help parents decide on steps they believed they should and could take related to each month's theme. All the materials, as well as the interpersonal interactions with the *promotoras*, were in Spanish or English, depending on participant preference; three-quarters of participants assigned to the micro condition chose Spanish. If participants asked to discontinue the home visits, they were given the option of receiving the newsletter and other materials by mail; 23 percent switched to that option at some point, most saying they did not have time for the home visits.

Booster calls

For all participants receiving the home intervention, the first year of monthly visits was followed by four booster calls over a two-year period. The *promotora* called the parent three times during the school year (in October/November, January/February, and April/May), and once more the following fall, to review points made during the home visits, ask about the family's experience with changes made and set further goals for improvement. A hand-written reminder of the new goals and the family's most recent accomplishments was mailed to the parent within a few days. In training sessions and printed guidelines, *promotoras* were instructed to tailor the calls, focusing on areas where each family had made improvement and/or needed improvement, and tailoring incremental goals to the family's readiness to change. The booster call training also included a session on motivational interviewing techniques, presented by a psychologist on the project staff (Miller & Rollnick, 1991). Continuity of promotora-family relationships was maintained wherever possible, and when promotora turnover required that a new promotora make the calls, she was given a folder with notes from the visits and the family's previously set goals.

School and community (macro) intervention

While the home intervention focused on influencing parents to change the child's home environment, the macro (school and community) intervention used various approaches to address the four realms of influence in the larger environment. In line with ecological theory, the intervention was designed to alter physical structures (e.g. playgrounds and salad bars), social structures and policies (e.g. teachers' discipline practices and public park maintenance), availability of protective or harmful products (e.g. physical education equipment and healthy children's menus in restaurants), and media and cultural messages (e.g. posters and newsletters). Some of the macro environmental changes were directly implemented by *Aventuras* staff and *promotoras*; some were aimed at the mediating adults who control children's daily environments, including principals, teachers, foodservice workers, restaurant owners, store managers and local government officials. A consistent theme across all macro intervention activities was an attempt to involve parents and local community members in making the changes, in hopes of increasing sustainability.

Unlike the home intervention, the macro *promotoras* and staff didn't specifically have contact with participating children or their families, or even know who they were. Information and programs were provided to the entire school, or at least the target grade levels, and to the community at large. All students and parents were invited to participate in macro intervention programs, regardless of their status as enrolled participants. Evaluation components of the study tracked whether the programs reached, attracted and/or impacted *Aventuras* participants.

The school programs and community change efforts lasted three years for each wave, building or at least maintaining strength over that period rather than tapering down to a "booster" level. The longer full-strength duration was deemed necessary because, compared to the home intervention, dose intensity for individual participants was much lower, many of the changes were harder to achieve, and less evidence was available of effective change strategies. Because of the innovative nature of this type of research and the need to adapt intervention strategies to the specific needs of many different organizations and settings, the macro intervention was modified throughout implementation to adjust the methods to the circumstances encountered.

The type of *promotora* work involved in changing school and community environments proved challenging for experienced *promotoras* who were accustomed to providing health education one-on-one or in small groups. Some *promotoras* were uncomfortable with the uncertainty associated with activities requiring interpersonal and group advocacy. Some of the best macro *promotoras* had no *promotora* or other job experience, but had outgoing personalities and a strong commitment to the project goals. The number of macro *promotoras* varied from six for the first wave of schools to nine with Wave 2 enrollment and finally a strong core group of four. They received an 8-session training at the outset, which included the same basic information on obesity, nutrition and physical activity that the micro *promotoras* received, as well as details of the project goals for the schools and an overview of community organizing techniques and possible community change goals, which were based on feedback from community members. Throughout the macro intervention, *promotoras* attended weekly meetings with a project coordinator for feedback, troubleshooting and continued training. They each worked 15-20 hours a week, and were paid hourly.

School intervention

As with the home intervention, the school intervention targeted policies and practices – as well as physical structures – that shape children's choices, For instance, methods of teaching Physical Education (PE) and the types of encouragement children received in making lunch choices were addressed, along with the physical availability of PE equipment and access to a well-stocked salad bar.

In formative and introductory interviews, school principals uniformly were concerned about intrusions into the tightly scheduled instructional day. That concern was amplified by almost all teachers at the schools assigned to the macro intervention, and became a guiding principle for selecting school intervention strategies with minimal demands on teacher time or class time. Academic content was incorporated wherever possible, to help teachers see the intervention as an enhancement rather than an interruption of the required curricula.

The school intervention included several previously developed programs: SPARK physical education training and equipment, Peaceful Playgrounds painted game designs, and Take 10!®, an in-class program of 10-minute activity breaks with academic content. *Aventuras* staff provided follow-up to reinforce the continued use of the programs. The *Aventuras* staff also developed a number of new school interventions: "Start with Salad" posters and stickers encouraging vegetable consumption at lunch, recess walking clubs and other structured physical activities, after-school parent and child walking clubs, physical activity and nutrition homework assignments, teacher training on "healthy classrooms", nutrition presentations, and a health newsletter sent home to parents.

Spark

In the six schools assigned to the macro and micro-macro intervention conditions, all teachers in grades K-2 received a shortened SPARK Physical Education curriculum and a 5- to 6-hour group training in PE teaching methods. The group trainings were followed by individual model teaching sessions, in which the trainer taught each teacher's PE class while the teacher observed, participated and asked questions. SPARK, which was originally developed at San Diego State University, emphasizes keeping more children active more of the time than in traditional PE classes, with minimal time spent listening to instructions or waiting for a turn (Mc Kenzie, Sallies, Kolody et al., 1999; Sallis, Mc Kenzie, Kolody et al., 1999). Teachers were encouraged to teach 30-minute PE sessions at least three and preferably five times a week. In the second and third years of the intervention, the training and model teaching was repeated for 3rd-grade and then 4th-grade teachers, as the participant cohort advanced into those grades. *Aventuras* gave each school a full set of the equipment needed for the K-2 abbreviated curriculum and another set for the upper grades, whose curriculum included more skill-based games such as basketball and soccer. The equipment included balls, beanbags, hula hoops, jump ropes, "parachutes," cones and spot markers; and for the upper grades soccer balls, soft balls, basketballs, Frisbee disks, relay batons, and hurdles.

Peaceful Playgrounds®

Before the intervention began, all the schools had some type of game markings outlined in white paint on the playgrounds, such as basketball and 4-square courts. The markings were sparse at some schools and rarely included any color. *Aventuras* purchased stencils, blueprints and school licenses for the Peaceful Playgrounds program, which was developed by a San Diego County educator as a method to keep more children occupied and out of trouble during recess (Stratton & Mullan, 2005). The *Aventuras* staff selected the most active games, tailored the designs with input from teachers, and worked with the principals and district staff to have the design outlines painted with striping machines. The *Aventuras* staff and *promotoras*, with the help of a few parents, then used rollers and brushes to paint 6-color shapes, numbers and letters to fill out the designs. All teachers were given a set of simple rules for active games using the newly painted designs.

Take 10!®

To give children an opportunity for vigorous movement during class time, *Aventuras* used the Take 10!® program developed by the International Life Sciences Institute in Atlanta (Stewart, Dennison, Kohl et al., 2004). Each teacher in grades K-2 – and in subsequent years, grades 3 and 4 – received a set of 30 grade-appropriate Take 10!® activity cards, along with a brief training and written instructions and tips. The letter-sized activity cards provide full scripts for 10-minute academic-oriented exercises that can be done in the classroom at any point during the day. To encourage and track implementation, *Aventuras* also developed and gave teachers monthly Take 10!® wall calendars and stickers to mark each day the class did one of the activities. The calendars were collected and new ones delivered at the end of each month.

Homefun

Although it was not an established program, the *Aventuras* component called "Homefun" was implemented based on physical activity homework ideas developed by an Illinois teacher (Gabbei & Hamrick, 2001). Teachers in the target grades were given colorful calendars for each student with simple activity suggestions on each day (e.g. *Crawl like an alligator around the house; Challenge your family to a "Limbo" contest; Put a toy on the floor and jump over it 15 times*) and a weekly nutrition assignment (e.g. *Try a red fruit this week; Look for blue or purple fruits and vegetables at the market*). Teachers handed out the calendars as homework, and students were told to have an adult initial each day they did the activity and bring back the calendars. Monthly calendars were used at first, but soon were switched to weekly based on teacher suggestions for improving the return rate.

Recess walking clubs and Super Aventuras

During the first two years of intervention, the macro *promotoras* organized "walking clubs" of children during the recess time following lunch. The children, sometimes accompanied by a *promotora*, walked laps around a designated area of the school grounds. At first, the *promotoras* tracked how many miles each child had walked over time; the second year, that cumbersome system was abandoned and they walked along with groups of children and simply tracked who had participated. Children received stickers, water bottles and other incentive prizes such as jump ropes and small balls, and those who walked most frequently received certificates of recognition at year-end school assemblies. During the 2005-06 school year (the third year of intervention for Wave 1 schools and the second year for Wave 2), the walking clubs were replaced by a new program called *Super Aventuras*, which was designed by staff to give children more interesting options for recess activity. This program allowed students to rotate between activity stations staffed by the *promotoras*. There usually were three stations at a time, including parachute games, aerobic dance or jump rope, and an exercise course of movements named for animals (e.g. bunny hop, cheetah chase, frog jump). Signs illustrating the movements, cones and other colorful markers were used to mark the circular course. Charts were mounted temporarily on a fence with the names of all students in the target grades, by class; each participating student was given a small sticker to place by his or her name. At the end of the year, students were given certificates and prizes for participation, but there were no other incentive prizes, which had become the focus of many students' participation in the walking clubs. *Super Aventuras* was held at each of the six schools twice a month, on a rotating basis, with all four macro *promotoras* working together. At one school, volunteer staff from a nearby sports equipment store came regularly to help. And other schools, the *promotoras* recruited several parents to help supervise the activities.

Start with Salad

All six macro schools already had salad bars available to children at lunch, and the districts had rigid district-wide rules about the contents. *Aventuras* provided training by a registered dietitian for foodservice workers at each school, on the importance of keeping the salad bars clean and well-stocked with fresh produce, and on prompting children to select and eat vegetables and fruit. Cafeteria workers also were asked to help the *promotoras* with a new program called "Start with Salad," in which children received large, colorful stickers as incentives to eat salad or vegetables first when they sat down to lunch. The program was developed from observations that children rarely selected vegetables from the salad bars and, even when they did, often threw the vegetables away after consuming the high-fat entrée. Using "Dole 5 a Day Friend" vegetable characters, with permission from Dole Food Co., Inc., posters were developed for cafeteria walls, and laminated character cutouts with messages like "Eat veggies first" were posted on the salad bars. The same characters (e.g. a smiling bunch of spinach on a skateboard, a broccoli crown wearing earphones and dancing, three radish buddies in sneakers) were used to create a series of 2.5-inch diameter stickers. Twice a month, on the same days as

Super Aventuras, the *promotoras* walked among the tables during lunch time for the target grades, giving stickers to all children who started lunch with at least one bite of salad or vegetables.

Poster contests

During the third intervention year, the Start with Salad posters were replaced or supplemented by student-designed posters. A poster contest was held at each school, with winners selected in each of the three target grades for two kinds of posters: one on eating vegetables and one on drinking water rather than sodas or other sugary drinks. As with Start with Salad, the emphasis was placed on vegetables because most children are more apt to eat fruit. Winning designs were enlarged for display in the schools, and all entrants received a gift bag with active toys such as jump ropes and frisbees. To kick off the contests, hands-on nutrition assemblies were held at each school, in which students measured the amount of sugar in various sizes of soda, tasted water with a squeeze of lemon or tangerine, identified displayed vegetables, voted on their favorites, and left munching on raw green beans.

Healthy classrooms

Teachers in the target grades received a brief training, followed by annual booster sessions, on ways to create a healthy classroom. The key topics included 1) rationale and ideas for nonfood rewards, rather than giving children candy to reward good behavior or completed work; 2) rationale and ideas for discipline methods that don't remove opportunities for physical activity (e.g. withholding recess); 3) ideas and encouragement to make healthy options available during class parties and other special events, and 4) the importance of encouraging children to drink water and allowing access to drinking water during the school day. Teachers also were given posters for their rooms that encouraged physical activity in healthy eating, including posters produced by the US Department of Agriculture and the 5-a-Day program.

Aventuras newsletter

Monthly newsletters were created describing *Aventuras* programs, inviting parents to participate, thanking school and community helpers and providing family health tips. They were tailored to each macro intervention school and printed in Spanish on one side and English on the other, and were sent home in the backpacks of every child in the school. During the second year of intervention, when the number of macro schools increased from two to six, the newsletters became bimonthly and were distributed only to the target grades.

Afterschool walking clubs

Efforts to start a Kids-Walk-to-School program, following the Centers for Disease Control and Prevention design, at the two Wave 1 schools, failed because parents declined to take responsibility for others' children on the way to and from school. Discussions with the parents instead resulted in afterschool walking clubs for parents and children together at the school track or a nearby park. Children received stickers and prizes for miles walked, but attendance was modest and the following year, at the Wave 2 schools, sparse. At two of the Wave 2 schools, parents were invited to participate in a "walk audit" to identify obstacles to walking in the neighborhood; two parents attended at one school and zero at the other.

Promotoras' role in the schools

During the first year of intervention, three *promotoras* were assigned to each of the two macro schools. In addition to working with parents and students at the schools, the *promotoras* were seen as the project's "eyes and ears". They were expected to implement or observe implementation of program activities and interact with each teacher at least monthly. They provided prompts to the teachers and feedback to project staff, in addition to delivering and collecting materials. However, it soon became clear that the *promotora* model was not appropriate for working with teachers, given differences in background and training. Language and cultural barriers impeded development of the peer relationships at the core of the *promotora* model, and monthly face-to-face contact was too time-consuming for teachers' schedules. Beginning with the second year of intervention, the School Coordinator, a public health graduate student, took over responsibility for all communications with teachers. To collect materials from the teachers, colorful plastic crates were placed in the teacher lounges with a hanging folder for each teacher. The number of macro schools increased from two to six that year, with Wave 2 enrollment, so that each *promotora* was now part of a team responsible for two or three schools rather than just one. However, with fewer school-based duties and a growing emphasis on the project's community intervention, the *promotoras* spent a much greater portion of their time working in the community at large.

Community Intervention

Community organizing for environmental change was expected to be a long-term effort. Initial challenges were inevitable given the lack of empowerment to create change among low-income immigrant community members. It is also possible that these parents were unable to prioritize their families' health because of other competing needs and perhaps lacked the health knowledge to feel an urgent need for a healthier community environment. In addition, many elementary school parents who expressed interest in *Aventuras* also had preschool children and were hampered by a lack of time and child care.

Community organizing

During the first and second year of intervention, parents were asked – through newsletters, meetings and face-to-face contact in front of the schools – what changes they would like to see in the community to increase their children's access to healthy food and physical recreation opportunities. Few parents responded. At one school, a group of parents expressed interest in getting crossing signs installed in front of the school, just the kind of physical environment change *Aventuras* was designed for. However, it became clear their motivation was to make it easier to wait in their cars when picking up their children, rather than making it easier for the children to walk to and from school. That goal was not pursued.

In the spring of 2005, during the second year of intervention, *Aventuras* offered free nutrition classes for parents, in Spanish, in an effort to boost awareness and spark interest in community change. A series of six classes was held during school hours at each of the six schools, with child care provided. The *promotoras* taught the classes, using selected basic lessons and activities from the California Latino 5 a Day's Toolbox for Community Educators. In hopes of generating activism, each session was to end with a discussion tying in nutrition and physical activity options available in the local community and how those options might be improved. Attendance at the classes ranged from 1 to 12, and no volunteers emerged to help with community change efforts.

Summer clubs for parents and children together were organized during the summer of the second year of intervention, in another attempt to raise awareness and rally interest. Led by the *promotoras*, the clubs met at a local park for active games, fruit and vegetable tastings and informal discussion of community needs. The clubs took hold at only two of the schools, and only a handful of families participated. That same summer, the project organized free soccer clinics for beginners and their parents, taught by a graduate student on the *Aventuras* staff who was a licensed soccer coach. The after-school clinics were specifically for children who had never played soccer, and were aimed at increasing their self-efficacy to get involved in the sport and connecting them to existing soccer leagues. Fifty-six boys and girls were registered for the six sessions offered, but only 23 attended. When the on-staff coach moved elsewhere, resources were not available to continue the clinics.

Ultimately, most of the community changes achieved by *Aventuras para Niños* were accomplished directly by the promotoras and project staff, working with owners and managers of local restaurants and grocery stores.

Restaurants

The *promotoras* visited virtually every locally owned restaurant within a one-mile radius of each of the six macro schools, and suggested a collaboration to create a healthy children's menu. When restaurant owners agreed, the *promotoras* worked with them to develop menus that fit with the existing menu and met the following guidelines: smaller portions than the regular menu, with lower prices; vegetable or fruit side dishes rather than french fries; fewer fried foods; and healthy beverages augmenting, or preferably replacing, the choice of sodas. The restaurants received colorful copies of the menus in both languages and various sizes, some laminated and some in tablestands, along with a wall certificate and laminated window signs announcing the new menus. The *promotoras* continued to visit the restaurants regularly to troubleshoot and check whether changes were needed in the menus. Participating restaurants received publicity in *Aventuras* school newsletters, in some cases a coupon, and a list and description of the restaurants circulated throughout the community. The effort focused on locally owned restaurants because managers of fast food and other chain restaurants said menu changes had to be decided centrally, and another local organization was working on persuading large restaurant chains to offer healthier menus.

Initial approaches to restaurants began in October 2004, and the effort intensified in summer 2005. As of February 2006, 36 restaurants were using *Aventuras* menus; another 8 had adopted the menus but later closed or changed owners. All served Mexican cuisine except for two Italian restaurants. Most had not had a children's menu previously; those that did had no side dishes except french fries listed for children.

Grocery stores

Aventuras para Niños staff and *promotoras* developed a program of "frequent produce buyer cards" for local grocery stores. Wallet-sized cards were created that shoppers could present at check-out to be marked each time they bought fresh fruits or vegetables. After nine purchases, the shopper received one free pound of fresh fruits or vegetables. In collaboration with Latino 5 a Day, the message "Eat fruits and vegetables and be active" and brief information about the food stamp program were printed on the back, in both languages. The *promotoras* proposed the program to the owners or managers of grocery stores near the macro schools, especially those where study participants had reported shopping. Again, the greatest response was from locally owned businesses. The program was implemented in five stores in fall 2005, with about 2000 cards distributed to parents at the macro schools, along with an explanation in the *Aventuras* newsletter. Another 2000 cards were given out at the stores, by store employees and by the *promotoras* during kickoff events featuring nutrition education, prizes, games and fruit and vegetable tastings.

Parks

Improvement of local parks to make them more accessible and attractive to local families was one of the first community goals identified. Several parks in San Ysidro, the southernmost portion of the City of San Diego, were in particularly bad condition, with few play structures, few picnic tables, broken and nonfunctioning playground equipment, non-functioning and graffiti-covered water fountains and bathrooms, and insufficient lighting. Two *promotoras* assigned to that region took photos of conditions in four parks, interviewed families and obtained more than 300 signatures on a petition for improvements. They created poster displays and made presentations to the San Ysidro planning and parks committees, and obtained a letter of unanimous endorsement from the San Ysidro Planning and Development Group. After the *promotoras* met with city council staff, the San Diego Park and Recreation Department made site visits to the four parks and prepared estimates for upgrading. With estimates ranging from $250,000 to $525,000 per park, the efforts stalled. However, the *promotoras* have enthusiastic support from a newly elected member of the San Diego City Council, who has agreed to pursue the issue.

Apartment complexes

Two apartment complexes were identified where a large number of *Aventuras para Niños* participants resided. Without contacting those participants directly, the *promotoras* worked with apartment managers to suggest easing restrictions on children's ability to engage in vigorous outdoor activity and adding healthy options to vending machines on the property. In addition, based on formative interviews with parents indicating they have little time to supervise outdoor play, the *promotoras* encouraged apartment residents to take turns accompanying each others' children to nearby parks.

Conclusion

A number of research trials throughout the developed world have targeted physical activity and/or dietary change to prevent childhood obesity; some have achieved behavior change in specific areas but none of the changes has been sufficient to impact weight gain (Lohman, Thompson, Going et al., 2003;

Summerbell, Waters, Edmunds et al., 2005). A review of 22 studies in Asia, Europe and the Americas concluded that no single program showed evidence of effectiveness in preventing childhood obesity, and that future research should employ comprehensive strategies incorporating both behavior change and the creation of supportive environments (Summerbell et al., 2005). By addressing multiple changes in children's home, school and community environments, the *Aventuras para Niños* intervention provides evidence of a feasible, comprehensive strategy that may help slow the obesity epidemic. While this intervention was designed specifically for a Mexican-American community, the process described could be modeled by other intervention researchers to develop materials and programs for other ethnic populations.

References

Candelaria, J. C., Lyons, G., Elder, J. P. & Villasenor, A. (1998). Strategies for health education: community-based methods. In S. Loue (Eds.), *Handbook of Immigrant Health* (S. 587-606). New York: Plenum.

Cohen, D. A., Scribner, R. A. & Farley, T. A. (2000). A strucural model of health behavior: a pragmatic approach to explain and influence health behaviors at the population level. *Preventive Medicine, 30*(2), 146-154.

Cossrow, N. & Falkner, B. (2004). Race/ethic issues in obesity and obesity-related comorbidities. *Journal of Clinical Endocrinology & Metabolism, 89*(6), 2590-2594.

Elder, J. P. (2005). View Point: conversation with John P. Elder, PhD. *American Journal of Health Behaviour, 29*(3), 269-279.

Elder, J. P., Ayala, G. X., Campbell, N. R., Slymen, D., Lopez-Madurga, E. T., Engelberg, M. & Baquero, B. (2005). Interpersonal and print nutrition communication for a Spanish-dominant Latina population: Secretos de la Buena. *Health Psychology, 24*(1), 49-57.

Flegal, K. M., Caroll, M. D., Ogden, C. L. & Johnson, C. L. (2002). Prevalence and trends in obesity among US adults 1999-2000. *The Journal of the American Medical Association, 288*(14), 1723-1727.

Flegal, K. M., Ogden, C. L. & Caroll, M. D. (2004). Prevalence and trends in overweight in Mexican-american adults and children. *Nutrition Reviews, 62*(7), 144-148.

French, S. A., Story, M. & Jeffery, R. W. (2001). Environmental influences on eating and physical activity. *Annual Review of Public Health, 22*, 309-335.

Gabbei, R. & Hamrick, D. (2001). Using physical activity homework to meet the national standards. *Journal of Physical Education, Recreation and Dance, 72*(4), 21-25.

Hedley, A. A., Ogden, C. L., Johnson, C. L., Caroll, M. D., Curtin, L. R. & Flegal, K. M. (2004). Prevalence of overweight and obesity among US children, adolescents and adults. *The Journal of the American Medical Association, 291*(23), 2847-2850.

Hill, J. O. & Peters, J. C. (1998). Environmental contributions to the obesity epidemic. *Science, 280*(5368), 1371-1374.

Jeffery, R. W. & Utter, J. (2003). The changing environment and population obesity in the United states. *Obesity Research, 11*(Suppl), 12-22.

Lohman, T., Thompson, J., Going, S., Himes, J. H., Caballero, B., Norman, J., Cano, S. & Ring, K. (2003). Indices of changes in adiposity in American Indian children. *Preventive Medicine, 37*(Suppl. 1), 91-96.

Mc Kenzie, T. L., Sallis, J. F., Kolody, B. & Faucette, F. N. (1997). Long-term effects of a physical education curriculum and staff develoment program:SPARK. *Research Quarterly for Exercise and Sport, 68*(4), 280-291.

Miller, W. R. & Rollnick, S. (1991). *Motivational Interviewing: Preparing People to Change Addictive Behaviour*. New York: Giulford Press.

Navarro, A. M., Senn, K. L., Kaplan, R. M., Mc Nicholas, L. J., Campo, M. C. & Roppe, B. (1995). Por La Vida intervention model for cancer prevention in Latinas. *Journal of the National Cancer Institute. Monographs*(18), 137-145.

Navarro, A. M., Senn, K. L., Mc Nicholas, L. J., Kaplan, R. M., Roppe, B. & Campo, M. C. (1998). Por La Vida model intervention enhances use of cancer screening tests among Latinas. *American Journal of Preventive Medicine, 15*(1), 32-41.

Ogden, C. L., Flegal, K. M., Caroll, M. D. & Johnson, C. L. (2002). Prevalence and trends in overweight among US children and adolescents. *The Journal of the American Medical Association, 288*(14), 1728-1732.

Sallis, J. F., Mc Kenzie, T. L., Kolody, B., Lewis, M., Marshall, S. & Rosengrad, P. (1999). Effects of health-related physical education on academic achievement. *Research Quarterly for Exercise and Sport, 70*(2), 127-134.

Stewart, J. A., Dennison, D. A. & Doyle, J. A. (2004). Exercise level and energy expenditure in the TAKE 10! in-class physical activity program. *Journal of School Health, 74*(10), 397-400.

Stokols, D. (1996). Translating social ecological theory into guidelines for community health promotion. *American Journal of Health Promotion, 10*(4), 282-298.

Stratton, G. & Mullan, E. (2005). The effect of multicolor playground markings on children's physical activity level during recess. *Preventive Medicine, 41*(5-6), 828-833.

Summerbell, C. D., Waters, E., Edmunds, L. D., Kelly, S., Brown, T. & Campbell, K. J. (2005). interventions for preventing obesity in children. *Cochrane database of systematic reviews*(3), CD001871.

II.
Overweight and obesity – Prevalence and Prevention

Chapter 7:
Facing Obesity: New Challenges for Government-funded Healthy Eating Campaigns

Anke Niederhaus

Abstract

Excess body weight is today the most frequent diet-related health impairment in children and adolescents in Germany. While some 10-18 % of children and youths in Germany are overweight, 4-8 % are heavily overweight (obese). The number of obese children and adolescents has soared over the past few years. This tendency can be observed in all Western industrialized nations. Therefore, the World Health Organization (WHO) already talks about an alarming epidemic.

As a main focus of food policy, i.e. to help prevent excess weight in children and adolescents, the Federal Ministry of Food, Agriculture and Consumer Protection (BMELV) launched the campaign "Eat better. Move around more. It's child's play" (*Besser essen. Mehr bewegen. KINDERLEICHT*) in summer 2003. The conference "Children and nutrition", that was held in Berlin, kicked off this campaign. Four interdisciplinary working groups were subsequently formed that worked out measures to prevent excess weight in children and adolescents. These measures to be implemented in the living environment of children and adolescents focus on improving the dietary education by involving parents, educators and teachers. In addition, advisory services for day-care centres and schools, specifically for all-day schools, make it easier for them to provide varied and wholesome food. Educational campaigns in the media and print media accompany these measures.

The problem of increasing overweight affects society as a whole. It does not only cause serious health impairments in children, adolescents and their families, but also places an increasing burden on the health care system. What matters now is to unite all social actors in pursuing one aim: To achieve effective and target-oriented prevention of overweight and obesity.

To this end, the "Platform Nutrition and Physical Activity" was established in September 2004 where alongside the BMELV, the food industry and the sports sector, other stakeholders from all relevant fields got involved.

Activities and measures in families, day-care centres for children, schools and the leisure sector should be networked as intensively as possible. These measures should serve dietary education and comprise initiatives that contribute to increased exercise and sports activities of children and adolescents.

Introduction

Apart from ensuring an adequate food supply, food policy needs to focus on a health-promoting diet which is adapted to the needs of consumers. Food policy measures such as providing consumers with dietary education and nutritional information therefore form an integral part of our consumer and agricultural policies.

The Federal Ministry of Food, Agriculture and Consumer Protection provides consumers with information

- on goods, markets and prices,
- on the production, labelling and proper handling of foods
- as well as on a balanced diet.

The dietary education schemes are mostly organised by government-funded information services for food and nutrition, e.g. consumer protection agencies, the German Nutrition Society or the aid infodienst. This service provides consumers with brochures and practical guides, for instance.

Efforts to prevent diet-related diseases, such as overweight, and to lay the foundations for a healthy lifestyle must start in early childhood. Preventing excess body weight in children and adolescents represents a key objective of food policy.

Obesity – A Global Epidemic

The World Health Organization states that non-communicable chronic diseases (NCD) are now the major cause of death and disability worldwide. These conditions include cardiovascular diseases, diabetes, obesity, cancer and respiratory diseases. They account for 59 % of 56.5 million deaths annually worldwide.

The WHO estimates that approximately one billion people all over the world are overweight – that is one sixth of the world's population. And more than 300 million people are obese. The World Health Organization (WHO) therefore already talks about an epidemic.

In 2004, the World Health Assembly adopted the Global Strategy on Diet, Physical Activity and Health. The strategy recommends a prevention-oriented approach in order to reduce the human and socio-economic costs of non-communicable diseases.

A healthy diet is essential for an individual's quality of life and the best foundation for developing one's physical and mental abilities to the full from early childhood to old age. Excessive energy supply, particularly in combination with low energy consumption, will cause excess body weight.

A connection is made between excess body weight and obesity, on the one hand, and the significant increase in various secondary diseases such as high blood pressure, coronary heart disease, type II diabetes and orthopaedic problems, on the other hand. Apart from the development of high blood pressure, arteriosclerosis and various kinds of cancer, type II diabetes is regarded as the most serious consequence of obesity. According to surveys conducted by the German Diabetes Society, more than 60 percent of the roughly four million cases of type II diabetes in Germany result from overweight.

Between five to ten percent of all healthcare costs in industrialized countries are spent on secondary diseases resulting from excess body weight. And diet-related diseases generate about one third of the total healthcare costs in Germany. In 2002, the total healthcare costs of diet-related diseases in Germany alone already amounted to approximately € 70 billion.

In Germany, approximately two-thirds of the male population and about 50 percent of the female population are overweight or obese according to the latest studies of the Robert Koch Institute. An increasing tendency to become overweight can also be observed in children and adolescents. While some 10-18 % of children and youths in Germany are overweight, 4-8 % are heavily overweight (obese). The number of overweight children and adolescents has increased dramatically in Germany and other industrialized nations. Scientific studies suggest that overweight children and adolescents will stay overweight as adults or become obese even.

As I have already mentioned before, overweight is caused by an imbalance between a high caloric diet and physical activity. The consequences of an imbalanced diet are further aggravated by the low level of physical activity. Children and young people spend many hours in front of the TV or playing computer games at the expense of physical activities such as playing games and engaging in sports.

Children entering school age are increasingly affected by impaired motor co-ordination. Since 1995, the physical fitness of ten- to fourteen-year-old children has decreased by more than 20 percent. This development could also have an adverse impact on the health of such children and adolescents as well as impair their quality of life, social behaviour or their ability to learn.

Excess body weight has become a socio-economic problem. Obesity has even become an indication of poverty in Germany nowadays. Children from socially disadvantaged groups or migrant families are disproportionately affected by obesity.

Government-funded Healthy Eating campaigns

What matters now is that we develop strategies to prevent overweight in children and adolescents. The course for future eating habits has to be set at an early stage. Dietary education and nutritional information must begin as early as possible, i.e. in nursery schools and schools. It is also crucial that children are encouraged to exercise more and that such exercise programmes are offered in schools and in the leisure sector.

In the light of the increasing overweight in children and adolescents, various initiatives have been launched by the Federal Ministry of Food, Agriculture and Consumer Protection to actively reverse this trend.

By holding our conference "Children and nutrition" on 8 July 2003, we have taken initial policy measures to enhance public awareness of this topic. Various scientists, the former EU Commissioner David Byrne and the WHO Regional Advisor for Nutrition, Aileen Robertson, demanded that comprehensive measures be taken to prevent overweight in children.

Right after this conference we launched the campaign "Eat better. Move around more. It's child's play" (*Besser essen. Mehr bewegen. KINDERLEICHT*). This campaign is aimed at improving the alarming situation through dietary education and initiatives for more physical exercise. Here, we focus on children and adolescents between three and twelve years of age in their respective living environments, i.e. at home, in day-care facilities and schools. Parents, educators and teachers are also directly involved in these activities. For more information, please refer to our website www.kinder-leicht.net.

The campaign will be pursued with several strong partners: the German Nutrition Society (DGE), the consumer protection agencies, aid infodienst, the Universities of Paderborn, Heidelberg and Flensburg, the Reading Foundation "*Stiftung Lesen*", the German Agricultural Marketing Board (CMA), FEZ Wuhlheide Berlin, and the initiative "Germany on the move" (*Deutschland bewegt sich*) set up by the health insurance company BARMER, the television broadcasting station ZDF and the magazine BILD am Sonntag.

It is intended that children learn from early on that a healthy lifestyle with a balanced diet and much physical activity is the most natural thing to do. Because most people maintain dietary patterns acquired in childhood throughout their entire life, "starting strong" must be the guiding principle for taking early action with regard to children.

Traditional dietary education only has a limited outreach with regard to our target group, the **families** concerned. With our activities in libraries "KINDERLEICHT in libraries", a project co-organised by the Reading Foundation, in the restaurant and catering sector "Make a Wish" (*Wünsch' Dir was*) in co-operation with the German Agricultural Marketing Board CMA), the itinerant exhibition in children's museums "Look at what you buy!" (*Guck mal was Du kaufst!*), with the tour "KINDERLEICHT on tour" – in conjunction with the tour around Germany's cities "Germany on the move!" (*Deutschland bewegt sich*) – we tread new paths in order to encounter families "in their everyday lives" without any wagging fingers and inform them about a healthy diet.

In addition to parents, it is especially the **day-care centres** which can lay the foundations of an independent, health-promoting and responsible dietary behaviour of children at an early stage. Starting points include communal catering, on the one hand, and the playful conveying of nutritional information and the encouragement to exercise more by nursery school teachers, on the other hand.

Our campaign "FIT KID - The healthy diet campaign in day-care facilities" (*FIT KID – Die Gesund-Essen-Aktion für Kitas*) takes both aspects into account. Nursery school teachers and the catering staff are being trained to improve meals. Sensory education with a view to a healthy diet is offered to parents and nursery school teachers.

The **school** of the future is a good and healthy school which conveys comprehensive basics. A healthy lifestyle and diet, exercise and the conveying of everyday skills are indispensable elements of a good and healthy educational establishment.

The issue of foods and a balanced diet is hardly dealt with in many schools. Quite often, old and in some cases even false teaching materials are used. Therefore, a pilot project we commissioned "Reform of nutritional and consumer education" (*Reform der Ernährungs- und Verbraucherbildung,* REVIS) formulated new and modern guidelines for teacher training in this field. School meals represent another important module to help children and youths to (again) enjoy a balanced diet. Our advisory campaign for schools "School + Food = Grade A" (*Schule + Essen = Note 1*) intends to improve the meals offered by schools.

A touring exhibition on non-alcoholic trendy beverages (*Die Mach-Bar-Tour*) visits schools all over the country and is intended for direct outreach to schoolchildren.

Apart from the KINDERLEICHT campaign, we have, for several years now, offered our touring exhibition "Enjoy the pleasure of a wholesome diet" (*Vollwertig essen und trinken mit Genuss*) to schools free of charge. This exhibition is designed to show students at the lower and upper secondary level the basics of a balanced diet in a clear and understandable way.

Within the scope of the 2005 campaign, a strategy competition had just been launched. **"Eat Better. Move around more. The contest"** (*Besser essen. Mehr bewegen. Der Wettbewerb*) encourages associations of local and regional initiatives to develop strategies to prevent overweight by promoting a balanced diet and sufficient exercise. The initiatives are to show in an exemplary way which methods, opportunities for access and which partners are suitable to prevent overweight in children on a permanent basis. To prevent obesity in the long term, it is of decisive importance that appropriate structures are created through local networks that will continue to function when government funding stops after three years. For more information, please refer to our website www.besseressenmehrbewegen.de .

Platform Nutrition and Physical Activity

Prevention is the key approach to solving the problem of "overweight in children", since the dietary and exercise habits of children are most decisively shaped at a very early age. In Germany, various actors had already seen to this matter and taken first measures. Yet, mostly they confined themselves to certain details of this topic and did not co-operate in networks. BMELV therefore took the initiative to set up the "Platform Nutrition and Physical Activity". The platform has by now been established as an incorporated society. It is to create a sustainable instrument to support and interlink the work of already existing initiatives and to develop and initiate new activities.

The platform is aimed at placing the topic "nutrition and physical activity" on a broad basis in society. The **founding members** of the "Platform Nutrition and Physical Activity" are

- the food industry, represented by the German Federation of Food Law and Food Science (BLL),
- the Federal Parents' Council (BER),
- the Federal Government, represented by the Federal Ministry of Food, Agriculture and Consumer Protection (BMELV),
- the central associations of the health insurance funds, represented by the Federal Association of Guild Sickness Funds (IKK),
- the German Agricultural Marketing Board (CMA),
- the German Society of Pediatrics and Adolescent Medicine (DGKJ),
- the German Sports Association/German Sports Youth (DSB/DSJ) and

- the Union of Workers in the Food and Catering Trades (NGG).

The founding conference of the "Platform Nutrition and Physical Activity" on 29 September 2004 showed the need for this holistic approach and for the participation of the greatest possible number of social actors. The platform is open to additional members. A wide variety of activities have already been initiated. Networking and development of assessment standards for these activities are required and are currently being developed. For more information, please refer to the website www.ernaehrungundbewegung.de .

Chapter 8:
Overweight in children and youth-determinants and strategies for prevention

Sandra Danielzik, Beate Landsberg, Svenja Pust & Manfred J. Müller

Introduction

The prevalence of obesity and its comorbidities has been steadily increasing over the last 50 years. Obesity, once established, is difficult to treat. Therefore prevention of obesity is a public health agenda as well as a high priority research goal (WHO, 2000; Dietz & Gortmaker, 2001; Kumanyika, Jeffery, Morabia et al., 2002; Ebbeling, Pawlak & Ludwig, 2002, IASO, 2004). Since the long-term consequences of childhood overweight are well documented there is need for early intervention. However there is only limited research on prevention of overweight in children (for reviews see IASO, 2004; Campbell, Waters, O'Meara, Kelly & Summerbell, 2002; Müller, Danielzik, Spethmann, 2004; James & Gill, 2004) and few strategies have been proved to work.

Determinants of weight gain

Preventive strategies aimed at childhood and adult obesity are based on the knowledge of risk factors and determinants of overweight. Risk factors of childhood obesity include parental overweight, a low socio-economic status (SES), high birth weight, early timing or rate of maturation, low physical activity/ high inactivity, dietary intake (including early infant feeding practices) as well as psychological factors (Ebbeling et al., 2002; IASO, 2004; Müller et al., 2004; James & Gill, 2004; Barker, Blundell, Dietz et al., 1996). In cross-sectional studies on prepubertal children most of the risk to become overweight is explained by SES and parental overweight (Danielzik, S., Czerwinski-Mast, M., Langnäse et al., 2004). The data also show that there are differences between boys and girls and also between overweight and obesity. The risk factors are related but their exact relationships are unknown at individual as well as at population level. Although most risk factors for obesity seem to be self evident, their confounding or cumulative effects on the development of obesity as well as their clustering and their effects over time on the causal pathway to the development of obesity remain unclear in children (as in adults).

Most experts agree that the causes of overweight are environmental, related to living in a world that allows easy access to food and encourages to inactivity (Hill & Peters, 1998). Besides environmental and behavioural determinants of body weight the importance of fetal nutrition, breastfeeding and genes for body weight and obesity has been demonstrated in animals and humans (Barker et al., 1996; Sherry, & Dietz, 2004). There is good evidence for a close association between nutritional status of parents and their children (Whitaker, Wright, Pepe et al., 1997; Birch& Krahnstoever-Davison, (2001); Danielzik, Langnaese, Mast et al., 2002; Müller, Langnaese, Danielzik, 2002). Overweight parents frequently have overweight children. Besides possible genetic links parents select environments that may promote overweight among their children. Detailed knowledge of interaction between children and adolescents of obese parents and the environment may add to future intervention programs. A low SES together with parental overweight is a considerable risk factor for childhood overweight (Langnaese, Mast & Mueller, 2002; Langnaese, Mast, Danielzik et al., 2003).

Based on the present knowledge of risk factors and determinants of childhood overweight new preventive measures should be developed which differ from the medical concepts. To tackle the impact of socio-economic status health inequalities should be reduced (e.g. by a better school education) or marginal groups should be supported. Because parental weight status had an important impact on the development of nutritional status of the children families must be counselled and/ or supported. To counsel pregnant women may normalise birth weight of the children. Individual as well as environmental preventive measures can influence lifestyle. These ideas may be considered as preferred intervention strategies.

Preventive strategies

Faced with the obesity epidemic this problem needs to be addressed by a public health approach as well as by interventions aimed at individual subjects. In practice different prevention strategies are used (WHO, 2000). First, intervention strategies are directed at everyone in a community with the aim to stabilise or to reduce mean BMI within a population (i.e. *universal prevention*). Second, *selective prevention* is directed at high risk individuals (e.g. children of obese parents). It is concerned with improving the knowledge and skills of people to increase competence and personal autonomy and, thus, to prevent excessive weight gain. Third, *targeted* or *secondary prevention* or *treatment* is directed at overweight and obese children and adolescents to prevent further weight gain and/or to reduce body weight. School-based intervention is considered as *universal prevention*, whereas family-based intervention may be considered as *selective* (in the case of health promotion and education) or even *targeted prevention* (in the case of a structured treatment program).

Interventions to prevent weight gain include school programs, correspondence programs, individual or group counselling including behaviour change methods and a public health approach. At present there are numerous uncontrolled activities in the area of prevention of childhood overweight. There are also some controlled and randomised studies. These studies differ with respect to strategy, setting (school, family, primary care, public health), focus, variables of outcome and statistical power. The studies also differ with respect to duration of intervention as well as of the observation period. We feel that follow up period should be at least 6 months but one family-based study reached a maximum of 10 years (Epstein, Valoski, Wing et al., 1990). The different authors used various outcome variables including BMI, fat mass, parameters of risks and comorbidities as well as indicators of health habits. Nearly all authors come out with mean values obtained in groups of children (intervention versus non-intervention group). At present there is a lack of detailed analysis within specific subgroups as well as data on the effect of intervention on the incidence and remission of overweight and obesity.

School- and family-based interventions: results of controlled studies

Families and schools represent the most important foci for preventive efforts in children (Dietz & Gortmaker, 2001; Kumanyika, Jeffery, Morabia et al., 2002; IASO, 2004; Summerbell, Waters, Edmunds et al., 2005). School health programs have the potential to influence health of nearly all children within existing institutional structures. In the US it has been suggested that one third of the health objectives for the nations can be significantly influenced by school health programs (US Department of Health and Human Services, 2000). However, feasibility of school-based obesity prevention programs has not been assessed systematically and most school-based trials addressing childhood overweight came out with some improvements in behavior but only minor or no effects on mean BMI (for reviews see Summerbell, Waters, Edmunds et al., 2005, Report of the World Health Organisation, 2004).

Studies on school-based interventions have been reviewed extensively (for reviews see IASO, 2004; Campbell, Waters, O'Meara, Kelly & Summerbell, 2002; Müller, Danielzik, Spethmann, 2004; James & Gill, 2004). One of the most frequently cited studies in this area is Planet Health (Gortmaker, Peterson, Wiecha et al., 1999; Wang, Yang, Lowry et al., 2003). Over a period of 2 years 1295 ethnically diverse grade 6 and 7 students from public schools (i.e. middle schools) participated in an interdisciplinary intervention aimed at (i) decreasing TV time as well as consumption of high fat foods and (ii) increasing vegetable intake and moderate to vigorous activities. Intervention units were developed with extensive teacher input and focus groups using a variety of methods including debates, case studies and projects. When compared with controls the prevalence of obesity among girls decreased but remained unchanged in boys. There were positive and sex-independent changes in TV-hours and nutrition. The reductions in body weight were related to reductions in time spent watching TV.

School-based interventions (as a measure of *universal prevention*) can thus not be considered as suitable intervention strategies to tackle the overweight and obesity epidemic. However faced with poor nutrition and sedentary lifestyle habits (see Ebbeling, Pawlak & Ludwig, 2002; IASO, 2004; Campbell, Waters, O'Meara, Kelly & Summerbell, 2002; Müller, Danielzik, & Spethmann, 2004) there is no doubt that health promotion within a school setting is also necessary.

The development of family-based prevention programmes for childhood overweight has been considered as a primary public health goal (IASO, 2004). At present most studies in this area had addressed obese children together with their parents. There are also some studies tackling parents only. Long-term effective management of overweight and obese children by a family-based intervention was reported by some authors (Müller, Langnaese, Danielzik et al., 2002; Flodmark, Ohlsson, Ryden et al., 1993; Epstein, Valoski, Wing et al., 1994). The data show that family therapy was effective to prevent the progression of severe obesity in 10 to 11-year-old children (Flodmark et al., 1993). The 1-year increase in BMI was 5 % in the group receiving family therapy vs. 12 % in the control group (p <0.02). However the groups differed with respect to the number of children with severe obesity (i.e. BMI >30kg/m^2; 1/20, 5/19, 14/48 in the three groups, respectively). Epstein and colleagues (Müller et al., 2002; Epstein et al., 1994) were most successful when children were treated together with their parents. The follow up period lasted up to 10 years. The effectiveness of these interventions was well documented by weight changes, a reduced prevalence of obesity as well as lifestyle changes. The 10-year decreases in percent overweight were –7.5 % versus +14.3 % in the control group. Nearly all family-based intervention studies resulted in long-term changes in health-related behaviours in obese children and adolescents but had no or only moderate long-term effects on nutritional status.

Bringing two strategies together (school-based and family based interventions) KOPS (i.e. Kiel Obesity Prevention Study) was started in 1996 and is planned to run until the year 2009 (Müller, 2004; Mueller, Asbeck, Mast et al., 2001; Danielzik, Pust, Landsberg et al., 2005; Müller, Danielzik & Pust, 2005). Up to now within KOPS three populations of 4.997 5 to 7 year (T0), 4.487 9 to 11 year (T1) and (up to now) 2.250 13 to15-year-old children (T2) were recruited. All study populations are part of the total population of all children born between 1990 and 1995 in Kiel (n = 12.254). Up to now 1764 children were measured twice (i.e. at T0 as well as T1). KOPS is mainly interested in prevalence, incidence and remission of childhood overweight as well as of its determinants.

Fig. 1 shows the prevalence of overweight in 5-7, 9-11- as well as 13-15-year-old children in Kiel. As reference triceps skinfold percentiles from the year 1978 were used (Reinken, Stolley, Droese et al., 1980). Compared with these reference data today, 23 %, 39 % and 49 % of the 5-7, 9-11 and 13-15-year-old children are overweight, respectively. This means the prevalence of overweight has greatly increased, especially in children after puberty.

Fig. 1:   Prevalence of overweight in 5-7 (n = 4.997), 9-11 (n = 4.487) and 13-15-year-old (n = 2.250) children in Kiel (according to triceps reference percentiles of Reinken et al., 1980)

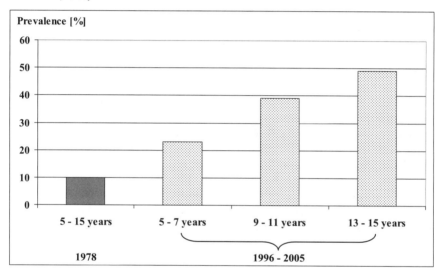

The 4-year follow up data showed a high persistence of overweight (79.1 % of children who were overweight at T0 remained overweight at T1). The cumulative 4-year incidence of overweight (i.e. children becoming overweight) was 10.8 % (i.e. 2.7 % per year). Spontaneous remission of overweight (i.e. children becoming normal weight) reached 5.2 % per year.

One part of KOPS assesses the long-term effects of "low level" interventions (i) at school for all children and (ii) within "overweight families" for overweight children. 780 children underwent a 6-hour curriculum of school intervention within the first year at school (i.e. at age 6-7 years) and 345 of these children could be re-investigated at age 9-11 years (i.e. in a 4-year follow up). These data were compared with 1.419 children from non-intervention schools also measured at age 5-7 as well as at age 9-11 years. In addition 92 families with overweight children and parents were offered a family-based intervention, which takes place within the family setting (i.e. 3-5 visits at home). A structured sport program was also offered to overweight children of this cohort. 52 families could be re-investigated 1-year later.

Outcome measures of KOPS are feasibility, nutritional status, lifestyle and risk factors for disease. Family history of diseases, parental weight and height, SES and parental smoking habits were also considered as confounding factors. Comparing the median of BMI or triceps skinfolds in the population of children in intervention (I) and non-intervention (NI) schools demonstrated a small but beneficial effect. However, the extent of overweight was lower in I than in NI (4-year changes in BMI-SDS was 0.07 in I versus 0.15 in NI, p <0.05). Prevalence of overweight increased by factor 1.8 in NI and 1.4 in I. Concomitantly cumulative 4-year incidence of overweight was reduced in I (9.3 % vs. 10.8 %, p >0.05, respectively). SES also had an effect on intervention. The effect was most pronounced in children of high SES families (3.6 % in I versus 7.6 % in NI, p >0.05). Cumulative 4-year remission of overweight was higher in I than in NI (41.7 % versus 27.0 %, p >0.05). The effect was most pronounced in children of normal weight mothers (61.5 % in I versus 26.2 % in NI, p <0.05) when compared with children of overweight mothers (20.0 % in I versus 23.3 % in NI, p >0.05). Comparing boys and girls a more pronounced effect was seen in girls (38.5 % in I versus 20.0 % in NI in girls, p >0.05, and 45.5 % in I versus 37.9 % in NI in boys, p >0.05). When compared with school-based intervention family-based intervention also showed some positive effects. Within a 1-year observation period family intervention was capable to normalise increases in BMI of overweight children. However a low SES served as a barrier against intervention measures (Langnäse, Asbeck, Mast et al., 2004).

Do we need more intensive interventions?

The majority of studies on school-based health promotion reported statistically significant effects on health knowledge, attitudes and behavior. By contrast only modest changes in nutritional status were observed within "real world" school settings. It can be questioned why school-based interventions had only minor effects on prevalence of overweight: perhaps the interventions were not intensive enough or they were not focussed on certain and simple key messages (e.g. eliminate soft drink consumption). Thus one may speculate that increasing intensity may also improve outcome. However high intensive interventions did not affect overweight; e.g. a 3-year school-based multicomponent intervention (with a classroom curriculum, food service, physical education together with a family intervention, strong support from tribal, educational and community authorities) for reducing percentage body fat in American Indian elementary schoolchildren (i.e. Pathways) did not reduce the prevalence of overweight (Caballero, Davis, Davis et al., 1998; Caballero, Clay, Davis et al., 2003). In addition concentrating on simple key messages did not show unique success outcomes. E.g. a cluster randomized controlled trial aimed to reduce consumption of carbonated drinks in 7-11-year-old children were able to reduce daily consumption of carbonated drinks and additionally decreased prevalence of overweight after 12 months (James, Thomas, Cavan et al., 2004). In this trial all three sessions of the intervention focussed on the key message (carbonated drinks). By contrast a Norwegian study to increase fruit and vegetable consumption in children which also concentrated on the key message could not influence the consumption of fruit and vegetables after a 1-year intervention at school (Bere, Veierod, Bjelland et al., 2005). Altogether when compared with KOPS these data suggested that more intensive or more focussed interventions did not improve effectiveness.

A more individualized approach may exceed the value of classroom education. In fact, the STRIP experience (Hakanen, Lagström, Kaitosaari, 2006) suggests that repeatedly given individualized dietary and lifestyle counseling during the first 10 years of life resulted in fewer overweight children. However the effect was significant in girls only (i.e. the prevalence of overweight was 10.2 % in intervention girls when compared to 18.8 % in controls, Hakanen et al., 2006). In STRIP, children and their families had been already recruited at the baby clinics. Families received individualized counseling at 1-3 months intervals until age 2 years which was followed by twice or once a year counseling up to age 7 and 10 years, respectively. The counseling was given by a nutritionist together with a physician. The major focus was on prevention of atherosclerosis, e.g. there was no focus on energy intake. The control children received routine health education at baby clinics as well as at schools. When compared with KOPS the STRIP data suggest that (at least for prepubertal children) repeated and individualized interventions result in better outcome than school-based health promotion offered in the first class only. Thus additional measures focussing on public health interventions are necessary.

Putting the findings into a public health perspective

It is evident that there is a spontaneous increase in the prevalence of childhood overweight which is explained by both, a high persistence plus a high incidence of overweight. The first long-term follow up data of the KOPS school intervention support the idea that prevention has some long term effects on childhood overweight. Family based interventions may add to school intervention. However there is evidence that there is a gender effect as well as an effect of parental weight status on outcome. In addition a low SES serves as a barrier against prevention and treatment. Thus the major determinants of overweight are confounders of the effect of preventive measures. Faced with the environmental contributors to the obesity problem societal rather than individual responsibilities are evident. This idea suggests that dissecting and tackling the obesogenic environment (Egger & Swinburn; 1997; Egger, Swinburn & Rossner, 2003) is necessary and has to complement school- and family-based interventions. This idea is sound. However it is based on theoretical thinking and systematic analyses of the macro- as well as the micro-environmental determinants of overweight. By contrast there are neither short- or long-term studies nor proven effects of environmental approaches to the overweight epidemic. Thus the public-health crisis demands increased funding for research into new and additive dietary, physical activity, behavioral and environmental approaches for prevention of obesity. There is clear need for more than action plans and frameworks.

Acknowledgement

KOPS was/is supported by grants from Deutsche Forschungsgemeinschaft (DFG Mü 5.1, 5.2, 5-3 und 5.5), WCRF, London, Wirtschaftliche Vereinigung Zucker, Bonn, Danone Stiftung, München, Deutsche Angestellten Krankenkasse (DAK), Hamburg.

References

Barker, D. J. P., Blundell, J. E., Dietz, W. H., Epstein, L. H., Jeffry, R. W., Remschmidt, H., Rolls, B. J., Rössner, S. & Saris, W. H. M. (1996). Group report: What are the Biobehavioral determinants of body weight regulation? In C. Bouchasel & G. A. Bray (Eds), *Regulation of body weight* (pp. 159-177). Chichester: Wiley Johnsons.

Bere, E., Veierod, M. B., Bjelland, M. & Klepp, K.-I. (2006). Outcome and process evaluation of a Norwegian school-randomized fruit and vegetable intervention: Fruits and Vegetables Make the Marks (FVMM). *Health Education Research*, 21 (2), 258-67.

Birch, L. L. & Krahnstoever-Davison, K. (2001). Family environmental factors influenceing. He developing behavioral controls of food intake and childhood overweight. *Pediatrical Clinics of North America, 48*, 893-907.

Caballero, B., Clay, T., Davis, S. M et al. (2003) Pathways: a school-based, randomized controlled trial for the prevention of obesity in American Indian schoolchildren. *American Journal of Clinical Nutrition, 78,* 1030-8.

Caballero, B., Davis, S., Davis, C. E., Ethelbah, B., Evans, M., Lohman. T., Stephenson, L., Story, M. & White, J. (1998). Pathways: A school-based program for the primary prevention of obesity in American Indian children. *Journal of Nutritional Biochemistry, 9,* 535-43.

Campbell, K., Waters, E., O'Meara, S., Kelly, S. & Summerbell, C. (2002). Interventions for preventing obesity in children. *Cochrane Database of Systematic Review, 2,* CD001871.

Danielzik, S., Czerwinski-Mast, M., Langnäse, K., Dilba, B. & Müller, M. J. (2004). Parental overweight, socioeconomic status and high birth weight are the major determinants of overweight and obesity in 5-7 y-old children: baseline data of the Kiel Obesity Prevention Study (KOPS). *International Journal of Obesity, 28,* 1494-1502.

Danielzik, S., Langnaese, K., Mast, M., Spethmann, C. & Mueller, M. J. (2002). Impact of parental BMI manifestation of overweight in 5-7 year old children. *European Journal of Nutrition, 41,* 132-138.

Danielzik, S., Pust, S., Landsberg, B., Müller, M. J. (2005). First lessons of the Kiel Obesity Prevention Study (KOPS). *International Journal of Obesity, 29 (Suppl. 2),* 78-83.

Dietz, W. H. & Gortmaker, S. L. (2001). Preventing obesity in children and adolescents. *Annual Review of Public Health, 22,* 337-353.

Ebbeling, C. B., Pawlak, D. B. & Ludwig, D. S. (2002). Childhood obesity: public-health crisis, common sense cure. *Lancet, 360,* 473-482.

Egger, G. & Swinburn, B. (1997). An „ecological" approach to the obesity pandemic. *British Medical Journal, 315,* 477-480.

Egger, G., Swinburn, B. & Rossner, S. (2003). Dusting off the epidemiological triad: could it work with obesity ? *Obesity reviews, 4,* 115-119.

Epstein, L. H., Valoski, A., Wing, R. R. & McCurley, J. (1990). Ten-year follow up of behavioural family-based treatment of obese children. *JAMA 264,* 2519-2523.

Epstein, L. H., Valoski, A., Wing, R. R. & Mc Curley, I. (1994). Ten year outcomes of behavioral family-based treatment for childhood obesity. *Health Psychology, 13,* 373-383.

Flodmark, C. E., Ohlsson, T., Ryden, O. & Sveger, T. (1993). Prevention of progression to severe obesity in a group of obese Schoolchildren treated with family therapy. *Pediatrics, 91,* 880-884.

Gortmaker, S. L., Peterson, K., Wiecha, J., Sobol, A. M., Dixit, S., Fox, M. K. & Laird, N. (1999). Reducing obesity via school-based interdisciplinary intervention among youth. Planet Health. *Archives of Pediatrics & Adolescent Medicine, 153,* 409-418.

Hakanen, M., Lagström, H., Kaitosaari, T., Niinikoski, H., Nänto-Salonen, K., Jokinen, E., Sillanmäki, L., Viikari, J., Rönnemaa, T. & Simell, O. (2006). Development of overweight in an atherosclerosis prevention trial starting in early childhood. The STRIP study. *International Journal of Obesity, 30,* 618-26.

Hill, I. O. & Peters, I. C. (1998). Environmental contribution to the obesity epidemic. *SCIENCE, 280,* 1371-1374.

IASO (2004). Obesity in children and young people. A crisis in public health. *Obesity reviews, 5 (Suppl.1),* 1-104.

James, W. P. T. & Gill, T. P. (2004). Prevention of obesity. In G. A. Bray & C. Bouchard (Eds.), Handbook of obesity. Clinical applications (pp. 75-96). New York: Marcel Decker.

James, J., Thomas, P., Cavan, D. & Kerr, D. (2004). Preventing childhood obesity by reducing consumption of carbonated drinks: cluster randomised controlled trial. *BMJ, 328,* 1237-42.

Kumanyika, S., Jeffery, R. W., Morabia, A., Ritenbaugh, C. & Antipatis, V. J. (2002). Obesity Prevention: the case for action. *International Journal of Obesity, 26,* 425-436.

Langnäse, K., Asbeck, I., Mast, M. & Müller, M. J. (2004). Influence of socioeconomic status on long-term effect of family-based obesity treatment intervention in prepubertal overweight children. *Health Education, 104,* 336-343.

Langnaese, K., Mast, M., Danielzik, S., Spethmann, C. & Müller, M. J. (2003). Socioeconomic gradient in body weight of German children reverse direction between ages 2 and 6 years. *Journal of Nutrition, 133,* 789-796.

Langnaese, K., Mast, M. & Mueller, M. J. (2002). Social class differences in overweight of
    prepubertal children in northwest Germany. International Journal of Obesity, 26, 566-
    572.
Mueller, M. J., Asbeck, I., Mast, M., Langnaese, K. & Grund, A. (2001). Prevention of
    obesity-more than an intention. Concept and first results of the Kiel Obesity
    Prevention Study (KOPS). International Journal of Obesity, 25 (Suppl. 1), 66-74.
Mueller, M. J., Langnaese, K., Danielzik, S., Spethmann, C. & Mast, M. (2002). Childhood
    obesity: the genetic-environmental interface. In A. Palou, M. L. Bonet & F. Serra
    (Eds.), Study on obesity and functional foods in Europe (pp. 193-204). Brussels:
    European commission.
Mueller, M. J., Danielzik, S. & Pust, S. (2005). School- and family-based interventions to
    prevent overweight in children. Proceedings of the German Nutrition Society, 64, 249-
    254.
Mueller, M. J., Danielzik, S. & Spethmann, C. (2004). Prevention of overweight and obesity.
    In W. Kiess, C. Marcus & M. Wabitsch (Eds.), Obesity in childhood and adolescence
    (pp. 243-263). Basel: Karger.
Reinken, L., Stolley, H., Droese, W. & van Oost, G. (1980). Longitudinale
    Körperentwicklung gesunder Kinder II. Größe, Gewicht, Hautfalten von Kindern im
    Alter von 1,5 bis 16 Jahren. Klinische Pädiatrie, 192, 25-33.
Report of the World Health Organisation (2004). Obesity in children and young people: A
    crisis in public health. Obesity reviews, 5 (Suppl.1), 1-104.
Sherry, B. & Dietz, W. H. (2004). Pediatric overweight : an overview. In G. A. Bray & C.
    Bouchard (Eds.), Handbook of obesity. Clinical applications (pp. 117-133). New
    York: Marcel Decker.
Summerbell, C. D., Waters, E., Edmunds, L. D., Kelly, S., Brown, T. & Campbell, K. J.
    (2005). Interventions for preventing obesity in children (Review). The Cochrane
    Database of systematic review, 3, CD001871.
US Department of Health and Human Services (2000). Healthy People 2010. Understanding
    and Improving Health. Objectives for Improving Health. Washington, DC: US
    Government Printing Office.
Wang, L. V., Yang, Q., Lowry, R. & Wechsler, H. (2003). Economic analysis of a school-
    based obesity prevention program. Obesity Research 11, 1313-1324.
Whitaker, R. C., Wright, J. A., Pepe, M. S., Seidel, K. D. & Dietz, W. H. (1997). Predicting
    obesity in young adulthood from childhood and parenteral obesity. New England
    Journal of Medicine, 337, 869-873.
World Health Organisation (2000). Obesity, preventing and managing a global epidemic.
    Report of a WHO Consultation. Geneva: WHO.

Chapter 9:
Nutrition, media consumption and obesity in children

Helmut Heseker & Anke Oepping

The importance of an adequate diet and of sufficient physical activities for health, well-being and performance are generally accepted. In developed countries non-transmissible nutrition-related chronic diseases are widespread and head the mortality statistics. Especially the prevalences of overweight, obesity and related chronic secondary diseases (e.g. type 2 diabetes mellitus, hypertension, joint diseases) have increased dramatically during the last 50 years. Significant social changes and modified life-styles have definite effects on the nutrition and exercise behaviour and make it more and more difficult to achieve a balanced energy metabolism. The World Health Organisation (WHO) therefore declared obesity to be the first global epidemic of the 21st century and attributes this to the dominating obesogenic environment.

Alongside to risk factors such as genetic predisposition, metabolic imprinting and nutrition, the imbalance of physical activity and inactivity in daily life plays a prominent role. In this context a causal relationship between media consumption and obesity has been established. The increasing prevalences of overweight and obesity in children and youth are especially alarming. For affected individuals this means a severe psychosocial and health burden, a long-term limitation of quality of life, and a reduced occupational outlook. For society it involves high follow-up costs for health and insurance systems. And expanding waistlines also contribute to higher fuel costs for airlines and cars.

Since nutrition and exercise behaviour usually become manifest in childhood, and once acquired the same pattern and habits are maintained lifelong, early learning of a healthy and active life-style is of great importance.

Nutrition recommendations for children

A well-balanced, diversified and wholesome diet including sufficient amounts of all nutrients that are necessary for growth, and physical and mental development. Such a diet is characterised by:

- a large of variety of food choices,
- the preference of low-fat food,
- consumption of whole grain products with a high content of dietary fibres,

- daily consumption of fruits and vegetables,
- regular consumption of low-fat milk and milk products,
- regular consumption of lean meat products,
- weekly consumption of fish,
- plenty of unsweetened beverages.

For children and adolescents a well-balanced diet includes a daily breakfast before school, appropriate snacks and sufficient beverages in school breaks and – in the case of all-day schools – a nutritious and tasty lunch.

Common nutritional problems

Severe disturbances of health caused by under-nourishment rarely occur in adolescence, but nevertheless unfavourable eating and drinking habits can result in considerable problems (Mensink, 2002; Heseker and Beer, 2004).

- Restricted school performance, lack of mental effort and fatigue occur if no breakfast or lunch is consumed.
- Caries, caused by frequent consumption of sweets and poor oral hygiene is prevalently observed.
- A high-fat and high-calorie lunch results in postprandial tiredness and reduced school performances ("plenus venter non studet libenter").
- A chronic positive energy balance caused by to much fat, sugar (e.g. fast-food, energy-drinks, soft-drinks, energy-dense snacks) in combination with inadequate physical activities result in the development of overweight and obesity.
- Further eating disorders such as anorexia nervosa, bulimia nervosa, binge eating are observed and may be associated with low, normal or overweight.
- Additionally, alcohol abuse by adolescents (drinking e.g. alcopops) represents a considerable challenge.

Definition of obesity

Overweight and obesity are defined as an excess of body-fat above the normal range. As the direct measurement of body fat is rather difficult, BMI (body mass index, a simple weight to height ratio (kg/m^2)), is typically used to classify overweight and obese adults. On this basis the World Health Organisation (WHO) has published international standards for classifying overweight and obesity in adults (Tab. 1).

Tab. 1:   Classification of overweight and obesity by criteria of WHO (2003)

BMI (kg/m²)	Classification	Risk of co-morbidities
<18,5	underweight	normal
18,5 - 24,9	normal weight	normal
≥25,0	overweight	
25,0 – 29,9	pre-obesity	increased
30,0 – 34,9	obesity class I	moderate
35,0 – 39,9	obesity class II	severe
≥40	obesity class III, (morbid obesity)	very severe

Overweight is defined as a BMI ≥25, obesity as a BMI ≥30 kg/m², but can be further sub-divided into classes I to III on the basis of the severity of the obesity.

In order to accommodate growth patterns BMI definitions for children and adolescents must be age and gender-specific. For this reason the classification of obesity for adults is not valid for the younger ones. A statistical approach is commonly used to define childhood obesity. Overweight and obesity for children and adolescents respectively are defined as being at or above the 90th and 97th percentile of the BMI of a German reference population (Kromeyer-Hauschild, 2005).

Prevalence of obesity

The prevalence of obesity is increasing in most parts of the world, affecting men, women and children. Furthermore, obesity is no longer just a concern for developed countries, but is becoming an increasing problem in many developing countries. Children are becoming increasingly vulnerable to overweight and obesity around the world (Seidell, 1999).

Using the BMI percentiles approach, 15 % of 3-17-years-old boys and girls in Germany are overweight, including 6.3 % who are obese (RKI, 2006). There is a sharp increase of overweight and obesity at primary school age in both sexes, whereas the rise is much slower in teenagers (Fig. 1).

During the last 20 years the prevalence of overweight has increased by 50 % and the prevalence of obesity has doubled. Especially the obligatory school enrolment examinations show a remarkable trend (Fig. 2). In Bavaria, due to the uninterrupted rise, prevalences of overweight and obesity increase by 0.3 % and 0.1 % respectively per year. A similar situation can be observed in North Rhine-Westphalia and other German states (Kromeyer-Hauschild, 2005). In specific risk groups (e.g. people from lower social classes, immigrants, etc.), cumulating problems arise (Kolip, 2004).

Fig. 1:   Prevalence of overweight and obesity in childhood and youth in Germany (RKI, 2006)

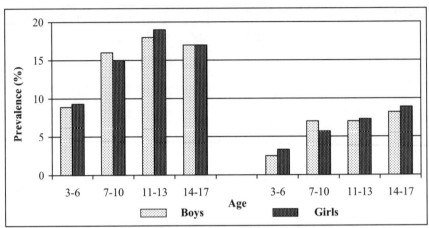

Fig. 2:   Prevalence of overweight and obesity in Bavarian school enrolment examinations
           (Koletzko et al., 2004)

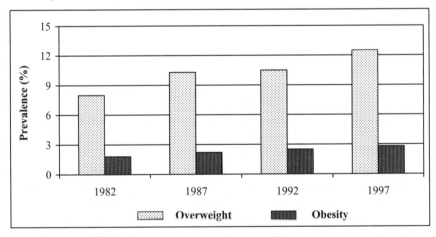

In adults an epidemic prevalence and high incidence of both overweight and
obesity are observed in Germany and in large parts of Europe. Men with normal
body weight are a minority from their 40's and women from their 50's (Fig. 3).

Many adverse health effects associated with overweight already are observed
in children and adolescents. Widespread consequences of childhood obesity are
psychosocial and have tremendous effects on quality of life. Obese children

easily become targets of early and systematic discrimination and often have a low self-esteem. Especially girls, who develop a negative body image, are at a greater risk for the subsequent development of eating disorders. As the obese children mature, the effects of discrimination may become more insidious. Many of the cardiovascular consequences that characterise adult-onset obesity are preceded by abnormalities that begin in childhood. Hypertension, hyperlipidemia, hyperuricemia, abnormal glucose tolerance as well as sleep apnoea occur with increased frequency in obese children and adolescents. Prevalence of overweight is reported to be significantly higher in children and adolescents with moderate to severe asthma compared to peer groups.

Fig. 3:   Prevalence of overweight (BMI >25) by sex and age in German adults (Stat. Bundes-amt, 2006)

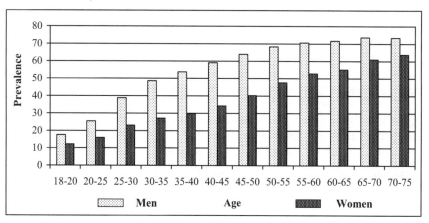

Among growing youth, bone and cartilage in the process of development are not strong enough to bear excess weight. As a result, a variety of orthopaedic complications occur in children and adolescents with obesity. In young children, excess weight can lead to bowing and overgrowth of leg bones. Increased weight on the growth plate of the hip can cause pain and limit range of motion.

In the Murnauer comorbidity study these secondary disorders were studied in detail. An imbalance of glucose metabolism was observed in 6 %, and type 2 diabetes in 1 % of an obese study group. A metabolic syndrome was diagnosed in 35 %, and steatosis hepatis in 30 %. In addition, 35 % had orthopaedic disorders. The youngest child (5-year-old boy) with type 2 diabetes and 55 kg weight (normal: ~20 kg) was found in Leipzig. It has been hypothesised that overweight during childhood and particularly adolescence is related to increased morbidity and mortality in later life. Today's children increasingly have typical adult disorders instead of childhood-diseases like measles or chickenpox.

Overall this dramatic development results in high health insurance and social costs, and furthermore in a long-term reduction in national opportunities in global economic competition.

The bane of genes

The fact that (nearly) all people have the ability to accumulate energy stores in form of adipose tissues is often ignored. The fat in a person's body is stored in fat cells distributed throughout the body. A normal person has between 25 and 35 billion fat cells, but this number can increase in times of excessive weight gain, to as many as 100 to 150 billion cells.

Over the long history of evolution, the capability to produce new lipocytes and to fill them quickly with fat in times of energy excess turned out to be an important advantage for survival and reproduction. Evolutionary genetic selection was driven by the necessity to survive hunger, but not overfeeding ("the gene trap"). The human genome and the metabolism it controls are excellently prepared to manage situation of hunger and deprivation, but not to tackle a situation of over-nutrition and energy affluence. It follows that the development of overweight and obesity are absolutely normal in times of food excess and lack of energy expenditure unless people deliberately control their energy balance. From this the development of obesity should be considered as a natural and physiological reaction to a chronic-positive energy balance.

There are many ways in which genes affect body weight, from the resting metabolic rate, to how calories are burnt during exercise, to how quickly and efficiently the brain generates satiety signals.

Causes of overweight and obesity

On the one hand, genetics play an important role. But on the other hand the gene pool has not changed significantly in the few decades during which obesity has become so prevalent. Genetics must be combined with an environment conducive to gaining weight. For the observed strong increase in both childhood and adult overweight and obesity the environment must have changed profoundly to an "obesogenic environment". The development of this obesogenic environment has been both rapid and multifactorial (Fig. 4).

As with adult-onset obesity, childhood obesity has multiple causes centring around an imbalance between energy intake (calories obtained from food) and energy expenditure (calories expended in the basal metabolic rate and physical activity). Childhood obesity most probably results from an interaction of nutritional, psychological, familial, and physiological factors.

Fig. 4:   The obesogenic environment (IOTF, 2004)

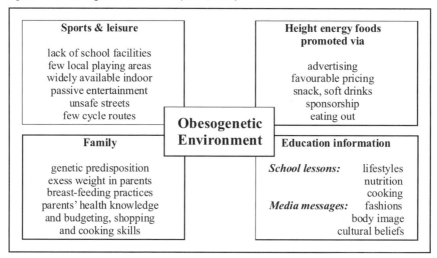

The main causes of overweight and obesity – summarised as "obesogenic environment" are relatively clear:

- An imbalance between energy intake and energy needs.

- Reduction in opportunities for recreational physical activity and increased sedentary recreation. Predominantly sedentary life-style with reduced physical activities during work and leisure time and excessive media consumption. Increased use of motorised transport, e.g. to school (Robinson et al., 2003; Ebbeling et al., 2002).

- Basic changes of eating habits and eating culture (Methfessel, 1999; Wabitsch, 2004).

- A lack of knowledge about food composition and a decreased competence to prepare appetising dishes from basic foods and to transfer nutritional guidelines into practice.

- Increased intake of refined foods/foodstuffs with high energy density and a reduced potential for a satisfying satiety (Prentice & Jebb, 2003; Popkin & Nielsen, 2003; Erbersdobler, 2005).

- More use of restaurants and fast food stores (Diliberti et al., 2004).

- Larger portions of food offering better 'value for money' (Ledikwe et al., 2005)

- High intake of fat/saturated fatty acids, carbohydrate-rich foods with a high glycemic index (Ludwig et al., 2003; Ebbeling, et al., 2003).

- Increased frequency of eating occasions (IOTF, 2004).

- Rising use of soft drinks to replace water, e.g. in schools (Ludwig et al., 2004; Dellavalle et al., 2005).

- More frequent and widespread food purchasing opportunities (Nielsen & Popkin, 2003).

- An aggressive marketing and advertising of food has a strong effect on children's diets and eating behaviour (Hastings et al., 2003; Becker et al., 2005).

Media consumption

The average child or adolescent spends several hours each day watching television; time which in previous years might have been devoted to physical pursuits. In Germany about 20 % of boys and girls view television to excess (Fig. 5). About 40 % of the boys and less than 10 % of the girls play GameBoy or computer games to excess (Fig. 6). A strong association has been established between the amount of time children spend watching TV and their body weight. Obesity more often occurs among children and adolescents who frequently watch television (Gortmaker et al., 1999; Suter et al., 2002), not only because little energy is expended while viewing but also because of the concurrent consumption of high-calorie snacks and soft-drinks. Not all children have weekly physical education at school, and not all of them have extracurricular physical activities after school. Carefully conducted interventions have shown that a reduction of children's media time results in weight loss and can protect children and youth from becoming obese (Robinson, 1999; Gortmaker et al., 1999).

Fig. 5: Excessive television viewing [>4 h/day] by age in Germany

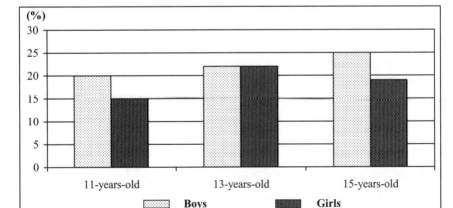

Fig. 6: Excessive playing video and computer games [> 4 h/day] by age in Germany

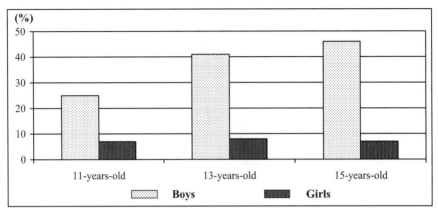

Many studies indicate that children's exposure to food advertising and marketing may be influencing their food choices. Careful studies document that children are exposed to a vast number of TV advertisements for food products such as sodas, sugared cereals, chocolate, candy, and fast food. Exposure to food commercials influences children's preferences and food requests. Advertisements can also contribute to confusion among children about the relative health benefits of certain foods.

Conclusions

Overweight and obesity are the normal consequence in times of food affluence. Overweight and obesity are mainly caused by a sedentary lifestyle, physical inactivity and a positive energy balance. Prevention and therapy of obesity need a reduction of media consumption, an increase of physical activities and an adaptation of the energy intake. This includes a good balance between inactive and active leisure activities, no snacks, sweets or fizzy drinks during media consumption. And, of course, responsible parents should not place television equipment in children's bedrooms.

Interventions at family or school level will need to be matched by changes in the social and cultural context so that the benefits can be sustained and enhanced. Such prevention strategies will require coordinated efforts between the medical community, health administrators, teachers, parents, food producers and processors, retailers and caterers, advertisers and the media, recreation and sport planners, urban architects, city planners, politicians and legislators.

References

Becker, C., Bizer, K., Führ, M., Krieger, N. & Scholl, J. (2005). Lebensmittelwerbung für Kinderprodukte - Strategieentwürfe für den vorbeugenden Verbraucherschutz. Forschungsprojekt im Auftrag des BLE. (http://www.bmelv.de from 1.11.2006).

DellaValle, D. M., Roe, L. S. & Rolls, B. J. (2005). Does the consumption of caloric and noncaloric beverages with a meal affect energy intake? *Appetite, 44,* 187-193.

Diliberti, N., Bordi, P. L., Conklin, M. T., Roe, L. S. & Rolls, B. J. (2004). Increased portion size leads to increased energy intake in a restaurant meal. *Obesity Research, 12,* 562-568.

Ebbeling, C. B., Sinclair, K. B., Pereira, M. A., Garcia-Lago, E., Feldman, H. A. & Ludwig, D. S. (2004). Compensation for energy intake from fast food among overweight and lean adolescents. *JAMA, 291,* 2828-2833.

Erbersdobler, H. (2005): Die Energiedichte, eine vernachlässigte Größe? *Ernährungs-Umschau, 52,* 136-139

Gortmaker, S. L., Peterson, K., Wiecha, J., Sobol, A. M., Dixit, S., Fox, M. K. & Laird, N. (1999). Reducing obesity via a school-based interdisciplinary intervention among youth: Planet Health. *Archives of Pediatrics and Adolescent Medicine, 153,* 409-418.

Hastings, G., Stead, M., McDermott, L., Forsyth, A., MacKintosh, A. M., Rayner, M., Godfrey, C., Caraher, M. & Angus, K. (2003). Review of research of the effects of food promotion to children. (http://www.food.gov.uk/multimedia/pdfs/foodpromotiontochildren1.pdf from 5.10.2006).

Heseker, H. & Beer, S. (2004). Ernährung und ernährungsbezogener Unterricht in der Schule. *Bundesgesundheitsbl - Gesundheitsforsch - Gesundheitsschutz, 47,* 240-245.

IOTF (2004). Obesity in children and young people: A crisis in public health. *Obesity Review, Suppl 1,* 4-104.

Koletzko, B. (2004). Herausforderungen bei der Charakterisierung und der Verbesserung der Ernährungssituation im Kindes- und Jugendalter. *Bundesgesundheitsblatt-Gesundheitsforschung- Gesundheitsschutz, 47,* 227-234.

Kolip, P. (2004). Der Einfluss von Geschlecht und sozialer Lage auf Ernährung und Übergewicht im Kindesalter. *Bundesgesundheitsblatt- Gesundheitsforschung-Gesundheitsschutz, 47,* 235-239.

Kromeyer-Hauschild, K. (2005). Definition, Anthropometrie und deutsche Referenzwerte für BMI. In M. Wabitsch, K. Zwiauer, J. Hebebrand & W. Kiess (Hrsg.): Adipositas bei Kindern und Jugendlichen (pp. 3-15). Berlin: Springer.

Ledikwe, J. H., Ello-Martin, J. A. & Rolls, B. J. (2005). Portion sizes and the obesity epidemic. *Journal of Nutrition, 135,* 905-909.

Ludwig, D. S. (2002). The glycemic index: physiological mechanisms relating to obesity, diabetes, and cardiovascular disease. *JAMA, 287,* 2414-2423.

Ludwig, D. S., Ebbeling, C. B., Peterson, K. E. & Gortmaker, S. L. (2004). Hard facts about soft drinks. *Archives of Pediatrics and Adolescent Medicine, 158,* 290.

Mensink, G. (2002). Was essen wir heute? In Robert Koch-Institut (Hrsg.): Beiträge zur Gesundheitsberichterstattung des Bundes. Berlin: RKI.

Methfessel, B. (1999). Ernährungserziehung, Selbstbewusstsein und Eigenverantwortlichkeit - Forderungen und Überforderungen. In Dr. Rainer Wild-Stiftung (Hrsg.): Gesunde Ernährung zwischen Natur- und Kulturwissenschaft (pp. 91-106.). Münster: Rhema-Verlag.

Nielsen, S. J. & Popkin, B. M. (2003). Patterns and trends in food portion sizes, 1977-1998. *JAMA, 289*, 450-453.

Popkin, B. M. & Nielsen, S. J. (2003). The sweetening of the world's diet. *Obesity Research, 11*, 1325-1332.

Prentice, A. M. & Jebb, S. A. (2003). Fast foods, energy density and obesity: a possible mechanistic link. *Obesity Review, 4*, 187-194.

Robinson, S. M., Crozier, S. R., Borland, S. E., Hammond, J., Barker, D. J. & Inskip, H. M. (2004). Impact of educational attainment on the quality of young women's diets. *European Journal of Clinical Nutrition, 58*, 1174-1180.

Robinson, T. N. (1999). Reducing children's television viewing to prevent obesity: a randomized controlled trial. *JAMA, 282*, 1561-1567.

Rolls, B. J. (2003). The Supersizing of America: Portion Size and the Obesity Epidemic. *Nutr. Today, 38*, 42-53.

Schaffrath Rosario, A. & Kurth, B. (2006). Die Verbreitung von Übergewicht und Adipositas bei Kindern und Jugendlichen. (http://www.KIGGS.de from 1.11.2006)

Seidell, J. C. (1999). Obesity: a growing problem. *Accta Paediatrica Supplement., 428 (Suppl.)*, 46-50.

Statistisches Bundesamt (2006). Ergebnisse der Mikrozensus-Befragung. (http://www.destatis.de/basis/d/gesu/gesutab8.php from 1.11.2006).

Suter, P., Bettoni, M. & Vetterm, W. (2002). Relationship between physical activity, TV-consumption, eating habits and BMI and fat distribution in Swiss. *American Journal of Clinical Nutrition, 75*, 378-379.

Wabitsch, M. (2004). Kinder und Jugendliche mit Adipositas in Deutschland. Aufruf zum Handeln. *Bundesgesundheitsblatt - Gesundheitsforschung - Gesundheitsschutz, 47*, 251-255.

WHO (2003). Diet, Nutrition and the Prevention of Chronic Diseases. Report of a Joint WHO/FAO Expert Consultation. Geneva: World Health Organization. WHO Technical Report Series, No. 916.

Chapter 10:
Overweight and obesity in children – are school-based interventions effective?

Christine Graf & Sigrid Dordel

Introduction

The prevalence of obesity among children and adolescents in developed and developing countries is increasing (Allison, Kaprio, Koskenvuo et al., 1996; Kavey, Daniels, Lauer et al., 2003). Excess weight is caused by an interaction of genetic and environmental factors including metabolic and behavioural components. In particular lack of physical activity, along with a high energy intake diet are contributors to the development of obesity (AGA, 2004).

The clinical consequences are most clearly seen in the increased risk of overweight children to develop various chronic diseases like hypertension, glucose intolerance or manifest diabetes mellitus type 2, orthopaedic and/or psychosocial disorders etc. (Power, Lake & Cole, 1997). In addition, obese children tend to become obese adults with its possible comorbidities (Whitaker, Wright, Pepe et al., 1997). The need for counter measures, therefore, is undoubtedly existing, but the most effective way to deliver interventions to children is still unknown (Summerbell, Ashton, Campbell et al., 2003; Summerbell, Waters, Edmunds et al., 2005).

School settings, in principle, are committed to provide measures to all children independent of their socio-economic status. Adequate interventions in primary schools may help to counteract this development at an early stage (AGA, 2004; Kavey et al., 2003). But up to now school-based programmes with an emphasis on a healthy lifestyle revealed inconsistent results (Müller, Mast, Asbeck et al., 2001; Nader, Stone, Lytle et al., 1999; Stone, McKenzie, Welk et al., 1998). In a recently published Cochrane review 22 studies were included, a minor but positive impact was found on BMI status and an improvement in diet or physical activity. Nevertheless, Summerbell et al. (2005) concluded that there is limited high quality data proving the effectiveness of obesity prevention programmes because of different samples, interventions and methods, so further research is needed.

The complete CHILT project (Children's Health InterventionaL Trial) is composed of sequent modules. In the first module or step (CHILT I) teachers are requested to initiate health promotion measures and to encourage children to enhance physical activity during everydays' school life. The main goal is to lower the prevalence of overweight as well as to positively influence the children's motor performance and to develop and/or maintain a healthy lifestyle. In the next step StEP TWO or CHILT II special focus was taken on risk groups, here overweight and obese children. The programme has been developed as a school- and family-based intervention consisting of extra lessons focussing on healthy nutrition and physical education (Graf, Rost, Koch et al., 2005). It is based on the modification of dietary intake, physical exercise, and behavioural therapy. The arising question is the impact of these measures on the body mass index (BMI), the BMI standard deviation score (BMI-SDS) and the blood pressure of the children. The third module (CHILT III) is an outpatient therapy programme for obese children from age eight and their families. This programme is conducted at the German Sport University Cologne; results thereof are not shown in this paper.

Within this article the role of school-based interventions in the universal and selected prevention of overweight and obesity shall be discussed in the following citing data from the first two modules of the CHILT programme.

CHILT-Programme

CHILT I

Programme and sample

The CHILT project is a professionally developed programme designed to promote a healthy lifestyle in primary schoolchildren (Graf, 2003). The primary aims of this intervention were to increase the total energy expenditure via physical activity during lessons and breaks, to optimise physical education lessons, to enhance pupils' health knowledge and to influence the prevalence of overweight and obesity.

Children of 12 primary schools took part in the intervention. The effects on their anthropometric data, the prevalence and incidence of overweight and obesity as well as their motor performance capacity (coordination and endurance) could be demonstrated compared with the children of 5 control schools. First data on the anthropometric measurements and on testing of performance capacity of the children were gained in the first classes at the beginning of the school year 2001/2002 (T1). Intermediate data was collected in June/July 2003. At this point of time the children were at the end of their 2nd class (results are not shown here). Final data was gained at the end of the 4th class at school in spring/summer 2005 (T2). 76 % of those who took part in the first measurements could be tested again at T2.

Anthropometric data

Height and weight were measured using the same free-standing seca-stadiometer. We deducted 500 grams for the clothes the children were wearing. BMI was calculated as weight in kilograms per height in metres squared and classified according to the German percentile graphs of Kromeyer-Hauschild et al. (2001). Overweight was defined as body mass index ≥90th percentile, but <97th percentile, using population specific data. Obesity was defined as body mass index greater than ≥97th percentile (Kromeyer-Hauschild, Wabitsch, Kunze et al., 2001).

Motor tests

The **6-minute run** was chosen to analyse endurance performance. It is valid for school children and correlates with results of treadmill testing ($r = 0.39$), the shuttle run ($r = 0.88$) and metabolic parameters such as lactate ($r = 0.92$) (Beck & Bös, 1995; Bös, 2001). The children had to run around a standard volleyball court (54 metres) in small groups of up to 8 children for 6 minutes. The children were allowed to walk but not to stop if they were exhausted. The number of rounds run were counted, the additionally run metres added and the exact distance covered by each child was determined in metres (Beck & Bös, 1995).

The **body coordination test for children (KTK)** was used to examine the gross motor development. It is valid for 5 to 14-year-old children (Schilling, 1974). The children were taken out of their classrooms in small groups. Each child completed each of the four KTK items (balancing backwards, one-legged obstacle jumping, lateral jumping and sideways movements). For each task, points were given that made up the overall motor quotient (MQ) under consideration of gender and age factor. Within this publication the MQ and the raw values of the four items are demonstrated.

Intervention

The teachers were asked to give one extra health education lesson per week (20-30 min). The main topics of the health education dealt with biological backgrounds, nutrition and self-management. Additionally, physical activity breaks (5 min each) should be interspersed during lessons once a morning. Furthermore, pupils were given physical activity opportunities during breaks and their physical education lessons were optimized by training the teachers. For this purpose the teachers were instructed during an intensive entrance workshops and yearly follow-ups dealing with the mentioned topics. The whole intervention was described in (Graf, Koch, Falkowski et al., 2005). In the first year site visits were made to all schools to ensure that all aspects were being applied as designed. Within the control schools the normal school programme took place.

After the intervention all teachers were asked to describe how intensive they fulfilled programme. In reality, health education lasting approximately between 20 and 45 minutes took place between once per semester up to twice a week. Physical activity during lessons took place between twice a week up to three times per morning. The attendance to the workshops were irregularly. The implementation of the whole programme decreased from the first to the fourth grade.

Main results: Anthropometric data

Within these results, only those children were included who underwent both BMI-classifications (n = 558).

The anthropometric baseline data for the intervention group (IS) and the control group (CS) are presented in Table 1 (entrance examination). All anthropometric data increased significantly due to growth (each p <0.001) during the period of follow-up (data not shown). No differences in the BMI were found between IS and CS (each p >0.05) at either examination.

Tab. 1: Entrance data, differences according to the anthropometric data between both groups; **IS** = intervention schools; **CS** = control schools.

		N	**mean**	**sd**	**p-value**
age (years)	IS	433	6.7	0.4	<0.001
	CS	178	7.2	0.4	
height (m)	IS	414	1.23	0.05	<0.001
	CS	172	1.25	0.05	
weight (kg)	IS	414	24.5	4.5	0.001
	CS	172	25.9	4.8	
BMI (kg/m²)	IS	414	16.2	2.2	n.s.
	CS	172	16.4	2.4	

m = mean; sd = standard deviation. n.s. = not significant

At the entrance examination, 6.6 % of all children in IS and CS were obese (n – 37), 8.1 % were overweight (n – 45), 77.8% were normal weight (n = 434) and 7.5 % were underweight (n = 42). At final examination 7.4 % were obese (n = 47), 11.3 % overweight (n = 63), 75.1 % normal weight (n = 419) and 5.2 % underweight (n = 29). No difference in the BMI-classification was found between IS and CS by χ^2 method (entrance examination p = 0.413; final examination p = 0.288).

The incidence of new onset obesity out of the normal and underweight population during the study period was 2.0 % in the IS (n = 7), and 1.6 % in the CS (n = 2). No difference was found by χ^2 method (p = 0.190).

23.2% of obese and overweight children from the intervention schools reached normal weight at final examination (13 of 56 children), and 19.2 % of the control school (5 of 26); p = 0.374 by χ^2 method.

Motor tests

Changes (= difference between T1 and T2) in the performance of the **6-minute run** are shown in Table 2. The increase of the intervention group tend to be higher (p = 0.055), adjusted by the influencing co-variables: age at the entrance examination, and by gender, initial test result at entrance and BMI classification at the final examination.

All of the four **KTK** items, without the MQ increase more in the intervention group, adjusted for all mentioned co-variables, but this was only significant in balancing backwards and lateral jumping (see Table 2).

Tab. 2:   Change in the raw values of the 6 min run, the four items of the KTK and the overall motor quotient from T1 to T2 between the intervention (**IS**) and the control schools (**CS**) calculated by analyses of covariance.

			N	mean	sd	p-value*
Change in motor test	**6 min run (m)**	**IS**	379	100,8	122,7	0,055
		CS	171	92,8	126,0	
	Balancing backwards (raw value)	**IS**	410	21,8	11,8	0,007
		CS	173	19,4	11,7	
	One-legged obstacle jumping (raw value)	**IS**	406	28,4	10,8	0,744
		CS	173	25,5	10,8	
	Lateral jumping (raw value)	**IS**	409	30,6	10,8	0,005
		CS	173	26,1	10,8	
	Sideway movement (raw value)	**IS**	410	12,2	7,7	0,169
		CS	170	11,3	7,3	
	MQ	**IS**	403	10,5	13,0	0,822
		CS	168	10,8	11,3	

* p-value adjusted for age at the entrance examination, and by gender, initial test result at entrance and BMI classification at the final examination

Subgroup analyses

In all tests the overweight and obese children of the intervention and control schools reached the worse results and the lowest increase independent of the group (data not shown).

CHILT II

Programme and sample

Based on the findings of CHILT I the outpatient programme, entitled StEP TWO was designed for overweight and obese children and aims to reduce body mass index by weight maintenance, increased physical activity, and improving motor abilities.

All overweight and obese children from three intervention schools were invited to take part (n = 121). 40 children completed the programme from November 2003 to July 2004 (intervention group = IG), albeit that 6 dropped out, 1 because of a change of school, and 5 for personal reasons. We recruited 2 children in February, but they were not taken into account. The other 74 overweight and obese children were informed about their weight and the necessity for intervention, but did not take part (non-participants = NP); one was lost because of unknown reason. Their parents were requested to respond to a questionnaire concerning the reasons for non-participation. 20 parents (27.0 %) responded to the questionnaire. Their main reasons were lack of time or interest. Overweight and obese children of four further primary schools were considered as control group (CG; n = 155) in order to verify the effect of the taken measures on BMI, BMI-SDS and on blood pressure. 71 non-participants and 144 control children could be followed.

Intervention

The intervention lasted approx. 30 weeks and took place twice a week. It started directly after school at each of the 3 participating primary schools.

In addition, nutritionists, gymnasts and medical doctors taught the children in each of their respective fields (see Table 3). The nutritionists cooked and ate with the children twice a week. After the meal, the children received a physical activity programme lasting between 60 and 90 minutes. Parents were involved in 6 information evenings and 2 family events. The complete intervention is described in Graf et al., 2005.

Main results

The anthropometric data of the three subgroups at T1 are shown in Table 4.

Height and weight increased significantly due to growth (each p <0.001) during the period of follow-up (data not shown). Body weight increased less in the children involved in intervention, but there were no differences between the non-participants and the controls (data not shown).

Tab. 3: Programme content with reference to the manual of the Konsensusgruppe Adipositasschulung (author's translation: consensus group obesity education and training; KGAS 2004; AGA 2004).

Medical contents (ca. 60x 5-10 min)	Nutritional contents (ca. 60x 5-10 min)	Physical education (ca. 60x 5-10 min)	Behaviour therapy (ca. 60x 5-10 min)
Children (2x/week; > 30 weeks)			
Expedition through the human body; (cardiovascular system)	Preparing and eating food together	Games for indoors and outdoors, activity games	Body perception
Importance of energy and appropriate suppliers thereof	Healthy/unhealthy food and drink	Endurance training	Relaxing
Importance of muscule and metabolism	Composition of food and drink	Strengh	Supervised mealtimes
Consequences of inactivity and high energy intake	"Traffic-light Systen" / Optimix*	Coordination and flexibility	Nutrition games, nutritional behaviour
Counteractive measures	Children's nutritional pyramid	Exercise in everyday life (e.g. way to school)	Rules for eating
Parents (Group meetings – in total 6 meetings lasting between 90 and 120 min)			
Co-morbidities	Importance and composition of a healthy diet	Effects of physical exercise	Nutritional behaviour
Improtance of physical exercise/nutrition/healthy lifestyle	Portion sizes, eating rules, pitfalls in the supermarket	Exercise alternatives/ supportive measures	Motor ability
Families			
Anamnesis, pre- and post examination of the children, spiroergometry (data not shown)	Shopping trip (1 morning), cooking together	Exercise together: Inline skating and Orienteering's hike (2 mornings)	Personal consultation upon request

*nutrition contents based on the OPTIMIX program/nutrition pyramid

37.5 % of the children undergoing the intervention, reduced their body mass index, compared with 33.8 % of the non-participants, and 28.5 % of controls. These differences were not significant (p >0.05).

Tab. 4:   Differences in the anthropometric data of the three subgroups at T1.

		N	m (sd)	p-value*	Range
age (yrs.)	IG	40	8.7 (1.3)	0.037	6.3 – 10.2
	NP	74	8.1 (1.2)		5.8 – 10.7
	CG	155	8.5 (1.3)		5.9 – 11.7
height (m)	IG	40	1.37 (0.10)	n. s.	1.20 – 1.57
	NP	74	1.33 (0.09)		1.19 – 1.54
	CG	155	1.36 (0.10)		1.15 – 1.59
weight (kg)	IG	40	43.6 (10.2)	0.011	26.7 – 70.2
	NP	74	38.1 (8.5)		25.7 – 63.5
	CG	155	40.8 (9.6)		25.1 – 80.3
BMI (kg/m²)	IG	40	22.8 (3.6)	0.012	18.5 – 37.2
	NP	74	21.2 (2.4)		18.1 – 29.4
	CG	155	21.8 (2.7)		18.1 – 35.2
BMI-SDS	IG	40	1.99 (0.52)	n. s.	1.30 – 3.81
	NP	74	1.82 (0.44)		1.24 – 2.98
	CG	155	1.87 (0.41)		1.25 – 3.39

* calculated by analyses of covariance, adjusted for age and gender; IG = intervention group;
NP = non-participants; CG = control group

The differences between T1 and T2 are shown in Table 4. Body mass index increased significantly in the non-participants and the control group compared with baseline measurements, but not in those selected for intervention. There were, however, no significant differences between the 3 subgroups in the increase in body mass index values throughout the study period. But the less increase was found in overweight and obese intervention children, the highest in the obese control children and non-participants. The overweight non-participants showed a markedly less increase than the obese ones, whereas these differences were unobvious in the other groups (see Fig. 1).

Body mass index-standard deviation score decreased in all groups, but most markedly in those chosen for intervention. There was a significant difference between those chosen for intervention and their controls (p = 0.028), but neither of these groups differed from the non-participants. The change in body mass index-standard deviation score was analysed separately in overweight and obese children. Normal development of body mass index-standard deviation score was demonstrated in the controls. Obese children involved in intervention reduced their body mass index-standard deviation score more markedly than overweight children. Among the non-participants, overweight children reduced their body mass index-standard deviation score more than the obese children. All these differences were not statistically significant due to the large standard deviation, although a consistent trend was demonstrable.

Fig. 1:   Body mass index increase from T1 to T2 in the IG, NP and control group, differentiated after overweight and obesity at T1.

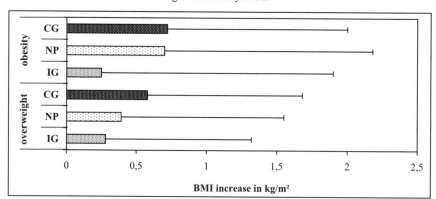

Heart rate and blood pressure

The differences between these parameters in the 3 groups are demonstrated in Table 5 and Fig. 2. Systolic blood pressure decreased significantly both in those selected for intervention group and non-participants, but not in the controls. The most marked decrease was seen in those selected for intervention. The difference between those chosen for intervention and their controls was significant, while there was no significant difference between the children undergoing intervention and non-participants (intervention versus control group $p = 0.002$; non-participants versus control group $p = 0.025$; each adjusted for age and gender). Diastolic blood pressure values and heart rate did not differ between the groups.

Discussion

As in numerous countries worldwide (Hedley, Ogden, Johnson et al., 2004; Kavey et al. 2003), the prevalence of overweight and obese children is rising in Germany (AGA 2004). Effective interventions are warranted, but an ideal strategy has not yet been developed (Summerbell et al., 2005).

Schools may play a key role in encouraging a healthy lifestyle among children in order to counteract this development (Kahn, Ramsey, Brownson et al., 2002). However, Summerbell et al. (2005) described in their review article only minor effects and inconsistent results of primary preventive investigations. Similar results were revealed in the present study. After nearly 4 years of school-based

Tab. 5: Difference in selected parameters between the final and the entrance examination; calculated by analyses of covariance, adjusted by age and gender.

		N	m	sd	p-value
difference BMI	IG	40	0.3	1.3	n.s.
	NP	71	0.5	1.3	
	CG	144	0.7	1.2	
difference BMI-SDS	IG	40	−0.15	0.26	0.028*
	NP	71	−0.09	0.31	
	CG	144	−0.05	0.27	
difference systolic blood pressure	IG	35	−9.5	19.6	0.002*
	NP	64	−5.3	15.6	0.025**
	CG	141	0.5	16.5	
difference diastolic blood pressure	IG	35	−3.3	14.6	n.s.
	NP	64	−1.7	12.6	
	CG	141	0.8	14.0	
difference heart rate	IG	34	1.1	16.4	n.s.
	NP	64	−2.4	16.0	
	CG	141	−0.5	13.4	

*intervention versus control group; **"non-participants" versus control group

Fig. 2: Change in systolic blood pressure (in mmHg) in the three subgroups.

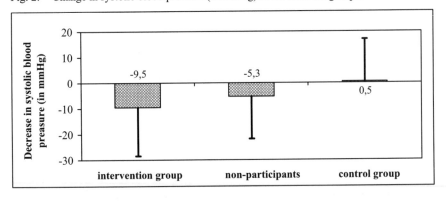

intervention, no positive effect on the incidence of overweight and obesity was found. There is a small trend in the intervention schools that more overweight and obese children reach normal weight. But this result was not significant. There was, however, an improvement in some motor tasks in the intervention schools. Greater skills were achieved in lateral jumping and balancing backwards and the increase was significantly higher than in the control schools; in all other tasks the increase of the values was higher but not significantly higher.

Therefore, solely school-based interventions do not seem to be intensive enough to cause essential improvements related to overweight and motor performance. We suppose that effects could be increased by a consequent implementation of the intervention contents into school day by the teachers. The realisation was clearly less intensive than predetermined. This reflects the poor possibilities of teachers during school day and their lack of skills in mediating healthy lifestyle. In this context, another aspect has to be added: In part, these findings can be led back to the insufficient inclusion of the parents. Parents, however, are responsible for nutrition and the dietary and activity lifestyle of the family (Flodmark, Lissau, Moreno et al., 2004), and are necessary participants in the successful transfer of any recommended changes in lifestyle.

This aspect is much more important in the care of overweight and obese children. In the framework of our StEP TWO programme experiences of primary prevention and therapy were bundled and the contents were put into practice as school- and family-based intervention for this special risk group. These measures were offered as additional units to regular school lessons. The purpose of our study was to document the effects of this multicomponent programme on children who completed the recommended intervention, and provide comparisons between them and children who were invited but did not participate, and age-matched controls.

At the beginning of the study the highest body mass index was found in those undergoing intervention. We speculate that parents of children who were more overweight than their peers presumably felt the need to participate in the intervention. The increase of body mass index was lowest, and the decrease of body mass index-standard deviation score was highest in those undergoing intervention. This was the case for both overweight and obese children. This development in the non-participants compared with the controls reveals that there is a positive effect of a screening programme which brings to the attention of the parents that their child is overweight or obese. While not significant, there was a consistent trend that this benefit was observed in overweight, but not obese children. Perhaps changes in lifestyle are easier to implement in overweight children and their families as opposed to obese children. To achieve an effect against obesity, an intensive interdisciplinary therapy is most likely necessary (AGA 2004; Epstein, Myers, Raynor et al., 1998).

Along with decreasing BMI-SDS a reduction of systolic blood pressure values in the intervention group could be detected and to a smaller extent in the group of the non-participants. It is obvious that the intervention lead to the most significant results though the screening measures provoked positive effects, too. The developing of the diastolic blood pressure values was similar, but not significant.

Therefore, our data reveal the effect of solely school-based programmes on overweight and obesity is small, and did not allow the development of final strategies, but an interdisciplinary multicomponent school- and family-based intervention seems to be effective. Basically, it has to be criticised that only one third of "intervention parents" attended the offered educational activities. Until now there is no strategy which attracts the parents to go in for the activities regularly and for a long-lasting period except on the basis of a financial participation. However, it is undoubtedly necessary to intensively integrate parents and those who belong to the educational setting of the children into the programme in order to achieve long-lasting effects thereof.

In conclusion, to implement effective preventive strategies it is necessary to include all participating occupational groups (teachers, paediatricians, nutritionists, sport scientists, governments) and to address all parts of children's environment, school, clubs, friends, and family.

References

Allison, D. B., Kaprio, J., Koskenvuo, M., Neale, M. C. & Hayakawa, K. (1996). The heretability of body mass index among an international sample of monozygotic twins reared apart. *International Journal of Obesity, 20,* 501-506.

AGA (Arbeitsgemeinschaft Adipositas im Kindes- und Jugendalter) (2004). Working group Obesity in childhood and adolescence. Guidelines. www.a-g-a.de

Beck, J. & Bös, K. (1995). Normwerte der motorischen Leistungsfähigkeitsfähigkeit (Standardised values of motoric performance). Köln: Sport und Buch Strauß.

Bös, K. (2001). Motorische Tests (motoric tests) (2nd edition). Göttingen: Hogrefe.

Epstein, L. H., Myers, M. D, Raynor, H. A. & Saelens, B. E. (1998). *Treatment of pediatric obesity Pediatrics, 101,* 554-570.

Flodmark, C. E., Lissau, I., Moreno, L. A., Pietrobelli, A., Widhalm, K. (2004). New insights into the field of children and adolescents obesity: the European perspective. *International Journal of Obesity, 28,* 1189-1196.

Graf, C. (2003). Das CHILT-Projekt (The CHILT-Project). *Deutsche Zeitschrift für Sportmedizin, 54,* 247.

Graf, C., Koch, B., Falkowski, G., Jouck, S., Christ, H., Bjarnason-Wehrens, B., Tokarski, W., Dordel, S. & Predel, H. G. (2005). Effects of a school-based intervention on the BMI and motor abilities in childhood (mid point data of the CHILT-Project). *Journal of Sport Science and Medicine, 4,* 291-299.

Graf, C., Rost, S. V., Koch, B., Heinen, S., Falkowski, G., Dordel, S., Bjarnason-Wehrens, B., Sreeram, N., Brockmeier, N., Christ, H. & Predel, H.-G. (2005). Data from the StEP TWO programme showing the effect on blood pressure and different parameters for obesity in overweight and obese primary school children. *Cardiology in the Young, 15,* 291-298.

Hedley, A. A., Ogden, C. L., Johnson, C. L., Carroll, M. D., Curtin, L. R. & Flegal, K. M. (2004). Prevalence of overweight and obesity among US children, adolescents, and adults, 1999-2002. *JAMA, 291,* 2847-2850.

KGAS (Konsensusgruppe Adipositasschulung) (2004). AID: Trainermanual Leichter, aktiver, gesünder. Interdisziplinäres Konzept für die Schulung übergewichtiger oder adipöser Kinder und Jugendlicher. Bonn: AID.

Kahn, E. B., Ramsey, L. T., Brownson, G., Heath, G. W., Howze, E. H. & Powell, K. E. (2002). The effectiveness of interventions to increase physical activity: a systematic review. *American Journal Preventive Medicine, 22,* 73-101.

Kavey, R. E.W., Daniels, S. R., Lauer, R. M., Atkins, D. L., Hayman, L. L. &Taubert, K. (2003). American Heart Association Guidelines for primary prevention of atherosclerotic Cardiovascular Disease beginning in childhood. *Circulation, 107,* 1562-1566.

Kromeyer-Hauschild, K., Wabitsch, M., Kunze, D., Geller, F., Geiß, H. C., Hesse, V., von Hippel, A., Jaeger, U., Johnsen, D., Korte, W., Menner, K., Müller, G., Müller, J. M., Niemann-Pilatus, A., Remer, T., Schaefer, F., Wittchen, H.-U., Zabransky, S., Zellner, K., Ziegler, A. & Hebebrand, J. (2001). Perzentile für den Body mass index für das Kindes- und Jugendalter unter Heranziehung verschiedener deutscher Stichproben. *Monatsschrift Kinderheilkunde, 8,* 807-818.

Müller, M. J., Mast, M., Asbeck, I. & Langnase, K. (2001). Grund A. Prevention of obesity-- is it possible? *Obesity Review, 2,* 15-28

Nader, P. R., Stone, E. J., Lytle, L. A., Perry, C. L., Osganian, S. K., Kelder, S., Webber, L. S., Elder, J. P., Montgomery, D., Feldman, H. A., Wu, M., Johnson, C., Parcel, G. S. & Luepker, R. V. (1999). Three-year maintenance of improved diet and physical activity: the CATCH cohort. Child and Adolescent Trial for Cardiovascular Health. *Archives of Pediatrics & Adolescent Medicine, 153,* 695-704

Power, C., Lake, J. K. & Cole, T. J. (1997). Measurement and long-term health risks of child and adolescent fatness. *International Journal of Obesity, 21,* 507-526.

Schilling, F. (1974). Körperkoordinationstest für Kinder. KTK. Manual (body coordination test for children, KTK, manual). Weinheim: Beltz.

Stone, E. J., McKenzie, T. L., Welk, G. J. & Booth, M. L. (1998). Effects of physical activity interventions in youth: review and synthesis. *American Journal of Preventive Medicine, 15,* 298-315

Summerbell, C., Waters, E., Edmunds, L., Kelly, S., Brown, T. & Campbell, K. (2005). Interventions for preventing obesity in children (Cochrane Review). Cochrane Database of Systematic Review, 3, CD001871.

Summerbell, C. D., Ashton, V., Campbell, K. J., Edmunds, L., Kelly, S. & Waters, E. (2003). Interventions for treating obesity on children. The Cochrane Library, 3, CD001872.

Whitaker, R. C., Wright, J. A., Pepe, M. S., Seidel, K. D., Dietz, W. H. (1997). Predicting obesity in young adulthood from childhood and parental obesity. New England Journal of Medicine, 337, 869-873.

III.
Active lifestyle – determinants and benefits

Chapter 11:
Active Lifestyles of Young People – Benefits and Outcomes

Antonin Rychtecký

In recent years the concepts of "lifestyle" and "active lifestyle" have become the focus of attention of the biological and social sciences and of their often different system approaches. The reason for this is due to the fact that the active lifestyle is closely related to significant human values, people's quality of life and health status. Social demographic and psychological characteristics such as age, gender, social and economical status, personal qualities, motivation and the position and values of the subject including his or her physical activities, all form part of the attributes of the lifestyle (Bouchard, Shepard, Stephens et al., 1990).

In general the specialists agree on the positive influence of an active lifestyle on the bio-psychosocial development of individuals. It is however much more difficult to identify and express precisely the extent of this influence. The reasons for this are differences in the explanation of the meaning of the term "active lifestyle" and the methodological problems found in the quantitative and qualitative evaluation of it. It is also difficult to diagnose precisely the physical activity that forms part of an active lifestyle even though the methods used have been continually improving.

The reason for the growing interest in the study of the relationship between physical activity, health and the quality of life is the assumption that a regular physical activity leads to positive somatic (BMI and fatness), physiological (aerobic fitness), medical (primary and secondary prevention), pedagogical (skill fitness and sport skills attitudes, values), mental (fitness, motivation, anxiety), social effects (socialization, integration) and economical impact (reducing money for health care, opportunities for labour in sport) etc. However the effects of physical activity may be both immediate (motor skills, decreasing of depression) and postponed, i.e. those that appear only after a long run and regular exercise (position, values, creation of a permanent active lifestyle, etc.). Apart from the biological approach which specially studies and defines the health or preventive effects of physical activity, social sciences introduce the term "quality of life" in which the benefits of active movement are assessed in a psychosocial context of personality and in social-psychological experiences and interpersonal relations.

Some assumptions should be revised in the evaluation of the relations between physical activity and its supposed benefits, for example the relationship linking physical activity and the improvement in health status (Lüschen, Abel, Cockerham et al., 1993). For example, mono-causal relations between these changing phenomena cannot fully explain the complexity of these relations. That is why the results and the assumed effects of an active lifestyle must be considered as a gradual identification and verification of the complicated biological, psychological and social variables that are always manifest in a complex way by the benefits of young people's active movement.

Can an active lifestyle be reduced to a mere physical activity and the practice of sports?

An active life is nothing new for people born with a competitive nature. Even though the term "activity" is associated with movement, it does not only mean a physical activity. An active lifestyle is also active in other leisure activities, such as cultural, social, educational, sports, charities and others. These may be competitive due to the participation in physical activities and sports but at the same time they can complement the development of young people's personality. Even though we refer to sports and physical activities in particular as an educational tool, it is important to know the role of sport and physical activities in the value spectrum of leisure activities and the importance which young people give them.

The results shown indicate the relationship between the answers of people of different genders and ages. As age increases there is a rise in listening to music, in having dates with folk of different sex, girls/boys, going to parties, dancing, relaxing, day dreaming, spending time alone, etc. On the other hand as age increases there is less interest in video and computer games, arts and handicrafts, helping in house work, visiting relatives and in organizing competitive sports. However recreational activities, organized and unorganized sports, watching TV/videos and reading of books and magazines are relatively independent of age.

We can observe the stable differences between boys on the one hand and girls on the other in the following activities: playing a musical instrument, singing in a choir, having dates with a boy/girl of the opposite sex, relaxing, day dreaming, spending time alone, recreational organized and unorganized sport. In the further course of ontogenesis the differences between boys and girls gradually disappear.

The answers received from the participants of all the age groups shows the active participation in recreational, organized and unorganized sports as important (always up to the fifth line of the assessment ladder)(see Tab. 1).

Tab. 1:   Participation in Leisure Time Activities in Czech Boys and Girls (%) (Rychtecký, 2002)

Activities	Boys				Girls			
	age/years				age/years			
	9-11	12-13	14-15	16-19	9-11	12-13	14-15	16-19
Listen to music	52	58	73	83	75	74	86	87
Play music or sing in a choir	15	14	12	14	30	23	24	27
Watch TV / videos	76	72	69	75	75	68	73	59
Earn some money	15	19	14	29	9	9	9	16
Hang around and talk with friends	57	42	45	50	57	52	61	63
Spend time with boyfriend/ girlfriend	13	20	30	43	15	21	28	45
Play cards, video games/ computer	69	61	49	56	25	37	22	15
Read (e.g. books, magazines)	57	49	37	47	66	58	66	68
Organized competitive sports	18	16	15	11	12	12	6	5
Visit sports events	17	37	39	37	25	28	21	21
Extra work for schools follows up on homework	20	17	12	8	31	23	18	9
Go to parties, dance	9	9	16	38	13	13	24	44
Arts and crafts (e.g. photo-graphy, sewing, making things)	17	16	12	8	33	27	18	15
Spend time alone (e.g. relaxing, day dreaming)	13	23	27	32	30	39	47	50
Go shopping	43	38	31	25	50	56	49	40
Go to movies, concerts and theatre	24	22	23	33	34	25	33	38
Volunteer work, social work	13	8	9	5	15	8	7	7
Help with housework	59	61	54	47	75	74	72	73
Go to youth club/ community centers	13	15	18	18	12	8	10	16
Visited relatives	55	44	38	38	62	52	48	45
Recreational/ unorganized sports	59	48	51	60	52	41	47	52
Others	8	6	6	4	7	5	5	4

The results of a factor analysis assessed the importance of leisure activities allowed the formulation and interpretation of five basic factors of leisure time activities (see Tab. 2): **F1**: socio-cultural activities (extraversion); **F2**: obligation towards society, one's family, oneself, self-education; **F3**: position concerning sports and physical activities; **F4**: audio video, multimedia, virtual reality; **F5**: individual cultural activities (introversion).

Tab. 2:   Factor analysis of leisure activities (Rychtecký, 2000)

Items /factors	F1	F2	F3	F4	F5
Spend time with boyfriend/ girlfriend	0.71				
Go to parties, dance	0.65				
Earn some money	0.46				
Hang around and talk with friends	0.44				0.30
Go to movies, concerts and theatre	0.38				0.33
Spend time alone (e.g. relaxing, day dreaming)	0.37				0.31
Go to youth club/ community centers	0.33				
Volunteer work, social work		0.58			
Extra work for schools follows up on homework		0.57			
Help with housework		0.55			
Go shopping		0.43			
Visited relatives		0.41			
Arts and crafts (e.g. photography, sewing, making things)		0.40			
Play music or sing in a choir					
Others					
Visit sports events			0.70		
Organized competitive sports		0.34	0.47		
Recreational/ unorganized sports			0.39		
Watch TV / videos				0.67	
Play cards. video games/computer				0.53	
Listen to music	0.35				0.43
Read (e.g. books. magazines)		0.32			0,42

Extraction Method: Principal Axis Factoring. Rotation Method: Varimax with Kaiser Normalization.
Rotation converged in 11 iterations.

Physical activities and their benefits

Physical activities are an important part of a healthy lifestyle. Well-chosen
exercise and sports contribute to improve the shape and posture of the body and
they increase the flow of energy by means of a active energy expenditure. The
reduction of the incidence of the diseases of civilization, mental and physical
wellbeing as well as a decrease in the symptoms of depression and distress
(Amisola & Jacobson, 2003; Thompson, Grouse, Goodpaster et al, 2001) are
some of the further expected consequences. Physical activities are much more
important in the life of children and young people than in adults. A good
physical activity is a necessary, stimulating and coordinating factor in the
ontogenetical development of most young people (Kucera, 1985).

Determinations of physical activities of youth

Several different studies focusing on the physical activities of young people were recently carried out in the Czech Republic. Both were based on questionnaires with a weekly registration of all physical activities and their transfer into percentage data of the basal metabolism (Rychtecký, 1993) by using the caltrack method (Frömel, Novosad & Svozil, 1999) and the international COMPASS questionnaire which observes the annual frequency of participation in several categories: from intensive to occasional; from organized to unorganized and the IPAQ questionnaire were used.

The results of the COMPASS study carried out in the Czech Republic in the year 2000 (see figure 1 & 2) show that two large groups of children and young people stand out from the total number of 2.953 respondents according to the annual frequency of physical activities. The first group includes individuals who train intensively several times a week, sometimes even twice a day. More boys than girls devote themselves to organized sports, even though in recent years the number of girls participating mainly in unorganized forms of physical activities has increased. 43 % of the boys and 34 % of the girls are engaged in all the existing organized forms of sports according to the COMPASS category. 30 % of selection of the sports changes as well. The "new sports", including adventure activities, are becoming more popular than the traditional ones. The second group includes children and young people who do not carry out any physical activity

Fig. 1:   Participation in Sports and Physical Activities According to Gender, Age and Annual Frequency of Participation in Males (Rychtecký, 2000)

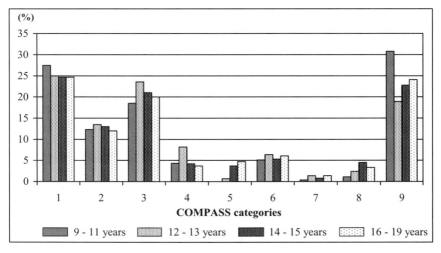

Fig. 2:   Participation in Sports and Physical Activities According to Gender, Age and Annual
           Frequency of Participation in Females (Rychtecký, 2000)

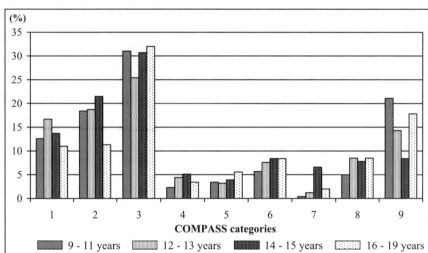

Legend to figures 1 and 2: 1. Competitive, organized, intensive (>120); 2. Intensive, competitive and /
or organized (> 120); 3. Intensive (>120), 4. Regular, competitive and / or organized (>60 <120); 5.
Regular, recreational (>60 <120); 6. Irregular (>2 <60); 7. Occasional (>1 <12); 8. Non-participant:
participation in other physical activities; 9. Non-participant: no physical activities.

(24 % of the boys; 15.5 % of the girls) This high percentage of young people who
do not practice any sport is alarming because of the prognosis of the possible
appearance of risk factors in individuals who are not active. In some age
categories the percentage of non-active individuals is even higher. The sports
organizations devoted to children's and young people's sports should concentrate
their attention on this group of young people who do not practice any sport.

Which sports and physical activities the young people select according to some COMPASS categories?

Boys:

Category: "Competitive, organized and intensive" Sports:

Football, Cycling, mounting bike, Basketball, Volleyball, Swimming, Table
tennis, Hockey in gym, Track and field, Roller skating, Tennis.

Other Physical activities: Exercising at home, Dancing, Fishing, Walking the
dog, Billiards, Work in the garden, Family trips.

Category: "Regular, recreational"

Sports: Cycling, mounting bike, Football, Basketball, Skateboard, Tennis, Swimming, Roller skating, Archery, Snowboarding, Body building.

Other activities: Walking, Jogging

Girls:

Category: "Competitive, organized and intensive"Sports:

Volleyball, Cycling, Mountain bike, Track and field, Basketball, Roller skating, Aerobic, Tennis, Swimming, Horse riding, Karate.

Other Physical Activities: Walking the dog, Disco dancing, Family trips, Exercising at home, Work in the garden or field.

Category: "Regular, recreational"

Sports: Cycling, Mountain bike, Aerobic, Roller skating, Basketball, Badminton, Swimming, Alpine skiing, Volleyball, Football.

Other physical activities: Home exercising, Billiards, Walking the dog, Disco dancing.

Physical activity during the week – IPAQ study

The Faculty of Physical Culture in Palacky University in Olomouc carried out the IPAQ study in the Czech Republic (Frömel & Sigmund, 2003; Frömel, 2004). The cooperating institutions were the Center for Disease Control and Prevention - The Karolinska Institute, Stockholm, Sweden, Canadian Fitness and Lifestyle Research Institute in Ottawa, U.S. Centers for Disease Control and Prevention, Atlanta, Prevention Research Center, School of Public Health, University of South Carolina, Department of Psychology, San Diego State University, Epidemiology Unit, University of New South Wales, Sydney, Australia. The aims of this study is to identify the mediators and moderators of the lifestyles of different ages, and other specific groups, of young and adult people and to find the relationship between physical activity and inactivity and other characteristics of the lifestyle of the people being investigated. From the results of this survey, which is still not fully evaluated, shows that the Czech boys in all the observed age categories (14 to 24-years-old) participate in intensive and moderately intensive physical activity more days in the week than girls. These differences continue with increasing ages of the boys and girls. The average daily time for intensive physical activity for boys is 51 minutes and 33 minutes for girls. No differences in the number of so called "walking days" between the boys and girls were registered (Fig 3, 4, 5, 6, 7).

Fig. 3:   Days with intensive physical activity during the week related to gender and age of Czech youth (Frömel, 2004)

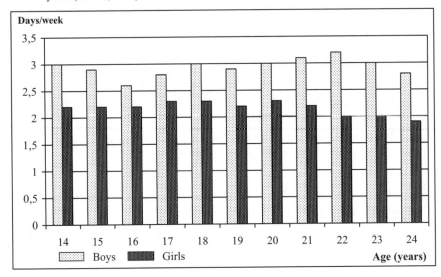

Fig. 4:   Intensive physical activity during the week in minutes according to gender and age of the Czech youth (Frömel, 2004)

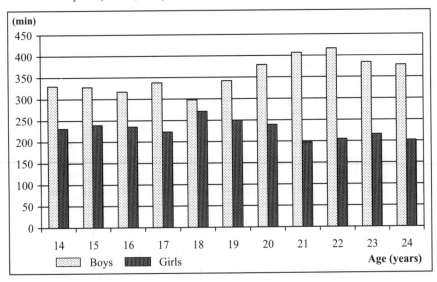

Fig. 5:   Days with middle intensity of physical activity during the week related to gender and age of Czech youth (Frömel, 2004)

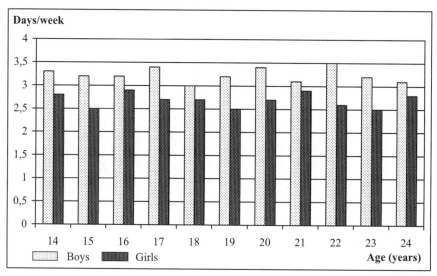

Fig. 6:   Days with walking during the week according to gender and age of the Czech youth (Frömel, 2004)

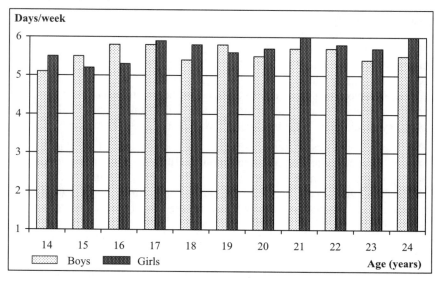

Fig. 7: Sitting in working days according to age and gender of the Czech youth (Frömel, 2004)

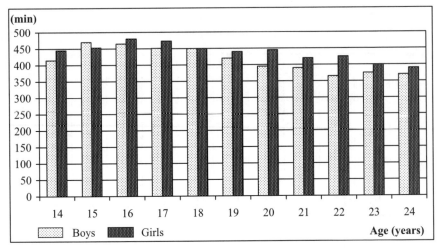

Habitual physical activities in childhood and adolescence

Technical progress and changes in cultural habits have significantly reduced physical effort in activities related to work as well as in every day life. This is evident, for example, in the fact that children make less effort on their way to and from school and that people in general have more passive activities in their leisure time, such as watching the TV and playing electronic and video games. It is therefore obvious that the amount of, intensity, and frequency of physical activities young people have (in leisure time as well as in the time spent at school) are not sufficient to have a decisive effect on their state of heath or to prevent health risk factors. (Naul, Rychtecký & Pauer, 1992; Naul, Neuhaus & Rychtecký, 1993; Rychtecký, 1994; Rychtecký, Naul & Neuhaus 1996; Frömel et al., 1999).

The habitual physical activities (regime) are characterized by the volume, intensity, frequency and time of their duration. Habitual physical activities occur both spontaneously and by rational intervention (sports, walking, etc.). Habitual physical activities can be observed in the spontaneous manifestation of movement in children, especially those of pre-school and early school age. Some theories (Gedda et al, 1981; Perussa et al., 1989) state that the tendency towards a spontaneous physical manifestation is caused genetically rather than by a rationally selected type of physical activity.

These hypotheses were partially confirmed in the Czech Republic by the experience resulting from the selection of children with a special talent for sports. In the regular physical activities of children and young people of medium and older school age, the importance of planned, principal physical activities increases. The choice of the day and week is determined by daily and weekly habits and social influences (Frömel et al., 1999; Frömel et al., 2004).

The research of Medeková, Šelingerová & Havlíček (2001) showed that spontaneously hyperactive children (very lively manifestations) have a significantly lower BMI index than hypoactive and normally active ones (see Fig. 8.). Thus hypo-activity, normal activity and hyperactivity probably have influence on the global manifestation of physical activity more than participation or non-participation in sports. Similarly no significant differences between children attending special sports classes on the one hand, and those studying in regular schools on the other, were found during observation of the weekly physical activities of primary and secondary school children. Even though the children studying in special sports classes have a higher load of physical effort in their training, they tend to choose sedentary kinds of activities in their leisure time.

Fig. 8:   Changes of BMI in Relation to Type of Spontaneous Physical Activity of Preschool and
            Young School Children (Medeková, Šelingerová & Havlíček, 2001)

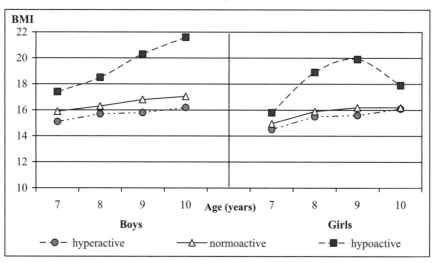

Aerobic fitness and physical activities

The positive biological effects of intensive physical activities and sport can be observed in some indicators of aerobic fitness. Physical fitness is a state of the individual which is determined not only by hereditary factors but also by social

life, education and exercising. Physical fitness is a product resulting from the
level of habitual physical activities (Blair, 1985).

Regular exercise may contribute both to the development of physical fitness
and indirectly to a better self-reflection of one's own health status. Thus for
example in our research in the middle of the 90's (Rychtecký, Pauer, Janouch et
al., 1995) the influence of physical activity on fitness and other physiological and
psychological indices was investigated. One group in this project was
completed from children with a high output of weekly intensity of physical
activity (more than 185 % of BMR) and the second one with a low output of
energy (less than 170 % of BMR). We found out that more active children and
young people achieved better statistically significant results in aerobic indices in
Ruffier's test, shuttle run test (Leger & Lambert, 1982) and bicycle ergometry
test as well. The results of these comparisons are presented in Table 3 (boys)
and Table 4 (girls).

Tab: 3: Results of observed indices in 11 – 12 years boys with high and low physical activity
         (n = 25 in each group) (Rychtecký, 1995)

Group with:	High physical activity – more than 185 % BMR		Low physical activity – less than 170 % BMR		Diffe- rences	Signi- ficance
INDICES:	Mean	SD	Mean	SD	t- test	p <
Body height (cm)	148.20	6.23	53.50	8.59	1.783	–
Body weight (kg)	41.54	5.87	46.41	8.67	3.009	**
Body fat (%)	14.65	2.46	20.05	4.71	3.634	**
BMI	18.91		19.69			–
Ruffier´s index (index)	8.65	3.28	17.67	3.47	6.736	**
20m shuttle run (VO₂/ml/kg*min⁻¹)	54.84	2.09	44.27	1.74	13.363	**
bicycle ergometry (VO₂/ml/kg*min⁻¹)	47.61	4.28	41.92	3.77	3.506	**
Total motivation (points)	48.50	7.69	46.00	10.60	0.677	–
Net motivation (points)	33.15	9.63	31.55	7.93	0.452	–
Extroversion (points)	14.92	4.89	16.50	2.53	1.896	–
Neurotic tendencies (points)	11.70	3.09	11.80	5.54	0.923	–

The evaluation of somatic data shows significant (p ≤0.01) differences in body
weight and body fat. Boys and girls with a low intensity of physical activity
have higher values of body weight (t = 3.009; t = 3.295) and body fat
(t = 3.634; t = 3.500). These findings correspond with the physiological results

obtained in estimating oxygen consumption in the multi-stage 20m shuttle run
test (t = 13.363; t = 7.765) and in the bicycle-ergometry test in the laboratory
(t = 3.506; resp. t = 2.700). The pupils (boys and girls) with a weekly regime of
high physical activities attained significantly (p ≤0.01; p ≤0.05) higher oxygen
consumption in both tests. The higher indices of oxygen consumption in the
multistage 20m shuttle run test can be explained by inter-individual
competition, which arises among the subjects during the testing procedures.
The better efficiency of the cardiovascular system of groups with higher
physical activity was confirmed also in the Ruffier's index (t = 6.736; t =
4.150). The positive effect of intensive physical activities is evident from the
parameters of physical performance. The results in tables 3 and 4 indicate that
a higher level of spontaneous physical activities constitutes an important part
in the structure of physical activities of the observed pupils and also have a
positive effect on their physical performance. The investigated differences are
in most cases (excluding standing broad jump and 50m dash for boys)
statistically significant. For example the differences in the 12-minute-run
(t = 4.579; t = 5.149), reflect not only the amount of persistence, but also the
influence on the need for achievement of the more active youngsters.

Tab. 4: Results of observed indices in 11 – 12 years girls with high and low physical activity
(n = 25 in each group) (Rychtecký, 1995)

Group with	High movement activity more – than 185 % BMR		Low movement activity – less than 170 % BMR		Diffe-rences	Signi-ficance
INDICES:	Mean	SD	Mean	SD	t- test	p <
Body height (cm)	155.20	9.84	159.50	6.42	1.277	-
Body weight (kg)	44.85	8.82	56.26	8.41	3.295	**
Body fat (%)	20.34	2.65	25.54	4.57	3.500	**
BMI	18.62		22.11		3.65	**
Ruffier´s index (index)	9.67	4.82	17.35	4.35	4.150	**
20m shuttle run (VO₂/ml/kg*min⁻¹)	51.38	2.33	42.96	3.07	7.765	**
bicycle ergometry (VO₂/ml/kg*min⁻¹)	40.30	6.07	33.00	6.90	2.700	**
Total motivation (points)	44.30	5,95	34.00	11.27	0.554	–
Net motivation (points)	42.84	7.17	37.07	10.13	0.452	–
Extroversion (points)	16.53	2.43	15.58	3.94	1.256	–
Neurotic tendencies (points)	13.92	5.32	15.15	4.62	2.212	–

The analysis of everyday physical activities of the observed youngsters confirms our hypothesis that spontaneous physical activities of children (playing with friends, physical activity, games and activities with their parents etc.) form the most important component of physical activities of their life and bring positive health and educational benefits. Other interesting results show that children with more intensive physical activities and better physical performance are smaller (not significant), weigh less and in particular have less body fat. These pupils (boys and girls) are probably not as advanced in their ontogenetic development, and obviously feel a higher need for physical activity in their everyday programme (they practice it more often) than children from the second group (with lower physical activity).

In other researches a significant relation between self-reflection on the state of health, physical fitness and physical activities in our other research was determined only in fifteen-year-old girls (Rychtecký, 1998).

Psychosocial effects of physical activities

An active lifestyle also has positive psychological effects. Some of the immediate effects are an improvement in the mood, a reduction of stress and tension. In the long run it increases self-assurance and influences the quality of life (Berger, 1996). Physical activity reduces anxiety and helps to react more adequately to different stress stimulations. Physical exercises potentially contribute to the quality of life by improving the mental state: good mood, self introspection (for example, reducing smoking) and by introducing new emotional experiences.

Physical activity – self-evaluation of the body image and of the body competence

Physical exercise influences the perception of the body. Individuals who practice sports intensively are more satisfied with their body but they control their weight in conformity with rational nutrition and health. The tendency to observe exaggerated diets is usually related to low physical activity. The general assumption is that there is a positive relation between physical activity and the evaluation of one's own physical competence. The following table documents the differences in self-evaluation between individuals who are more active in sports activities and those who are less active in them, and between physically fit and less fit persons.

The results in the table 5 show that physically active and physically fitter young people evaluate their own physical competence more positively than physically inactive individuals. Nevertheless no significant relation between physical activity and physical fitness was determined. The differences between physically more active and physically less active individuals were found in girls more often than in boys. Especially fifteen-year-old girls who were more engaged in physical and sports activities were significantly more self-confident in almost all the observed parameters.

Tab. 5: Differences in the self-evaluation of Czech respondents carrying out more intensive and less intensive physical activities, more and less physically fit (Rychtecký, 2002)

Competence	12-year-old boys	12-year-old girls	15-year-old boys		15-year-old girls	
	More Fit	Higher PA	Higher PA	More Fit	Higher PA	More Fit
Athletic abilities.		0.01 +	0.01 +	0.01 +	0.01 +	
Gracefully		0.05 +			0.05 +	
Flexibility		0.01 +	0.01 +		0.01 +	
Fitness	0.05 +	0.01 +	0.01 +		0.01 +	
Fastness	0.05 +	0.05 +	0.01 +		0.01 +	0.05 +
Strength	0.01 +			0.01 +	0.05 +	0.05 +
Courageousness					0.01 +	
Height					0.01 +	
Weight	0.05 +					
Appearance				0.01 +		

+: Significant difference in persons with high physical activity

Motivation towards physical and sports activities – the basis of the quality of life

Young people who regularly participate in physical activities will continue to do so when they grow up and become adults if they are consistently internally motivated. A consistent internal motivation is influenced by how the motivation towards physical activities is satisfied. Pleasant experiences as a product of participation in competitions play an important role in strengthening internal motivation and are essentially a positive emotional reaction to a sporting experience.

Much attention is devoted to the question of motivation towards physical and sports activities in research studies. Internal motivation has its biological basis in the need of movement and in the need of competition and self-determination (Deci & Ryan, 1985). These needs lead individuals to seek an optimal challenge – incentive, a co-acting stimulation from the environment. Motivation is a key psychological process which influences the decision about the frequency, intensity and duration of the participation in sports and in the same way the quality of life of young people and their life styles when they become adults (Van Reusel, Renson, Lefevere et al., 1990). The persistence and the efforts made are an indication of the motivation and are decisive for the effectiveness of their participation in sports (Singer, 1984). An opposite phenomenon, the decision to stop participating in sports is also a part of the motivation.

Tab. 6:   Motivation towards physical and sports activities (Rychtecký, 2002)

Variables	12-year-old boys	12-year-old girls	15-year-old boys	15-year-old girls
	Rank	Rank	Rank	Rank
My fiend do it	14	13	13	13
I want to make a career of it	8 +	10 +	14 +	14
I meet new people	11 +	8,5	10 +	5,5
I can do something that is good for me	2 +	1,5	1	1
I enjoy competition	3	5 +	4 +	7 +
I want to be physically fit	1	3 +	2 +	2 +
It relaxes me	12 +	11	7	8 +
I enjoy exercise	6	1,5	9 +	3 +
I like being part of the team	4	8,5	6 +	5,5 +
My family wants me to participate	15 +	15	15	15
I can get my body in shape	5	4	3	9
I can make money in it	16	16	16	16
It is exciting	9	14	11 +	11
It makes me physically attractive	13	12 +	12 +	12
I can meet friends	7	6 +	5 +	4 +
It gives me the opportunity for self expression	10 +	7 +	8 +	10 +

+: Significant difference in persons with high physical activity

The results (see Tab. 6), independently of the gender and age of the respondents show a significant agreement in the motivation to participate in sports. This agreement is mostly evident in the motivations which are assessed as important (I can do something that is good for me, I enjoy competition, I want to be physically fit, I can get my body into shape). On the contrary, we find significant differences in less preferred motivations Thus for instance a career in sports is evaluated as more important by young respondents rather than by older ones (rationalization of the position). Meeting new acquaintances is more important for girls than boys. Identical results were also found in other European countries (Telama, Naul, Nupponen et al., 2002). The motivation towards physical activity is influenced by various sources: by the family (the fact that the father practices sports has a stronger influence than if the mother practices sports), by the mass media, by the school and sports environment, by the sport's cultural traditions etc.

The results of finding out of the motivation include the answers of young people who do not practice sports. The answers are imaginative and they are influenced by received information and sources of publicity and even by the evaluation of past personal experience obtained in personal contact with sport.

The main reason why young people do not practice sport is explained by the lack of time and other obligations.

Goal orientation, need for achievement and physical activities

The analysis of goal orientation contributes to the understanding of how an individual obtains and interprets experiences and values pertaining to physical and sports activities. The research of goal orientation is usually classified as an inseparable part of projects studying participation in sports.

Goal orientation is closely related to the need of motivation for achieving performances and to the creation of motivation in sports. Their specific attributes are: feeling competitive, effort, the selection of tasks, performance, persistence etc. The challenge of the competition, the overcoming of internal and external obstacles is very important in sport. People show their competence by using goal orientation of the kind "task" and "ego". A subject oriented on the task "task orientation" concentrates this disposition on the development and training of new abilities and activities. He demonstrates his success by mastering them and at the same time strengthens his internal motivation (self discipline) and is a favourable factor for participation in sport.

On the other hand an individual with a predominating "ego orientation" has higher dispositions for and is more successful in activities in which he overcomes others with a minimum of effort. He strengthens his external motivation which depends on the social environment (Duda & Nicholls, 1992; Fox, 1996; Papaioannou, 1995; Guivernau & Duda, 1995; Walling & Duda, 1995).

The results in the table 7 shows that the order of the items are in better agreement among respondents of the same age than amongst those of the same gender. Preferences in "task orientation" are higher than in "ego orientation" but they become lower as the age increases. Practice in sports only deepens these tendencies in some cases. The worsening of the relation ego/task orientation (higher value of the index) may show that sports and school physical education are organized more as a competition (inter-individual comparison) than as an intra-individual comparison which is a more positive factor for the development of long term participation in sport.

A. Rychtecký

Tab. 7: Task and Ego orientation in physical and sports activities of the Czech youngsters (Rychtecký, 2002)

Items	12-year-old boys	12-year-old girls	15-year-old boys	15-year-old girls
	Rank	Rank	Rank	Rank
I am the one who can do the play or skill (Ego)	7	7	7	8
I learn a new skills and it makes me want to practice more. (Task)	3,5	3	9	3
I can do better than my friend (Ego)	5	6	5	7
The others don't do as well as me (Ego)	10	9	10	10
I learn something that is fun to do (Task)	2	2	1	1
Others mess up and I don't (Ego)	12	12	11	11
I learn a new skills by trying hard (Task)	9	8	12	12
I work really hard (Task)	6	5	8	9 +
I score the most points/goals etc. (Ego)	8 +	10	4	4
I am the best (Ego)	11	11	6	5
A skill I learn really feels right(Task)	3,5	4 +	3 +	2
I do my best (Task)	1	1	2	6
Rate: Ego / Task	0,76	0,77	0,93	0,91

+: Significant difference in persons with high physical activity

Conclusion

The evaluation of the all benefits of an active lifestyle is a very complicated task. The very rich literature in this area documents both identical and controversial results in the evaluation of the effects of physical activities, especially in cases in which the relation between physical activity and its supposed benefits are assessed as mono-casual and not in a bio-cultural context. The different methodological approaches, methods etc. are also a problem. At present two bio-cultural models predominate in research oriented on health. The first one tries to integrate the biological and environmental and cultural variables. The second one is a multi-segment model and judges biological data as the primary ones and environmental data as the secondary ones (McElroy, 1990).

We may find the same trend in the topic we are researching, inactivity in young people. Due to the fact that the effects of inactivity are often associated with the obesity of children and young people, biological data are predominantly studied. Nevertheless the cause of obesity can be determined by social factors which lead to a sedentary way of life and to obesity. Genetic influences, physical activities, nutrition, the family and social environment also play a very important role. It would be very useful to have a common European project which would compare national systems in the bio-cultural area both qualitatively, which is our present task, and quantitatively. It should not only deal with participation in sports, but also document and verify good examples which could be applied successfully in the European context of youth sport. The sports organizations devoted to children's and young people's sports should concentrate their attention on this group of young people who do not practice any sport.

References

Amisola, R. V. B. & Jacobson, M. S. (2003). Physical activity, exercise, and sedentary activity: Relationship to the causes and treatment of obesity. *Adolescent Medicine*. 14 (1), 23.

Berger, B. (1996). Psychological benefits of an active lifestyle: What we know and what we need to know. *Quest, 48*, 330-353.

Blair, S. (1985). Physical activity leads to fitness and pays off. *The Physician and Sports medicine, 11*, 87- 94.

Bouchard, C., Shepard, R. J., Stephens, T., Shutton, J. & McPherson, B. D. (1990). *Excercise, Fittness and Health: A Consensus of Current Knowledge*. Champaign, IL: Human Kinetic.

Deci, E. L. & Ryan, R. M. (1985). *Intrinsic motivation and self-determination in human behavior*. New York: Plenum Press.

Duda, J. & Nicholls, J. (1992). Dimensions of achievement motivation in schoolwork and sport. *Journal of Educational Psychology, 84*, 290-299.

Fox, K. (1996). Physical activity promotion and the active school. In N. Armstrong (Ed.), *New directions in physical education. Change and innovation* (pp. 94-109). London: Cassel.

Frömel, K., Novosad, J. & Svozil, Z. (1999). *Pohybová aktivita a sportovní zájmy mládeže*. (Physical activity and sporting interests of young people). Olomouc: Palacky University.

Frömel, K. & Sigmund, E. (2003). A komplex approach to the evaluation of the educational process in physical education. In R. Bartoszewicz, T. Koszczyc & A. Nowak (Eds.), *Kontrola i ocena w wychowaniu fizycznym* (pp. 83-89). Wroclaw: Wrocławskie Towarzystwo Naukowe.

Frömel, K. et al. (2004). Physical activity of men and women 18 to 55 years old in Czech republic. In F. Vaverka (Ed.), *Movement and Health* (pp. 169-173). Olomouc: Palacky Univerzity.

Guivernau, M. & Duda, J. (1995). Psychometric properties of a Spanish version of the task and ego orientation in sport questionnaire (TEOSQ) and beliefs about the causes of success inventory. *Revista de Psicologia del Deporte, 5*, 31-51.

Kučera, M. (1985). *Kvantitativní změny bipedální lokomoce (Qualitative changes in bipedal locomotion)*. Praha: Universita Karlova.

Leger, L. A. & Lambert, J. A. (1982). Maximal multistage 20-m shuttle run test to predict VO2 max. *European Journal of Applied Physiology, 49*, 1-12

Lüschen, G. L., Abel, T. L. Cockerham, W. L. & Kunz, G. (1993). Kausalbeziehungen und soziokulturelle Kontexte zwischen Sport and Gesundheit. *Sportwissenschaft*, 23 (2), 175-186.

McElroy, A. (1990). Biocultural Models in Studies of Human Health and Adaptation. *Medical Anthropology Quarterly, 4 (3)*, 243-265.

Medeková, H., Šelingerová, M. & Havlíček, I. (2001). Ontogenéza telesného rozvoja deti z hladiska pohybovej aktivity. In P. Tilionger, A. Rychtecký & T. Perič, *Sport v České republice na začátku nového tisíciletí (pp. 84-88)*.

Naul, R., Rychtecký, A. & Pauer, M. (1992). Daily Physical Activities and Motor Performance of West German and Czechoslovakian School Children. In J. Standeve, K. Hardman & D. Fischer, *Sport for All into 90 s* (pp. 204-211). Aachen: Meyer & Meyer Verlag.

Naul, R., Neuhaus, W. & Rychtecký, A. (1994). Daily Physical Activities and Motor Performance of West German and Czechoslovakian Schoolchildren. In R. C. Wilcox (Ed.), *„Sport in the Global Village"* (pp. 477-492). Morgantown: Fitness Information Technology.

Papaioannou, A. (1995). Motivation and goal perspectives in children's physical education. In S. J. H. Biddle (Ed.), *European perspectives on exercise and sport psychology* (pp. 245-269). Champaign, II.: Human Kinetics.

Perussa, L. & al (1989). Genetic and environmental influences on level of habitual physical activity and excercise participation. *American Journal of Epidemiology, 128 (5)*, 1012-1022.

Rychtecký, A. (1998). *Pohybová aktivita, motorická výkonnost a olympijské ideály evropské mládeže.* (Physical Activity, Movement performance and Olympic ideal of Euroepean Youth). Charles University report.

Rychtecký, A. (1993). Motivation of school youngsters for a lifelong physical activity. In *Proceedings of VIIth World Congress of Sport Psychology*, 803-806.

Rychtecký, A.(1994). The Contribution of School Physical Education to Life Long Activity. *Journal. of ICHPER-SD, 30*, 38-44.

Rychtecký, A., Pauer, M., Janouch V., Sýkora B. & Stejskal, F. (1995). Effect of Different Physical Activities on Physical Performance and Some Psychophysiological Characteristics of Youngsters aged 11-14 Years. *Kinesiologia Slovenica, 2 (1)*, 44-49.

Rychtecký, A., Naul, R. & Neuhaus, W. (1996). Physical Activity and Motor Performance of Prague and Essen School Children. *AUC-Kinanthropologica, 32 (2)*, 5-21.

Rychtecký, A. (2000). *Monitorování účasti ve sportu a pohybové aktivitě v České republice a v evropských zemích.* (Monitoring of participation in sport and physical activities in the Czech Republic and in the European countries). Ministry of Education, Youth and Sport report 149.

Singer, R. (1984). *Sustaining motivation in sport.* Tallahasse: Sports Consultants International.

Telama, R., Naul, R., Nupponen, H., Rychtecký, A. & Vuolle, P. (2002). *Physical Fitness, Sporting Lifestyle and Olympic Ideals: Cross-Cultural Studies on Youth Sport in Europe.* Sport Science Studies 11. Schorndorf: Verlag Karl Hofmann.

Thompson PD, Grouse SF, Goodpaster B, et al (2001). The acute versus the chronic response to exercise. *Med Sci Sports Exerc* 33(suppl): pp. 438-445,.

Van Reusel, B., Renson, R., Lefevere, J., Beunen, G., Simons, J., Claessens, A, Lysens, R., Vanden eynde, B. & Maes, H. (1990). Sportdeelname. Is jong geleerd ook oud gedaan? *Sport, 32 (3)*, 68-72.

Walling, M. & Duda, J. (1995). *Goals and their associations with beliefs about success in, and perceptions of, the purposes of Physical Education, Educational Psychology*, Champaign, Illinois: Human Kinetics.

Chapter 12:
Peculiarities of young people's lifestyle in the Baltic States

Skaiste Laskiene

Introduction

An overview of the scientific research and statistical data available in Lithuania and Latvia points to the fact that the physical activity of children and adolescents is widely studied, but not in depth. The abundance of scientific methods and methodologies used in research makes it difficult to compare the data, consequently, contradicting conclusions and evaluations of the data are made. Contradictions are also present in the assessment of children's physical activity. The majority of researchers tend to acknowledge that children's physical activity is not satisfactory. However, the international study of health behaviour in school-aged children (HBSC) has, after nearly ten years of research, confirmed that the change in criteria for assessing physical activity significantly changes the results of the research. Accordingly, depending on the chosen criterion for assessing physical activity, the results in Lithuanian and Latvian studies of school-aged children, within the international scale of data comparison, ranges from the lowest to the highest, so one of the main problems in this field of research is the low validity of research methods.

Despite their cultural differences children and adolescents have similar demands – appropriate home, care, healthy nutrition, education, and, finally, physical exercise. Therefore, strategic goals to improve children's and adolescents' health across countries are also similar: to implement health care programs by emphasizing regular medical examinations and promoting physical education. The promotion of physical education, physical exercise and fitness is an important and demanding task.

Attitude towards Physical education and sports in educational systems

Since the reestablishment of independent Lithuania on 11th of March 1990, a change in the attitude towards physical education has taken place. Physical education is treated as a holistic (unified) trend with a particular emphasis on the physical nature of a young person, his or her health, physical abilities, age, sex, lifestyle, and right to one's free choice, but not on the mere recording of results of certain physical capacities (Lietuvos respublikos Švietimo ir mokslo ministerija, 1999). Physical education is seen as a tool to achieve personal physical, mental and spiritual harmony, i.e. to improve young people's health. It is essential that physical activity in schools would inspire the joy and pleasure of movement, self-confidence, and respect to the activity of others. Such activity should make young people realise how important exercising is to their health and, thus, instil in them the habit of regular exercising. For this purpose four new educational curricula of physical education have been introduced in Lithuania since 1990 on this purpose (Lietuvos respublikos Švietimo ir mokslo ministerija, 1997).

Latvian Ministry of Education and Science is a leading public administration institution in the field of education and science. In compliance with the regulations of the Ministry of Education and Science and the Education Law, the Ministry implements a unified national policy and development strategy in education, develops policies in education, science, sport, youth and state language.

On 24 October 2002 the Saeima adopted the Sport Law. According to the Law the Ministry of Education and Science and the Sport Department have to implement a unified state policy and development strategy in the field of sport. The purpose of the Law is to provide general and legal basis for the organization and development of sport, interrelation among sports organizations, state and municipal institutions and their basic tasks in sport development, as well as to provide a basis for sports funding (Latvian Ministry of education and science, 2004).

The fourth Sports Congress held on 14 January 2001 evaluated the recent progress of the sport developments, underlying importance of inter-sectoral co-operation in favour of sports. The three main objectives of the Latvian sports policy are firstly to provide legal, economical and social conditions for every individual to participate in sport irrespective of one's age, sex, nationality, race, religion, mental and physical abilities, secondly to determine public responsibility for providing physical education programmes for children and young people at every educational institution and thirdly to promote participation of most talented athletes at Olympic and Paralympic Games, World and European Championships (Council of Europe, 2002).

The third Sports Congress of Lithuania that took place on 27 June 2000 charted the strategy of the country's physical education and sports. It noted that ten years of independence saw few changes in society's attitude towards physical activity and sports; consequently, there was little progress in improving physical activity of young people. On the contrary, an increase in poor health, drug addiction, violation of law by young people was observed (Lietuvos sporto taryba, 2000).

Congress has set the strategic goal of Lithuanian physical education: "To create an efficient system of physical education that would encourage the need for physical fitness, health improvement, secure, healthy and productive lifestyle, would provide joy of life, conditions for physical, spiritual, moral and cultural development of a child, a teenager, a student, a soldier or any working or handicapped person" (ibid., p. 34). The Department of Physical Education and Sports under the Government of the Republic of Lithuania works in close cooperation with the Ministry of Education and Science, Ministry of National Defence, Ministry of Health, the Lithuanian National Olympic Committee and other organizations in order to implement the goal. However, the analysis of causes for physical inactivity of young people demonstrates that the cooperation between institutions should have a common action strategy with clear directions for analysis of the situation set and clear distribution of areas of responsibility in order conditions for young people to live an active and healthy lifestyle would be guaranteed. This is partly implemented through the strategy of Lithuanian physical education and sports for the period 2000 – 2012 (Lietuvos sporto taryba, 2000). Yet the strategy emphasizes the implementation of sports directions and aims rather than those of physical education. This could be explained by the fact that physical activity of school-aged children is a prerogative of the Ministry of Education. It should be mentioned that school physical education is currently undergoing crisis as an unattractive part of education due to outdated teaching methods and loss of touch with everyday realities.

As we mentioned before, the Ministry of Education and Science is responsible for providing physical education at schools. Law on Education, which determines physical education classes 2-3 times a week in schools, regulates compulsory organization of physical activities. In parallel with compulsory physical education, different out-of-class sport activities are organized by school clubs, regional/city sports schools, School sport federation, Youth Sports Centre. 14 % out of the 342.000 schoolchildren take active part in optional sports activities.

It should be emphasised that the subject of PE/sport in Latvia has the same problem as in many other European countries, that even if the legal status of the subject is the same as other subjects taught in the schools the actual status of the subject compared to other curriculum subjects is inferior. Careful efforts have to be made to find reasons for that and to try to improve the importance and position of physical education and sport (Council of Europe, 2002).

According to the law of Physical education and sport three lessons of P.E. weekly should be introduced in primary, secondary and higher educational institutions and not less than one hour per day in pre-school institutions since the 1995 (Lietuvos Respublikos Kūno kultūros ir sporto įstatymas, 1995). One of the reasons preventing schools from increasing schoolchildren's physical activity or introducing the third lesson of physical education per week is insufficient availability of facilities and equipment.

The publication of the Sports Congress of Lithuania (Lietuvos sporto taryba, 2000) states that 347 secondary and primary schools lack sports halls. A group of 3-4 grades simultaneously use sports facilities available in schools that points to the shortage of facilities. Therefore, the school network should be restructured in such a way that general school would have a sports hall and outdoor sports facilities. These would be minimal requirements.

Kardelis, Kavaliauskas & Balzeris (2001) research shows that 12.4 % of secondary schools in Lithuania do not have any sports hall. Schools in cities and towns are better equipped; however some of them lack outdoor sports facilities. 37.7 % of schools have 2 sports halls, 31.5 % have a training hall, 21.3 % have an aerobics hall (traditionally it is a school meeting hall) and 52 % of schools have other sports facilities. Very few schools can afford to allow only one group (grade) of schoolchildren use their sports hall, especially in cities/towns where schools are large. On average 2.04 groups (grades) simultaneously train in sports halls in cities/towns and 1.6 groups (grades) in villages. This number for outdoors sports facilities is 2.3 and 1.7 respectively.

Unlike other countries, Latvia spends more money from its education budget to cover regular maintenance and upkeep of school buildings (Latvian Ministry of Education and Science, 2000).

Economical and social situation in Lithuania and Latvia with regard to physical education

Current economic and social situation in Lithuania calls for new, updated and effective ways and means to reinforce physical education and fitness of school-aged children.

Department of Statistics has carried out a survey on relative poverty rate in Lithuania (Fig. 1). According to the study, households with children under 18 dominate in the group of the households that are classified as living below relative poverty level[1]. Relative poverty rate[2] among the households with children in 2002 was 19.5 % (the country's average is 16.6 %). In comparison to 2001 the poverty rate increased insignificantly (0.1 %). The poverty rate among the households with children under 18 increased by 1.1 %.

The study also shows that the relative poverty rate depends on the number of children in the family (Statistikos departamentas, 2002).

The results of a study conducted by the Economics Institute of the Latvian Academy of Sciences, "The Family in Latvia" showed if the family has more children more of the household expenses (over 40 – 50 %) are for groceries which points to the relative low standard of living. What is very disturbing is

[1] Relative poverty level is 50 % of the average of consumption expenditure
[2] Poverty rate is the rate of inhabitants that live below poverty level. Their consumption expenditure is lower than the estimated poverty level for that year.

the fact that in families with more children, the average amount spent to feed each child is much less. Health related expenses show the same pattern.

Fig. 1:   Relative poverty rate (%) in households with children in 2002

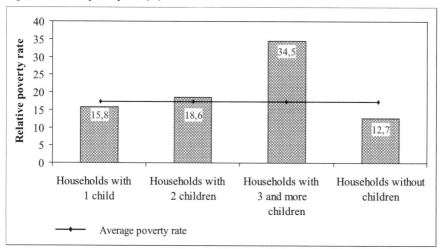

The greatest part of a family's income is spent on food, clothing and shelter – up to 75 %. That means that there is less to spend on other necessities, including education. Children's talents and abilities are not realized to their fullest potential due to financial hardship (Latvian Ministry of education and science, 2000).

The research data on household budget in Lithuania indicates that in 2002 monthly disposable income of households with children under 18 was 362 Litas per person (this is 86 % of the country's average). In comparison to the previous year, the disposable income increased by 1.5 %, however taking inflation into consideration, the disposable income increased by 1.2 %. The biggest amount of income (Table 1) is expended for food and non-alcoholic beverages. (Statistikos departamentas, 2002).

Almost 60 % of respondents (Lithuanian State Department of Physical Education and Sports, 2002) cannot allocate any finances for sports services. The results are presented in Table 2.

Transformation to a free market economy and democratic society has showed how difficult it is to change a traditional attitude towards health, fitness, physical activity and sport. Health care and education reforms in Lithuania and Latvia still leave open questions of how to organize physical activity and physical education in order to ensure physical fitness and good health in school-aged children.

224   S. Laskiene

Tab. 1: Consumption expenditure structure in households with children in 2002 (%)

	Households with children under 18	of these:			Households without children
		with 1 child	with 2 children	with 3 and more children	
Total consumption	100,0	100,0	100,0	100,0	100,0
Food and non alcoholic beverages	39,9	38,1	40,3	48,6	41,4
Alcoholic beverages	1,9	2,0	1,8	1,5	2,2
Tobacco	1,7	1,8	1,6	1,5	1,6
Clothing and footwear	7,5	7,6	7,6	6,9	5,4
Housing, water, electricity, gas and other fuel	12,6	13,3	12,3	9,6	15,3
Furnishing, household equipment and routine maintenance of the house	5,6	5,9	5,6	3,7	4,3
Health care	2,8	2,9	2,8	2,4	6,7
Transport	7,6	7,3	8,0	7,3	6,3
Communication	5,2	5,3	5,3	4,2	5,3
Recreation and culture	5,1	5,3	4,8	4,4	3,6
Education	1,0	1,1	0,9	0,4	0,3
Hotels, restaurants, cafes, canteens	5,2	5,0	5,4	5,6	4,1
Miscellaneous goods and services	4,0	4,3	3,7	3,9	3,5

Physical activity of school-aged children

National health scientists and specialists of physical education have long been discussing what standard norms for length and intensity of physical activity should be applied. Despite the diversity of opinions, it is jointly agreed that a medium intensity physical activity, similar to adults, is the most appropriate for young people. Scientific evidence confirms that this kind of moderate and regular physical activity has the greatest benefit for health (Physical activity and Health, 1996).

In 1997 an international team of experts formulated the main recommendations of physical activity for young people (Biddle, Sallis, Cavill, 1998). The document states that young people should be physically active for at least an hour a day. It is considered that sufficient physical exercise means an increase in intensity of heartbeat, breathing, and body heat. Intensive walking, playing basketball, etc.

Tab. 2:   The amount of finances that family can allocate for sport services (What biggest amount of finances do you allocate per month paying for sport services?).

	Replied		Among them							
			Girls		Boys		City residents		Village residents	
	In total	%	In total	%	In total	%	In total	%	In total	%
Do not allocate	278	59,40	130	62,20	148	57,14	180	52,63	98	77,78
Up to 50 Lt	165	35,26	70	33,49	95	36,68	139	40,64	26	20,63
Up to 100 Lt	23	4,91	8	3,83	15	5,79	21	6,14	2	1,59
Up to 200 Lt	1	0,21	1	0,48	—	0,00	1	0,29	—	0,00
200 Lt and more	1	0,21	—	0,00	1	0,39	1	0,29	—	0,00

achieves such conditions. In addition, physical activity for bone and muscle system should be introduced two or more times a week. The new recommendations differ entirely from those formulated in 1994 (Sallis & Patrick, 1994) that set a standard of 20 minutes physical activity three or more times a week.

Scientists from different fields of study participate in the assessment of physical activity of school-aged children in Lithuania and Latvia. The institutions of physical education, education and health conduct most of the research. Although they use different methodology and the results of their research cannot always be compared, they come to a single conclusion that physical activity is not sufficient for the normal physical condition of school-aged children in two Baltic States. The number of schoolchildren involved in school sports activities in villages is statistically higher (p <0,001) than those in towns, yet the number of students engaged in sports activities outside the school curriculum (sports schools, clubs) is higher in cities/towns than in villages. This is because there are more sports facilities available in cities/towns than there are in villages. For example, in 1999 there were 798 sports organizations in cities/towns and 529 in villages (Lietuvos sporto statistikos departamentas, 1999). The most active in this respect are the boys who are both physically active in schools and engage in extra curricular activities. In general boys are more active than girls and this has been confirmed by a number of researchers (Zuozienė, 1998; Levickienė & Kardelis, 1999). 21.3 % of girls participate in school sports activities and 10.3 % attend sport schools and clubs (30.8 % and 20.2 % of boys respectively). Senior boys do not change their sporting habits (Zaborskis, 1996; Zuozienė, 1998), yet senior girls become more passive.

A statistical report of the Ministry of Education in Lithuania (Lietuvos respublikos Švietimo ir mokslo ministerija, 2000), asserted that 51,949 school-children attended sports schools, i.e. 9.3 % of all schoolchildren: 37.7 % of all primary schoolchildren and 20.9 % of all 11-18-year-old gymnastic adolescents. The percentage of school-aged children who attended school sports clubs were: 37.7 % in primary schools; 29.3 % in secondary village schools; 24.1 % in secondary town and city schools and 20.9 % in gymnasiums. This report pointed to the decreasing number of primary schoolchildren involved in sports: 11 % of 7-year-old schoolchildren, 17 % of 8-year-old schoolchildren, 18 % of 9-year-old schoolchildren, and 25 % of 10-11-year-old schoolchildren. In the group of adolescents, those attending sports clubs ranged from 22 % to 29 %.

The research of Kardelis et al. (2001) shows that 33.2 % of village schoolchildren and 37 % of city/town schoolchildren consider themselves as physically active, i.e., they exercise daily. Another part of the respondents (25.6 % of village schoolchildren and 28 % of city/town schoolchildren) exercise only at weekends, whereas the rest of the participants of the research (26.7 % of village schoolchildren and 33.2 % of city/town schoolchildren) do not exercise at all. Schoolchildren are more physically active during their holidays and boys are more physically active than girls. Morning exercises are mostly disliked by senior schoolchildren; furthermore, it is ignored by 62.9 % of city/town male adolescents and 42.5 % female adolescents.

Fig.. 2:   Participation in sports activities after school hours

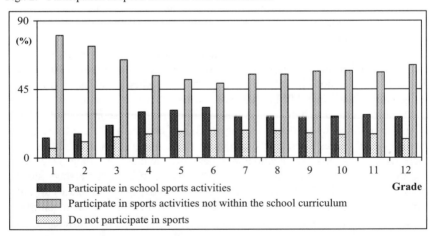

More than half of schoolchildren do not participate in any additional sports activities (Figure 2). Therefore, the necessity to have the third lesson of physical education per week for schoolchildren is essential.

The number of 1-4 grade schoolchildren involved in school sports activities is smaller than that of senior grades, however, the total number involved increases up to grade 6 (from 13.3 % to 33.1 %), then it shows no rise in the group of grades 7-12 and remains within 27.7 %. The number of students involved in sports activities outside the school curriculum rises in grades 1-7 (from 6.3 % to 18.8 %), after that it decreases to 12.4 % in grade 12.

One of the latest research initiated by the Lithuanian State Department of Physical Education and Sports was carried out in 2001. The respondents were asked about the frequency of exercise individually and attending organised sports practices (free training sessions in educational institutions, paid sport practices, supplementary education sport practices at the educational institutions, practices in health clubs, sports clubs). Figures 3 and 4 show the results for both groups of exercise.

Fig. 3:   The frequency of exercise by Lithuanian schoolchildren individually (hours per week)

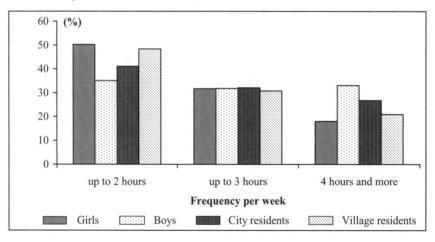

Insufficient physical activity has been determined in 50 % of school children aged 6-8, 60 % of teenagers aged 6-12, and 75-80 % adolescents in Latvia. Statistical data convey that 80% of all school-aged children have bad posture because of sedentary lifestyle, unbalanced nutrition, TV or computer addiction (Lazda, 1982; Kokina, 2002).

Fig. 4:   The frequency of attending organised sports practises by Lithuanian schoolchildren
(hours per week)

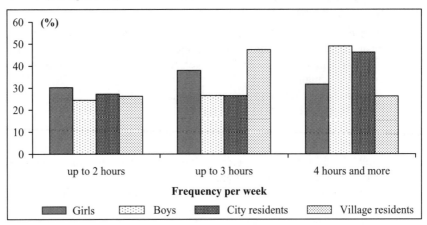

Latvian researchers (Latvijas jaunatnes sporta centrs, 2003; LR Veselības
veicināšanas centrs, 2004) were interested in the frequency of sports activities
for school children during the school year (the results are presented in Table 3)
and during their summer holidays (Table 4).

Tab. 3:   Time per week spent on sports activities for school children aged 11-14 during the
school year, including PE lessons

Age	9 hours/week	6 – 8 hours/week	4 – 5 hours/week	3 hours/week	0 – 2 hours/week
11 – 15	5%	12%	24%	38%	21%
15 – 25	2%	7%	12%	17%	62%

Tab. 4:   Sports activities of young people during their summer holidays in 1998 (according
to Grabovska, 1999)

Sports activity (%)	Girls (7 – 16-years-old)	Boys (7 – 16-years-old)	Comparison
do not take part in any sports	45.9	54.2	8.3
occasionally (twice a week, at least 45 min.)	32.3	20.4	11.9
several times a week	18.4	19.3	0.9
every day	3.4	6.1	2.7

Health and fitness

Health assessment of children and adolescents is based on the surveys of their physical and psychical development, the data about mortality rate, health condition, and a healthy lifestyle. Due to specific development factors of adolescence period (10-19 years of age) additional assessment should be carried out that takes into consideration the adolescent's attitude to his/her personal health, emotional problems, self-destructive behaviour, aggression, violence, smoking, drugs and alcohol abuse. This information proves essential when analysing physical activity and the fitness of adolescents. The following is based on selected data about the physical development, health and fitness of children and adolescents in Lithuania and Latvia. This data will allow us to inter relate physical activity, health, fitness, and the quality of life.

As in many other countries, in the Baltic States, over the past decades, an accelerated process of reaching puberty is observed (physical, sexual and psychological development at an earlier age compared to previous generations) (Balčiūnienė et al., 1991; Tutkuvienė, 1995).

Since 1965, the height of children and adolescents in Lithuania has increased on an average of 2 to 8 cm, but their chest, waist and hip measurements have become relatively smaller along with their weight, lung capacity and physical strength, in other words, asthenization has taken place. This effect in accelerated puberty is caused by reduced physical activity and disproportionate growth of internal organs. Fast physical development does not always coincide with physical development causing a gap between the physical and social growth of an individual. This is the cause of psychological and pedagogical problems (Nacionalinės sveikatos taryba, 2000).

The changes in the height and weight of Latvian schoolchildren aged 7 to 15 years have been recorded in Aboltina's (1998) and Valtneris' (2001) research. The change observed in boys' height (aged 7-10) is about 3 cm and has a tendency to decrease, while the change observed in boys aged 11-15 years is 2-3 cm and has a tendency to increase (Table 5). The changes to girls' height show similar tendencies.

Analysing the results of the weight of the 7-15 age male group (Table 6) the tendency to gain weight averages 2-4 kg. This can be seen particularly in the 13-14 age group. The greatest difference in weight change is seen in the girls aged 7-8 and the change of weight of older girls is around 1 kg.

Considering a healthy lifestyle, most of Lithuanian schoolchildren take an interest in unhealthy pursuits, sexual activity, and healthy nutrition (Figure 5). 80.2 % of the city/town schoolgirls and 78.3 % of the village schoolgirls are interested in

Tab: 5:   Changes in height of male and female, ageing from 7 to 15 years

Age (years)			7	8	9	10	11	12	13	14	15
Height (cm)	1991	Male	129	133	141	145	147	153	161	167	171
		Female	126	133	138	145	149	152	161	163	168
	2001	Male	126	134	138	135	148	155	165	170	173
		Female	124	130	138	141	147	155	159	163	167

Tab. 6:   Changes in weight of male and female, ageing from 7 to 15 years

Age (years)			7	8	9	10	11	12	13	14	15
Weight (kg)	1991	Male	26,4	27,5	28,9	31,9	35,3	42,2	44,6	51,1	57,5
		Female	24,4	27,7	29,3	35,4	37,3	41,0	49,6	53,7	56,2
	2001	Male	26,3	28,1	30,1	34,0	38,2	43,3	50,1	56,0	61,9
		Female	22,8	25,1	30,9	33,6	37,4	42,9	50,0	55,8	57,0

the question of overweight. Also 76.3 % of the city/town schoolgirls and 63.3 % of the village schoolgirls pointed out the necessity of discussions about unhealthy pursuits (p <0.05). Girls are less interested in questions of sexual activity than boys. 51.3 % of the city/town school adolescent females and 46.6 % of the village adolescent females think these questions are important, while 72.8 % of the city/town adolescent males and 69.5 % of the village adolescent males were interested in the questions of sexual activity. The next most interesting item for boys is unhealthy pursuits (66.1 % and 63.2 % respectively) (Kardelis, Kavaliauskas & Balzeris, 2001).

Fig. 5:   Health related topics that schoolchildren take interest in

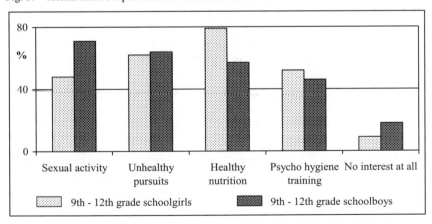

The analysis of primary medical care reports on children aged between 0-14 years shows a rise in the number of health problems in this age group. In 1990 730 children in 1,000 were diagnosed with various health problems, in 1998 the figure increased twofold (LR Sveikatos apsaugos ministerija, 2002). Respiratory problems are among the most frequent health problems (65 %). Bad posture is the cause of wide spread bone and muscle system disorders: 25-30 % of all school-aged children have bad posture; another 6-8 % suffer from scoliosis (Saniukas, Aleksejevas, 1991). Research has shown that the first sign of spine rotation – FBT asymmetry – is manifested at the pre-school stage, at the age of 3-4 11.6 % of children suffer bad posture, and 16.3 % are diagnosed with FBT asymmetry (Petravičius, 2000). Medical examination of 6-7 year old children at the Institute of Hygiene testifies that half of the examined children had asymmetrical posture (Juškelienė, 1998). To prevent the onset of scoliosis, the doctors recommend muscle exercise such as remedial gymnastics, swimming and water treatment. Emphasis on physical activity, training of back and abdomen muscles, mental control of posture are the means of healthy development of the spine (Juškelienė & Dailidienė, 1999).

In Latvia in 1996 6.9 % of school-aged children were admitted completely healthy. Signs of depression were observed in 20 % of cases, regular agitation, nerviness and bad moods was felt by 45 % of students, 15 % of teenagers complained they felt lonely and ignored, and only 7 % felt happy and satisfied. This showed evidence of mental health problems.

The state of Latvian children's health today is getting worse in many respects. According to medical statistical data, this is how children judge their own health: 'I am completely healthy' – 25 %; 'I am quite healthy' – 64 %; 'I am not healthy' – 11 % (LR Veselibas ministrija, 1996). Girls at the age of 13 acknowledge having most health-related problems. Only 7.1 % of them do not mention a pathological symptom in answering questions about their health. Comparing personal assessment of their health in school-aged children and medical examination data it is seen that only 6.9 % of Latvian school-aged children are completely healthy. The most frequent health problems are caused because of unhealthy food, bad teeth-cleaning habits, deficiency of physical activity, drug abuse, and insufficient knowledge about sexual behaviour (Veselības veicināšanas centrs, 1999).

Most Latvian doctors acknowledge that bad posture and insufficient physical activity in childhood and adolescence could cause disability in adulthood (Rubana, 1998; Knipše, Baumanis & Kokina, 2001; Diržine, 2004). Z. Kasvande (2004) has carried out research in the Health and Medical Rehabilitation Centre, which demonstrates that 11 % of pre-school and primary school children have minor deviations in their posture, 26 % have average deviations in their posture, and 63 % have serious deviations in their posture. As a result, additional corrective gymnastics in schools have been recommended to the Ministry of Education.

Alcohol consumption and smoking

Teenage alcohol abuse is especially hazardous as the transitional period between episodic alcohol abuse and alcoholism is short. Alcohol addiction and abstinence syndrome develop much faster in adolescents than in adults. The deterioration of health and degradation of personality in young alcoholics also develops fast and the risk of traumas increases. Alcohol abuse is a frequent cause of juvenile delinquency. It is also recorded that children try alcohol for the first time during family holidays with the encouragement of their parents (Davidavičienė, 1996). The ESPAD (European School Project of Alcohol and Other Drugs) has researched alcohol and other drug abuse thoroughly among 15-16-year-old adolescents (ESPAD, 2000; Davidavičienė, 1996). 30 countries, including Lithuania, participated in the research. Research in 1999 found that 15-16-year-old Lithuanian adolescents used alcohol more frequently than was established by the HBSC (Curie, Samdal, Boyce et al., 1998) research. For instance, 81.2 % of boys and 65.5 % of girls said they had been intoxicated by alcohol at least once. According to the HBSC research in 1998 the percentage for boys and girls was respectively 58.8 % and 45.7 %, that is, considerably less than in the ESPAD research.

Various research data ascertain the relationship between alcohol intake and the habit of smoking, progress at school, and hobbies of adolescents. ESPAD (Davidavičienė, 1996; ESPAD, 2000) confirms that nearly everyone who takes smoking-based drugs also smokes cigarettes. That is why smoking is hazardous to health; furthermore, it is a form of addiction and should be treated as a drug addiction risk.

Physical activity and risk behaviour

Numerous studies in Lithuania and in other countries focus on the behaviour of adolescents that have a positive or negative influence on their health (Wold, 1989; Pate, Heath, Dowda et al., 1996). L. Jaruševičienė (2000) has done research involving 3,000 15-16-year-old schoolchildren. The research reveals the relationship between alcohol abuse, smoking and indiscriminate sexual behaviour. Any form of risk behaviour – alcohol abuse, smoking or drug addiction – is related to a more intensive sexual activity. 78.3 % of sexually active adolescent girls are frequent smokers; in comparison, only 4.6 % of girls who do not have a sexual relationship smoke frequently. All sexually active girls try some smoking and 63.6 % of girls who do not have sexual relationship have never tried smoking. The same tendencies are observed among boys, yet the relationship between smoking and sexual activity is less expressed: 22.2 % of sexually active adolescent boys smoke frequently and 6.8 % of boys who do not have sexual relationship smoke frequently. Sexually active adolescents consume more alcohol than those who do not have sexual relationship. No obvious relationship between physical activity and early or indiscriminate sexual behaviour has been noted. That explains the fact that not all forms of behaviour harmful to one's health have yet been thoroughly researched.

It is thought that physical activity and sport might balance activities that are harmful to one's health or even bring such behaviour to an end. The research on school-aged children's health conduct helps to substantiate this statement. The relationship between risk behaviour (smoking and alcohol abuse) and physical activity is most expressed in the group of 13-year-old girls. The more physically active the girls are, the less frequently alcohol abuse or the habit of smoking is noted. The research carried out in 1998 did not detect such relationship, whereas the research of 1994 proved the opposite tendency in boys, that is, physically active boys smoked and consumed alcohol more frequently than those who were physically passive (Zaborskis, 1996; Zaborskis ir kt, 1996).

Some authors explain the correlation between positive and negative behaviour of adolescents by referring to their socializing model (Wold, 1989; Pate et al., 1996). The conclusions based on the research of these authors and on our own investigations show that the physical activity of Lithuanian adolescents is currently not completely health oriented. Therefore, the promotion of more intensive physical activity must draw attention to sport as the source of health, and therefore incompatible with smoking or consumption of alcohol.

Scientific research in Lithuania demonstrates that the health improvement program 'Let's grow healthy' (Zaborskis ir kt., 1995; Zaborskis ir kt, 1993), currently implemented in primary schools of Lithuania, could bring beneficial results in encouraging physical activity (Zaborskis & Šumskas, 1993, 1995; Zaborskis, 1997). In addition to all other means of enhancing health, fitness, and physically active lifestyle such a program could also be implemented in other age groups.

Physical activity, motivation and environment

The research done by K. Kardelis (1993) testifies that ambitions to engage in sports and be physically active are conditioned by a complicated system of various factors. The research, based on rich material collected from school-aged children and university students of Kaunas, draws the conclusion that the closest psychosocial environment of school-aged children, like family, school, classmates, and friends, are the components that influence school-aged children's physical activity. Other factors, such as personal psychological qualities, information about physical activity and health, geographical conditions, and climate also influence the choice of a particular physical activity, but are of indirect influence and are dependent on the former (Figure 6).

Fig. 6:   Physical activity of school-aged children and sources of aspiration to exercise

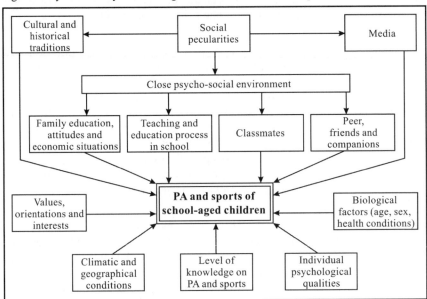

The most popular motive for physical activity among the school-aged children in Lithuania was the improvement in their health, such an answer was provided by 67.7 % of respondents, 60.6 % of boys and 68.7 % of girls (p <0.001). Other equally important motives were fitness, a beautiful body, encouragement by parents, and the experience of achievement (Table 7)[†].

S.Vainauskas (1998) has explored how school-aged children assess their own health. 6-, 9-, 11-, 13- and 15-year-old school children were tested. The author researched the attitude of school-aged children to the physical education lessons and their incentives for physical activity. 80.8 % of respondents replied they enjoyed the physical education lessons. A positive evaluation of physical education lessons was given by 89 % of boys and 72.9 % of girls (p <0.001).

[†] *p <0.05; **p <0.01; ***p <0.001, comparison of the groups according to sex and place of residence

Tab. 7:   Motivations for engaging in physical activity (according to Vainauskas, 1998)

Motive	Average	Boys	Girls	Town/City	Village
Health improvement	64.7	60.6***	68.7	65.8	63.8
Fitness	58.6	56.9**	60.2	60.6**	56.7
Body enhancement	48.3	39.6***	56.6	48.3	48.3
Please parents	45.5	44.5	46.5	44.1*	46.8
Achievement	42.7	47.6***	57.9	42.8	42.6
Control of the body	39.9	40.0	39.9	40.7	39.3
Results	38.8	42.1***	35.6	40.6**	37.1
New friends	33.8	30.0***	37.5	33.4	34.2
Become a star	30.5	34.2***	26.9	30.0	30.9
Meet friends	25.0	24.5	25.5	24.3	25.6
Enjoyment	13.8	13.7	13.9	15.3**	12.5

Questions of motivation are raised in the Master thesis by I. Lapinska (2000). The author of the research reveals that 22.11 % of respondents engage in sports because they want to feel good and be healthy; 20.05 % of the respondents intend to improve their posture; 11.82 % of the respondents wish to be fit, and 18.77 % of the respondents find sport a method of fighting stress. The research of J. Porozov (2004) aims at relating the physical activity of children and the habits of physical activity of their families. 34.5 % of respondents indicated that one of their parents engaged in some physical leisure activity. The research revealed that if the father of the family enjoyed physical activity, the chances that the children would be physically active went up by 1.5 times (CI 95 %: 1.28–1.69).

The assumption that physically active parents motivate their children is also confirmed by Lithuanian researchers (Viliūnienė & Jankauskienė, 2002). The aim of the research was to determine how physically active and passive parents treated the physical fitness and physical activity of their children. The results of the research reveal that physically active parents pay much more attention to physical fitness and health than physically passive parents; they read specialised literature and frequently attend sports events. Physically passive parents justify their inactivity by stating that they would rather spend time with the family. Physically active parents often play games and go in for sports with their children, buy sports goods. Children of physically active parents are more physically active than those of passive parents. The research also calls for a further investigation of the family as a source of motivation for children's physical activity.

The participants of the research initiated by the Department of Physical Education and Sport stated the joy of exercising as their main motive for engaging in physical activity (50.79 %). 40.13 % admitted that it was their personal decision to start some physical activity; 16.67 % were encouraged by their parents, 14.5 % by their teachers, and 18.35 % by their friends (Figure 7). Among the most frequently mentioned driving forces behind the decision to go in for sports were the wish to improve one's physical fitness, health and work efficiency (72.61 %), and the possibility to enjoy achievement over other contestants (Lithuanian State Department of Physical Education and Sports, 2002).

Fig. 7:   People who influence going in for sport

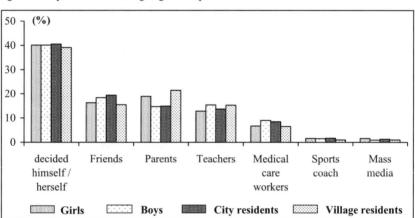

The book also includes the analysis of motives for physical inactivity. The main reasons for school-aged children's physical inactivity were as follows (Figure 8): 29.48 % blamed the lack of energy and will, 27.49 % indicated bad health state.

Types of passive leisure

During the period of 1992-1994 V. Volbekienė ir G. Mikaitienė (1998) assessed the physical activity of 4,493 Lithuanian boys and 4,916 girls. The research revealed that only 10-15 % of all participants chose sport as their leisure activity. Only 9 % of the girls and 16 % of the boys were sufficiently active.

In assessing physical activity it is important to know what other leisure activities, apart from sports and games, school-aged children have, for example, how much time they spend watching TV, videos, or playing computer games. Such types of passive leisure make the person spend time in isolation.

Fig. 8: Reasons not going in for sport

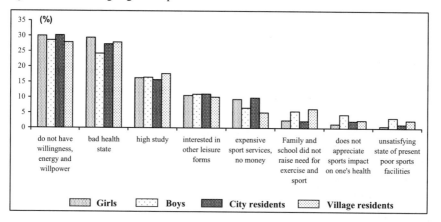

The passive leisure activities of school-aged children in Lithuania and Latvia in the years 1985-1990, were researched by K.Kardelis' (1993) who found that 1/3 (33.6 %) of 8-18-year-old Kaunas schoolchildren and adolescents spent their leisure time learning, reading or visiting cultural events. 45.3 % of girls and 21.9 % of boys devoted their time for these types of passive leisure. Passive types of leisure were also needlework, knitting and crochet work (5.2 %), listening to music (3.9 %), and watching TV (2.3 %). It is interesting to mention that, despite the statistical figure stating that 2.3 % of the children spent time watching TV, this was the most popular type of activity (boys watched 7.5 ±0.34 hours, girls – 6.6 ±0.26 hours). The author of the research stated that the older the school child, the more passive leisure he/she enjoys. Moreover, in comparison to the research data from the years 1966 and 1976, the number of physically passive school aged children increased.

There is more research in Lithuania which demonstrates that schoolchildren, girls in particular, frequently choose physically passive type of leisure activities like watching TV or video, playing computer games, reading, and etc. (Baubinas & Vainauskas, 1998; Zuoziené, 1998). Levickiené and Kardelis' (1999) research shows that schoolgirls devote 26.7 % of their time to reading, 31 % – listening to music, and 29.1 % – meeting friends. The dominating passive leisure activity among boys is playing computer games (24.8 % of the respondents). I. Zuoziené (1998) states that among the designated types of leisure activity 56.2 % of those selected by boys and 47 % of those selected by girls are active types of leisure. Regrettably, a large group of schoolchildren do not participate in any extra curricula sports activity. This group is by 12.8 % larger in villages than it is in cities/towns. This is confirmed by the 1998 research conducted by A. Baubinas and S. Vainauskas who make the conclusion that 63.3 % of schoolchildren in villages and 15.3 % of schoolchildren in cities/towns do not exercise sufficiently. TV watching is one of the most popular leisure time activities in Latvia also. Only 24 % (Table 8) of all respondents regularly spend their leisure time physically actively while the number of pupils regularly watching TV is bigger by a factor of two.

Tab. 8: How school pupils spend their leisure time

Leisure time activities	Regularly	Frequently	Rarely	Never
Sports activities	24%	51%	21%	4%
watch TV	41%	32%	26%	1%
Computer activities	24%	26%	33%	16%
going to cinema	2%	11%	58%	29%
watch video tapes	3%	16%	61%	17%
reading	17%	34%	46%	3%
other hobby	3%	21%	33%	43%

Conclusions

As was mentioned before, since regaining its independence in 1990, the social and economic changes in Lithuania have had a direct impact on the development of physical education and sport. New sports organizations have been set up and more attention is now being paid to the physical education of youth and school children. Sport for all events, which are intended for all age groups, is being promoted as well. It can be stated, that more and more public organizations join together their physical education and sport initiatives to prevent young people from being drawn into a street culture such as a TV programme "Winner's League", contest "The Healthiest of All", "Best School-Aged Athletes and Their Coaches of the Republic of Lithuania", "The Most Sporty School", etc. One of the initiatives to make physical education (sport) lessons more attractive in Latvia is a creative sport lesson open for the general public who can watch, get involved and discuss it. As another example, could be mentioned the sport lesson led by an invited Olympic athlete.

More initiatives could be listed which seek to encourage youths' physical activity, but there is not enough scientific evidence that would confirm the effectiveness of the above-mentioned initiatives and identify the factors and determinants which affect participation forms in sport and physical activity in contrast to idleness and inactivity such as psychological determinants, social determinants, organizational/institutional determinants and sociohistorical determinants.

The most neglected and the least studied research area in Lithuania and Latvia is psychological motivation of youth to get involved in physical activity or to be more physically active. On the other hand, the attempt to determine relations between:

1) Sport and PA/sedentariness and psychosocial competence (well-being, selfconcept, self-esteem),

2) Sport and PA/sedentariness and risk behaviours and

3) Sport and PA/sedentariness and emotional stability (coping with stress, psycho-somatic complaints, depression, anxiety) is carried out at Bachelor or Master level. This means that the surveys involve only unrepresentative sample and it is not rational to refer to this data trying to influence the solution of problems related to physical activity for youth.

References

Āboltiņa, M. (1998). *Kā aug mūsu bērns*. Rīga: Datorziņibu centrs.

Balčiūnienė, I., Nainys, J. V., Pavilonis S., Tutkuvienė, J. (1991). *Lietuvių antropologijos metmenys*. Vilnius: Mokslas.

Baubinas, A. & Vainauskas, S. (1998). Lietuvos moksleivių požiūris į kūno kultūrą ir savo sveikatą. *Sporto mokslas, 2,* 65-68.

Biddle, S., Sallis, J. & Cavill, N. (1998). Policy framework for young people and health-enhancing physical activity. In S. Biddle, J. Sallis & N. Cavill (Eds.). *Young and active? Young people and health-enhancing physical activity – Evidence and implications*. London: Health Education Authority.

Councile of Europe (2002). *Report of the advisory visit to Latvia on the European sports charter and physical education*. Retrieved on February 06, 2006 from http://www.coe.int/T/E/cultural_cooperation/Sport/Monitoring_fulfillment/European_ Sport_Charter/2.Latvia.asp#P76_15692

Currie, C., Samdal, O., Boyce, W. & Smith, B. (1998). *Health Behaviour in School-Aged Children: a WHO cross-national survey (HBSC). Research protocol for the 1997/98 survey*. Edinburgh: University of Edinburgh.

Davidavičienė, A. (1996). *Sveikos gyvensenos įtvirtinimas mokyklose.Tyrimų medžiaga*. Vilnius: Pedagogikos institutas

Diržine, D. (2004.) *Bērna stāju var labot, ja vien vēlas*. Newspaper - Zemgales Ziņas, 3210.

Grabovska, L. (1999). *Skolēnu kustību aktivitātes vasaras brīvlaikā*. Unprinted master's thesis, Rīga: Latvijas Sporta pedagoģijas akadēmija.

Hibell, B., Andersson, B., Ahlström, S., Balakireva, O., Bjarnason, T., Kokkevi, A. & Morgan, M. (2000). *The 1999 ESPAD Report. Alcohol and Other Drug Use Among Students in 30 European Countries. The Swedish Council for Information on Alcohol and Other Drugs (CAN) and The Pompidou Group at the Council of Europe.* Stockholm: The Swedish Council for Information on Alcohol and Other Drugs (CAN) and The Pompidou Group at the Council of Europe

Jaruševičienė, L. (2000). *Paauglių lytinė elgsena ir reprodukcinės priežiūros sveikatos galimybių vertinimas*. Unprinted doctoral dissertation, Kaunas: Kauno medicinos universitetas.

240   S. Laskiene

Juškelienė, V. (1998). *Asimetrinės laikysenos rizikos veiksniai ir pokyčiai tarp 6–8 metų vaikų.* Unprinted doctoral dissertation, Kaunas: Kauno medicinos akademija.

Juškelienė, V. & Dailidienė, N. (1999). *6 – 8 metų vaikų asimetrinės laikysenos rizikos veiksniai ir jos pokyčiai.* Vilnius: Higienos institutas.

Kardelis, K. (1993). Informacinio pobūdžio poveikio priemonių moksleivių požiūriui į fizinį aktyvumą keisti vertinimas. Kn.: *Visuomenės sveikata: Dabartis ir ateitis.* Kaunas: Kauno medicinos akademija, pp. 179-183

Kardelis, K., Kavaliauskas, S. & Balzeris, V. (2001). *Mokyklinė kūno kultūra: realijos ir perspektyvos.* Kaunas: Lietuvos kūno kultūros akademija.

Kasvande, Z. (2004.). Prevention and early diagnostics of manifested supportive – locamotor apparatus disturbances for kindergarten and school age children, Theory and practice in teacher training II. *The International scientific conference,* 447 – 454.

Knipše, G., Baumanis, J. & Kokina, I. (2001.) *Kustību aktivitāte, tās ietekme uz bērna fizisko attīstību un fizisko sagatavotību.* Rīga, Latvia: Papers presented at the 4th World Latvian Art congress.

Kokina, I. (2002.) *Fiziskās aktivitātes sirds un asinsvadu slimību profilaksē.* Unprinted master's thesis,Rīga: Latvijas Sporta pedagoģijas akadēmija.

Lapinska, I. (2000.) *Ārpusstundu fiziskās audzināšanas saturs. Unprinted master's thesis.* Rīga: Latvijas Sporta pedagoģijas akadēmija.

Latvian Ministry of education and science (2000). *National report of Republic of Latvia: education for all.* Retrieved on February 06, 2006 from http://www2.unesco.org/wef/countryreports/latvia/rapport_2_3.html

Latvian Ministry of education and science (2004). *Development of education: national report.* Retrieved on February 06, 2006 from http://www.izm.gov.lv/dokumenti/izglitibas_politika/zinojums_2004_en.doc

Latvijas jaunatnes sporta centrs (2003). *Sporta izglītības rādītāji – 2003./ 2004.māc. g.* Rīga: LJSC, p. 7 – 21.

Lazda, A. (1982). *Mazkustība.* Rīga, Zinātne, pp. 36.

Levickienė, G. & Kardelis, K. (1999). Moksleivių fizinės saviugdos komponentų ir socialinių bei edukacinių veiksnių sąsaja Socialiniai mokslai. *Edukologija, 4 (21),* 91-97.

Lietuvos Respublikos sveikatos apsaugos ministerija (2002). *Lietuvos gyventojų sveikata ir sveikatos priežiūros įstaigų veikla 2001 m.* Vilnius: LR sveikatos apsaugos ministerija.

Lietuvos Respublikos Švietimo ir mokslo ministerija (1997). *Lietuvos bendrojo lavinimo mokyklos Bendrosios programos. I-X klasės.* Vilnius: Lietuvos Respublikos Švietimo ir mokslo ministerija (Government printing office).

Lietuvos Respublikos Švietimo ir mokslo ministerija (1999). *Išsilavinimo standartai.* Vilnius: Lietuvos Respublikos Švietimo ir mokslo ministerija (Government printing office).

Lietuvos Respublikos Švietimo ir mokslo ministerija. (2000). *2000-2012 metų vaikų ir jaunimo kūno kultūros ir sporto strategija.* Retrieved on April 29, 2004 from http://www.smm.lt/veiklos_planai_ir_programos/docs/stratg1.htm

Lietuvos sporto statistikos departamentas (1998-1999). *Lietuvos sporto statistikos metraštis.* Vilnius: Informacijos – leidybos centras.

Lietuvos sporto taryba (2000). *III Lietuvos sporto kongresas.* Vilnius: Lietuvos Sporto taryba (Government Printing Office)

Lithuanian State Department of Physical Education and Sports (2002). *Attitude of 7-80 Years old Inhabitants of Lithuania towards the Physical Exercises and Sport as well as their Participation Level: year 2000l survey results abridgment.* Vilnius: Lithuanian State Department of Physical Education and Sports, Lithuanian Sports Information Center.

LR Veselības ministrija (1996). *LR medicīniskās statistikas gada grāmata*. Rīga: LR Veselības ministrija.

LR Veselības veicināšanas centrs (2004). *Latvijas iedzīvotāju veselību ietekmējošo paradumu monitorings 1998 – 2002*. Rīga: LR Veselības veicināšanas centrs.

Nacionalinė sveikatos taryba (2000). *1999 m. Nacionalinės sveikatos tarybos metinis pranešimas*. Vilnius: Nacionalinė sveikatos taryba (GPO).

Pate, R. R., Heath, G. W., Dowda, M. & Trost, S. G. (1996). Associations between physical activity and other health behaviors in a representative sample of US adolescents. *American Journal of Public Health*, 86 (11), 1577-1581.

Petravičius, A. (2000). Naujas požiūris į idiopatinę vaikų skoliozę. *Medicina, 36*, 420-422.

Physical activity and health: a report of the Surgeon General. (1996). Atlanta, GA, Centers for Disease Control and Prevention, U.S. Department of Health and Human Services, National Center for Chronic Disease Prevention and Health Promotion,. Retrieved on April 15, 2004 from http://www.cdc.gov/nccdphp/sgr/sgr.htm.

Porozov, J. (2004). The self estimation of sport activities, life style and health level of the young people. Theory and practice in teacher training II. *The International scientific conference Rīga, Latvia*, 390 – 398.

Rubana, I. M. (1998). *Tava veselība*. Rīga: RaKa.

Sallis, J. F. & Patrick, K. (1994). Physical activity guidelines for adolescents: consensus statement. *Pediatric Exercise Science, 6*, 302–314.

Saniukas, K. & Aleksejevas, E. (1991). *Stuburo iškrypimai (klinika, gydymas)*. Vilnius: Statistikos departamentas prie LR Vyriausybės (Government printing office).

Statistikos departamentas (2002). *Lietuvos vaikai: metinis statistikos rinkinys*. Vilnius: Statistikos departamentas prie LR Vyriausybės (Government printing office).

Tutkuvienė, J. (1995). *Vaikų augimo ir brendimo vertinimas*. Vilnius: Meralas.

Vainauskas, S. (1998). *Lietuvos moksleivių gyvensenos ir požiūrio į savo sveikatą įvertinimas*. Unpublished doctoral dissertation. Vilnius: Vilniaus universitetas.

Valtneris, A. (2001). *Bērnu un pusaudžu fizioloģija*. Rīga: Zvaigzne ABC, pp.160

Veselības veicināšanas centrs (1999). *Projektu pārskati*. Rīga: Veselības veicināšanas centrs.

Vilūnienė, A. & Jankauskienė, R. (2002). Skirtingo fizinio aktyvumo tėvų požiūris į fizinę saviugdą bei vaikų fizinį ugdymą ir jo sąsaja su vaikų fiziniu aktyvumu. Ugdymas. Kūno kultūra. *Sportas, 4 (45)*, 109-114

Volbekienė, V. & Mikaitienė, G. (1998). Lietuvos moksleivių fizinis aktyvumas ir pajėgumas. Sveikata ir kūno kultūra: republic conference presentation. Kaunas: Lietuvos kūno kultūros institutas.

Wold, B. (1989). *Lifestyle and physical activity. A theoretical and empirical analysis of socialization among children and adolescents. Doctoral thesis*. Bergen: University of Bergen.

Zaborskis, A. (1997). *Lietuvos moksleivių sveikata ir jos stiprinimas. Unpublished doctoral dissertation*. Kaunas: Kauno medicinos akademija.

Zaborskis, A. (1996). Kiek Lietuvos moksleivių vartoja alkoholinius gėrimus? Socialiniai mokslai. *Sociologija, 3 (7)*, 71-74.

Zaborskis, A., Černiuvienė, V., Šumskas, L., Levinienė, G., Prasauskienė, A., Milčiuvienė, S., Stanikas, T., Kudzytė, J., Laskienė, S. (1995). *Aukime sveiki. Sveikatos ugdymo kursas. Pradinių klasių mokytojo knyga*. Kaunas: Šviesa.

Zaborskis, A. & Šumskas, L. (1993). Sveikatos mokymo programa pradinėms mokykloms "Aukime sveiki". Kn.: *Visuomenės sveikata: Dabartis ir ateitis*. Kaunas: Kauno medicinos akademija, p. 176-179

Zaborskis, A. & Šumskas, L. (1995). "Let's Grow Up Healthy": A Health education pilot
    Project for primary schools in Lithuania. *Journal of Baltic studies, 26 (3),* 243-252.
Zaborskis, A., Žemaitienė, N., Šumskas, L. & Diržytė, A. (1996). *Moksleivių gyvenimo būdas
    ir sveikata: pasaulinės sveikatos organizacijos 1994 m. tarptautinės moksleivių
    apklausos rezultatai.* Vilnius: Leidybos centras.
Zuozienė, I. (1998). *Kūno kultūros ir sveikos gyvensenos žinių įtaka moksleivių fiziniam
    aktyvumui. Unpublished doctoral dissertation.* Kaunas: Lietuvos Kūno kultūros
    akademija.

Chapter 13:
Physical and motor development, sport activities and lifestyles of Slovenian children and youth – changes in the last few decades

Janko Strel, Marjeta Kovač & Gregor Jurak

Introduction

Modern trends in the lifestyles of Slovenian children and youth, and the significance of sport, are presented in this paper on the basis of over 30 years of systematic research. Despite the methodical approach applied to education [new curriculum, there are over 1,500 hours of PE in the education programme for each individual (Kovač, 2001); PE being the most popular school subject (Strel et al., 1996, 2004a); with parents believing PE has a particular importance for the future life of their children (Strel, Kovač, Štihec et al., 1996; Strel, Kovač, Jurak, 2004a; Kovač et al., 2004) and sports fields (an ever growing number of sports programmes and sports surfaces), it can be seen that some goals in sports for children and youth are only partly, or not at all, being fulfilled (Strel, Kovač & Jurak, 2004b). Teachers in practice, and research findings, revealed some particular problems that also occur in Slovenia, as in all modern societies.

It can be seen that the intensive development of information technology, and a pluralist society, are having significant negative pedagogically functional effects on the motor, physical and psychosocial development of children and youth. New and so far unmanageable factors affecting young people's socialisation in today's affluent and hedonistic modern societies lead to many problems in education. Television and other forms of entertainment are available at the press of a button and occupy the free time of many young people. As a result of trends in fashion, young people are joining in the new features of social life, which are unfortunately often connected with the pathology of various social groups. When deciding between easily available entertainment and a healthy lifestyle young people too often tend to choose the former.

It is important to understand the changes and needs of young people and to listen to the problems facing teachers, coaches and parents. Public institutions and the civil sphere should be involved in the process of looking for solutions which should derive from actual situations and can be carried out realistically.

In Slovenia changes have been monitored systematically for decades. The first data on physical development of Slovenian children and youth were published in

1903, while representative data on motor and physical development for Slovenia were collected for the first time in 1970 (Šturm & Strel, 1985), and have since been collected approximately every ten years (Cross-study of the physical and motor development of children aged 7-19 in the period 1970-1983-1993-2003 – Strel, Kovač, Štihec et al., 1996, Strel et al., 2004a; Kovač, Jurak, Strel, & Bednarik, 2003). Some physical characteristics and motor abilities of the whole population of children and young people have been monitored since 1987 as part of the "Sports Educational Chart" – a longitudinal study of physical and motor development (Strel et al., 1997, 2001, 2003).

More information about the methods used and the detailed research findings are published on the web page www.sp.uni-lj.si/didaktika/english.htm. Major ongoing research has been carried out during the last two years and new research findings will be added as they emerge.

Physical development in the past few decades

A cross-study for the period 1970 to 2003 (Šturm & Strel, 1985; Strel et al., 1996, 2003, 2004a, b) reveals that young people in 2003, compared with those in 1970, experienced their biggest growth spurt a year earlier. Girls grew nearly 7 centimetres between the ages of 10 and 11 years, whereas boys had their biggest growth spurt of 8 centimetres between the ages of 12 and 13 years. Boys finish primary school at the age of 14 more than 5 centimetres taller than 30 years ago, while girls are nearly 4 centimetres taller. Most of these changes were recorded in the period 1970 to 1983, whereas in the last ten years a stagnation or even retardation can be noticed. These changes might just be a coincidence or could be the result of migratory tides involved in the formation of the new state.

Changes in weight are significant, especially when considering that the gain in height is moderate, and young people today, in particular girls, have less subcutaneous fat than 30 years ago. This can be seen as a result of changed dietary habits (Gabrijelčič Blenkuš, 2001), more sports activity (Jurak et al., 2003a; Strel et al., 2004; Kovač, Starc, & Topič, 2005), fashion trends (Starc, 2003) and, perhaps, artificial food additives. It has to be mentioned that 14 year old boys in 2003 were 20 % (more than 8 kilograms) heavier than those in 1970, yet these same children of both genders in 2003 were lighter than those of 10 years ago. In girls this may be seen as a result of a smaller amount of body fat and, for both genders, it could also be a sign of slightly reduced height than in 1993. Secondary school girls in particular have worse dietary habits than boys as they eat less than three times a day, consume less milk and dairy products, meat and meat products, fish, eggs and hot meals and eat less frequently in the evenings (Gabrijelčič Blenkuš, 2001).

It needs to be stressed that the upper arm skin folds of children younger than 10 years have increased in the last few decades. The largest of these values were measured in 2003 and show a more than 30 % increase for 8-year-old children (see Figure 1). This is probably a result of an insufficient amount of motor stimulation and increased concern for the comfort of the youngest children, as is also reflected in the excessive amount of inappropriate, yet tempting food.

Fig. 1:   Changes in upper arm skin folds for the period 1970-2003 for boys aged 7 to 14 years (Strel et al., 2004b)

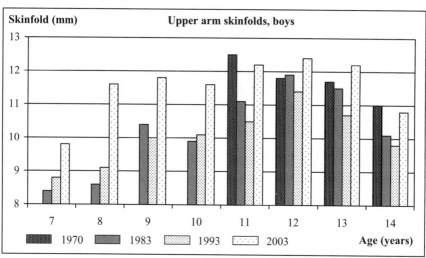

In contrast, there has been a tendency for a gradual reduction of body fatness in the last few decades for older children of both genders (Strel et al., 2003). Values of upper arm skin folds for 14-year-old girls have been reduced by 10 % in the last few decades; also noticeable is the reduction of values for boys of the same age, which were at their highest in 1970. It can also be seen that the number of girls with extremely low weight and inadequate amounts of skin folds is on the increase (Strel et al., 2004a), which could be an indication of dietary problems (anorexia and bulimia). These problems are probably influenced by fashion and media, which promote low weight as the desired fashion ideal of young people.

Overweight and obesity

In order to determine appropriate weight, overweight and obesity, the following indicators have been calculated: Body Mass Index (BMI) according to the IOTF standard (Cole & Rolland Chachera, 2002), percentage of body fat (according to

Slaughter, 1988 and based on skin fold values on the triceps and the back) and the percentage of children and youth with upper arm skin folds above 30 mm (Strel et al., 2004a). Different comparisons have been used due to the significant gain in weight (approximately 8 kilograms) over the last 20 years, especially in boys older than 12 years, and the simultaneous decrease in upper arm skin fold, in particular for girls. Due to the BMI not being sensitive enough to detect the quality of mass (muscular or fat tissues), other comparisons were used to more realistically evaluate the problem of overweight and obese children and young people.

Analysis of the BMI values for the population of children aged 7-19 in the period 1983-2003 (Strel et al., 2004a, b), shows an oscillation between 74.6 % for 12-year-old and 87.4 % for 16-year-old boys who had the appropriate weight in 2003 (see Figure 2). The same data indicates a range between 75.1 % for 8-year-old and 89.3 % for 19-year-old girls with the appropriate weight. In comparison with 1983, 10 % less of 8 to 12-year-old children had the appropriate weight in 2003, which is in line with findings that the biggest increase in body fat occurred precisely during this period. The percentage of 15 to 19-year-old girls with appropriate weight in 2003 exceeded 85 % and was slightly lower for boys. The appropriate weight of young people in reality 4 achieves even better values as a result of increased muscular tissue, which is itself a positive indicator of an active lifestyle.

Fig. 2:   Percentage of girls aged 7-19 with the appropriate weight in the period 1983-2003 (Strel et al., 2004b)

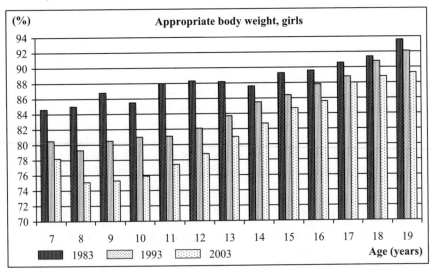

The biggest percentage of overweight children according to BMI (25-30 kg/m^2) is in between the ages of 9 and 14 for boys (see Figure 3), and 8 and 13 years for girls. The values for younger and older children are lower (Strel et al., 2004a, b). The significantly bigger number of overweight children in 2003 in comparison to 1983 requires a detailed analysis of the environment in which young people lived during their puberty. When explaining the percentage of overweight children, it has to be considered that certain adjustments of BMI, as determined by the IOTF, are needed from the age of 14 onwards. Namely, the increase of BMI in 2003 is mainly a result of an increase in the amount of muscular tissue and less in the amount of body fatness.

Fig. 3:   Percentage of overweight boys aged 7-19 in the period 1983-2003 (Strel et al., 2004b)

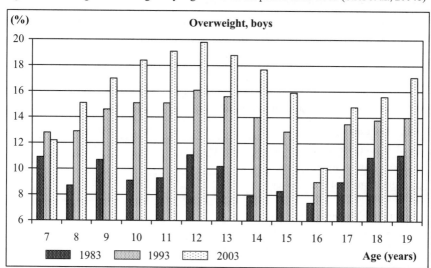

The percentage of obese children and youth, calculated with the BMI and according to IOTF standards, was significantly bigger in 2003, especially in the younger age groups (Strel et al., 2004a, b). Tendencies of change in the BMI, which are greater than 30, are very similar to those for overweight. 1.8 % of girls and 2.2 % of boys are obese by the age of 19.

The percentage of body fat, according to Slaughter (1988), is continually increasing from the age of 7 to 14 in all three periods (1983-1993-2003). This changes only slightly in 2003, when a decrease in 14-year-old boys and girls is noticed, compared with 13-year-old children, by as much as 1.5 % in boys (Strel et al., 2004a, b).

Conclusions can be drawn that, particularly for girls, the percentage of body fat is increasing with age due to specific developmental characteristics. Analyses show a worrying increase of values of BMI, percentage of body fat and values of upper arm skin fold in the period 1983-2003, especially for children aged 9 to 12. Puberty is an especially sensitive time, therefore suitable strategies should be produced to prevent any increase in obese children. In addition to school and sports areas, the sales of food of doubtful quality should be questioned, while youths should be encouraged to pursue correct dietary habits and active lifestyles thereby stimulating greater participation in sport.

Motor development in the past few decades

Motor abilities are key factors allowing an individual to learn different sports skills and are a prerequisite for quality, suitable and safe sports participation. This kind of participation enables a relaxed approach to games and enjoyment, together with achieving a high level of positive health.

Tab. 1:   Indexes of average changes in the motor abilities of school children aged 8-19 years in the period 1990-2000 (Strel et al., 2003)

Area of measuring	Male	Female	Both
speed of alternate motion (arm plate tapping)	+0.6 %	+0.9 %	+0.75 %
explosive power (standing long jump)	−1 %	−2 %	−1.5 %
co-ordination of body movements (polygon backwards)	+3.9 %	+7.2 %	+5.6 %
strength of abdominal muscles (sit-ups)	+10.2 %	+14.0 %	+12.1 %
flexibility (bend forward on the bench)	+1.6 %	+1.3 %	+1.45 %
muscular endurance of the shoulder girdle and arms (bent arm hang)	−9.8 %	−1.5 %	−5.65 %
sprint speed (60-metre run)	−1.1 %	−1.1 %	−1.1 %
general endurance (600-metre run)	−5.7 %	−5.7 %	−5.7 %
motorics (average of all 8 motor tests)	+0.2 %	+1.6 %	+0.9 %

Individual motor abilities of children and youth in Slovenia aged 8-19 years in the period 1990-2000 reveal some very diverse developmental trends (see Table 1; Strel et al., 2003). Positive changes in the endurance of the abdominal muscles are very noticeable in both boys and girls (boys +10.2 %, girls +14 %); positive changes in the co-ordination of whole body movements are also noticeable in girls (+7.2 %). Negative changes are manifested in boys for muscular endurance of the shoulder girdle and arms (−9.8 %) and a decrease in general endurance of both genders can also be seen (−5.7 %).

Fig. 4:   Index of changes of the "average of 8 motor variables" of children and youth in
Slovenia aged 8-19 years in the period 1990-2000 (Strel et al., 2003)

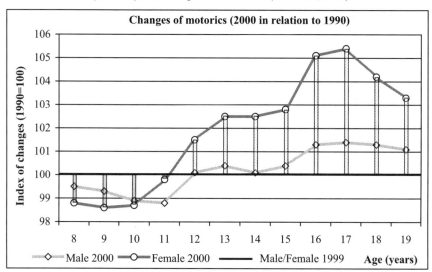

Figure 4 illustrates the index of changes in motor status according to the age of
the measured subjects in the period 1990-2000. Several findings deserve
comment:

- The developmental tendency has the same direction in both genders;
  however, the development of girls (1.6 %) is greater than the development of
  boys (0.2 %).

- The biggest positive changes in motor development happen in secondary
  schools. Presumably the better financial circumstances in secondary schools
  – construction of more sports halls, gyms, dance studios, fitness rooms,
  outdoor courts and certain athletics stadiums – have a significant impact on
  motor development. At the same time, with the improvement of such
  conditions, the number of PE hours also increased from two to three hours a
  week at the beginning of the 1990s. Further, the number of free-time sports
  programmes has increased. The new curriculum introduced in 1998 and
  favourable rules, which enable groups, in most schools, to consist of around
  20 pupils, are also important. Strel et al. (2003) found, for the first time, that
  in a period of ten years the largest positive changes occurred during the time
  of secondary school education. The results achieved are even more important
  as secondary schools were accessible to 98.5 % of the population in 2000,
  therefore it also encompassed pupils with a lower level of motor ability.

- The biggest improvement (more than 5 %) is found in girls aged 15-18 years, whereas boys improved by slightly more than 1 %. A study of the adult populations' participation in sports reveals that women's attitude to sport has changed significantly (Petrović et al., 2001); a good number of leisure sports programmes (fitness, aerobics) are aimed solely at girls and women; another key factor involves fashion trends which promotes sport as a way of achieving a beautiful figure.

- Negative changes in motor development (–1 %) occurred between the ages of 8 and 10 years, when in the majority of schools class teachers teach PE. This deterioration is present despite the construction of many new sports halls, modernisation of the school curriculum, introduction of additional programmes, reduction of numbers of children in classes and the improved qualification of class teachers. Obviously, after modernisation of the curriculum, class teachers focus more on other subjects and neglect the planned work in PE. Changing tendencies become positive (by more than 1 %) immediately after PE teachers started teaching children.

Changes in four tests of motor abilities detected in the period 1970-2003 (Strel et al., 2004a) will be demonstrated. In other motor abilities, such as flexibility, speed of alternate movement, power strength and sprint speed, no critical changes were observed.

The motor ability muscular endurance of the shoulder girdle and arms, measured with the test bent arm hang, has changed most in the last thirty years in children and youth. These changes are significantly negative, however, they are diminishing over the decades (see Figure 5). This can be seen to be a result of the reduction in everyday physical work, the absence of gymnastic skills in PE and changed morphological structures. According to Strel (1976), the results of this test also depend on height, length of the arms, weight and upper arm skin fold. These factors have a negative correlation with the above test; therefore, these negative changes are also a consequence of increased height and a greater amount of body fat in 10-year-old children.

Negative changes are less apparent in girls, whose way of life changed less significantly in the period 1970-2003; they also participate in sport more often and have gained less body fat than boys from the commencement of puberty. The decrease in the muscular strength of boys and girls aged 7-9 years is more worrying as the results for the above test fell by more than 50 % in the period 1970-2003. Factors for this decline are undoubtedly the 30 % increase in upper arm skin fold, the permissive education in school and at home and changes in free-time activities, where computer, television and mobile phone technology have replaced spontaneous movement activities.

Fig. 5:   Changes in the "bent arm hang" test for boys aged 7-14 in the period 1970-2003 (Strel et al., 2004b)

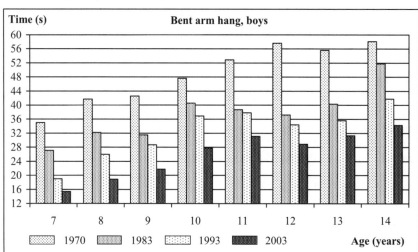

Tab. 2:   Changes in the "polygon backwards" test for boys and girls aged 7-14 in the period 1970-2003 (Strel et al., 2004b)

Age (years)		7	8	9	10	11	12	13	14
Polygon backwards		seconds							
1983	boys	25.39	22.29	20.02	19.06	18.28	17.26	15.88	14.60
	girls	29.25	26.12	22.82	22.17	21.03	19.75	17.29	17.52
1993	boys	25.62	20.51	18.12	16.05	15.08	14.63	13.91	13.28
	girls	30.87	24.85	21.03	18.76	17.19	16.44	15.08	14.57
2003	boys	28.33	22.31	19.80	17.89	15.98	15.28	14.01	13.11
	girls	32.81	25.74	21.88	20.35	17.66	16.97	16.29	15.05

Changes in whole body co-ordination, measured with the test 'polygon backwards', were positive up until 1993, whereas in the last decade these changes have mainly been negative (see Table 2). Particularly negative tendencies can be seen in children aged 7-10 years, especially in boys. Negative differences between the ages 11 and 14 years are smaller in different periods; 14-year-old boys in fact achieved the highest level of development of whole body co-ordination in 2003.

Somewhat surprising is the poor state of movement co-ordination of girls in 2003, in particular for 8-10-year-old girls. Presumably PE lacks complicated movements and a focus on aesthetic expressions and enjoyment in less demanding sports activities. Similarly, Štemberger (2003) reports a lack of preparation and consequently insufficient comprehension of demanding contents at the end of the first three years of school.

The abdominal muscular endurance of children aged 7-10 years was slightly better in 2003 than ten years before. Positive changes between the ages of 11 and 14 years show a 10 % improvement, in particular for girls, (see Figure 6). Annual improvements are quite gradual; these positive changes are mainly a result of fashion trends which, in the last couple of years, have decreed that bare stomachs should be displayed ('abdominal cult').

Fig. 6:   Changes in the "sit-up" test for girls (F) aged 7-14 in the period 1970-2003 (Strel et al., 2004b)

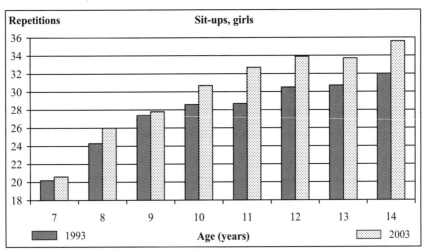

The described changes are a result of material conditions, expertise of teachers, amount and quality of PE, organisation of sports at local and national levels, the enlightenment of parents and their guiding of young people in sports development and other factors. The presented comparisons are a sign of the important changes in the motor status of children and youth seen in the last decades; however, additional interpretations are needed, especially with the help of other available indicators (economic situation of a region, health status of children and youth, attitudes of children and parents to sport, number of sport surfaces per individual, daily routines etc.).

Aerobic fitness and cardiovascular status

Aerobic fitness can be estimated by various measurements among which VO_2max proves to be the most appropriate from a physiological aspect. However, this measurement also has its drawbacks, because the generalization of the findings is problematic, because of accompanying organisational and other problems due to a smaller number of subjects.

According to the findings about correlation of results in VO_2max, velocity at VO_2max and duration of the treadmill test (Škof & Milić, 2002; Kropej, Škof & Milič, 2002) the results of the 600-m running test are reliable indicators of 12-year-old children's aerobic fitness that can be, in the Slovenian case, compared longitudinally over the last thirty years. Nevertheless, it should be stressed that this interpretation is limited from the perspective of metabolic and respiratory parameters and cardiovascular parameters, as well as body mass, which can also influence running velocity.

Fig. 7:   Changes in the "600-metre running" test for girls aged 7-14 in the period 1970-2003 (Strel et al., 2004b)

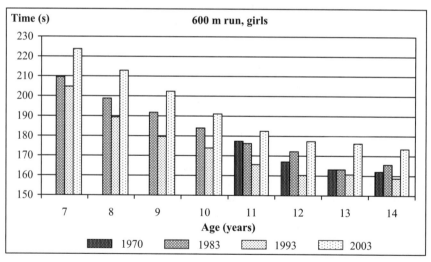

A study by Strel et al. (1996, 2004a) has been monitoring the 600-metre distance run, for over 30 years. Results of this test depend mainly on the capacity of cardio-vascular and respiratory systems and have, as a rule, been stagnating in the past, while in the last decade they have significantly deteriorated. There are no significant differences between genders, a greater disparity can be seen between different age groups of children and youth. The results of 14-year-old children (see Figure 7) have decreased by 10 % since 1993 and by a staggering 20 % in even younger children. This suggests changes in both the family environment and the school system, along with the unsuitability of the effect of physical education regarding endurance ability.

It is necessary to shed light on attitudes towards the overcoming of efforts and the realisation that systematic work leads to the desired effects. The deterioration in results of the 10-year-olds is partly a consequence of the 10 % or more increase in body fat. The findings of Škof, Kropej and Milič (2002) indicate that the factor that most positively correlates with the 600-m running is body height while the biggest drawback is caused by body fat. The two parameters alone explain the 76 % inconsistency in the test results.

After children start school the improvement of the 600-m results is observable each year. These positive changes are not as significant in the period of accelerated growth, when muscular mass and cardio-vascular and respiratory systems adjust to big changes in body height (over 7 centimetres annually).

This deterioration could also be a result of the bad habits of young people during the summer holidays, when too many children fall prey to sports inactivity (Strel, Novak, Pisanski et al., 1993; Jurak, Kovač, & Strel, 2002b, c). This has been confirmed by comparing measurements of motor abilities in September, December, May and again the next September (Strel et al., 1993). Positive changes in motor status were detected between September and May, whereas a significant decline in motor abilities was seen from May to September. The measurements shown in figure 7 were carried out in September.

Sports skills and theoretical knowledge of sport

Young people's leisure activities also impact on their mastery of sports skills and understanding of sport. The introduction of new PE curricula in Slovenia determines specific standards of knowledge in educational content in primary schools at the end of every three years, and at the conclusion of secondary education. A review of standards achieved at the end of the compulsory nine years of education assists in the final assessment of PE knowledge at the national level.

Approximately 15 % of all pupils choose PE as a third optional subject. In past years, boys achieved significantly better overall results than girls, indicating they had more interest in different aspects of this subject (Kovač, 2003). Practical knowledge of basketball, football and handball is very good (average scores of between 4.25 and 4.29 points out of 5), whereas the results of athletics (3.76 points) and dance (3.92 points) are slightly lower. A significant differentiation between genders, in favour of girls, can be seen only in dance (Kovač, 2003), otherwise there are no differences in boys' and girls' mastery of sports skills.

For the eleventh year running, the swimming skills of primary school pupils have also been systematically assessed in Slovenia. Through systematic annual testing in the 6th year of primary school, and by subsidising swimming courses and summer outdoor activities incorporating swimming courses, the number of non-swimmers[1] was reduced from 27.7 % in 1995 to 17.4 % in 2002 (Jurak & Kovač, 2002).

The young generation's lifestyle

The organisation of schoolwork, leisure activities and time for rest and sleep are important for the typical living pace of children and youth.

In addition to going to school, older children in primary schools spend another 75 minutes per day on studying and schoolwork (Strel et al., 2004a, b). For the rest of the time they mostly watch TV or participate in sport (Erjavec, 1999; Jurak et al., 2002b; Strel et al., 2004a, b).

During the school year 60 % of primary school children spend their weekends at home (Strel et al., 2004a). Nevertheless, a fair share of children is active in sport during the weekend (above 20 %), or go for a walk outside in nature or into the mountains (above 20 %). Recently, an increasingly popular alternative for spending one's weekend in Slovenia is to visit big shopping centres, where a variety of activities are on offer for all members of the family.

Children are physically and mentally more active during the school year than in the holidays (Strel et al., 1993, 2004a). During the school year primary schoolchildren are active in sport for around five-and-a-half hours a week, with PE at school being included in this amount (Strel et al., 2004a). Therefore, summer holidays can present a critical period from the point of view of health, since young people spend too much time lying in bed, in front of TV sets and computer screens and only more rarely do they take part in systematic sports activities (Strel et al., 1993, 2004a; Jurak et al., 2003a). Such lifestyles mean that the motor abilities of pupils diminish during the summer holidays (Strel et al., 1993, Strel et al., 2004a). This is not surprising if we take into account that within the education system obligatory and optional sports programmes account for half of all sports activities (Kovač, 2001) since it cannot be expected that sport will occupy such a place in the value system of all children and their parents (Strel et al., 2004a) that they would go in for it regularly even in their free time. The daily rhythm of secondary school children during the summer

---

[1]Jumping into water and swimming a distance of 50 metres in an optional style determines the knowledge of swimming skills in Slovenia. During swimming a special safety exercise has to be performed by the swimmer.

holidays is specially worrying. The rave culture, followed by a lot of youngsters in their spare time, requires a nocturnal rhythm of life. Roughly one-fifth of them quite often go to sleep after 1 o'clock in the morning, and they start their day relatively late so they also have less time for sport (Jurak et al, 2002c).

In primary schools Slovenian children are most active in sport (Jurak et al., 2003a). Up to the age of 12 their sports activity increases, while it falls after the age of 14, as a result of physical and mental changes in adolescence. More recently, some new and still uncontrolled factors of youth socialisation, in modern affluent and hedonistic societies, have appeared and are causing a series of educational problems. The intrusive offer of the mass media and information technology (Erjavec, 1999; Nadoh, 2001; Jurak et al., 2003a; Strel et al., 2004a) provides easy and immediate satisfaction, and encourages children and youth to choose activities where they mainly sit, increasingly they are choosing fewer sports activities.

The variety of free-time activities and fashion trends today indicate how primary school pupils (young people aged 7 to 15) spend their summer holidays in a slightly different way to some years ago.

Tab. 3:   Comparison of the sports activity of young people during their summer holidays in
          1993 – 2000 – 2003 (Strel et al., 1993, 2004a; Jurak et al., 2003a)

Sports activity (%)	Strel et al. (1993)		Jurak et al. (2003a)		Strel et al. (2004a)
	primary school	secondary school	primary school	secondary school	primary school
do not take part in any sports	11.2	10.6	7.7	13.6	3.9
occasionally (twice a week, at least 45 min.)	14.9	24.8	26.8	36.6	19.4
several times a week	40.9	38.4	32.4	27.7	48.5
every day	33.1	26.2	33.2	22.1	28.1

Primarily, positive changes during the last twelve years (see Table 3) can be attributed mainly to the systematic process of PE in schools, the widening of voluntary sports activities and organisations at that level; and also to the greater number of sports that children can now participate in (skateboarding, inline skating). As a result of other free-time activities, which in the modern world of electronic games entertainment compete with sport, the proportion of children participating daily in sport has fallen.

Even bigger changes can be seen in the selection of sports which primary school children participate in during their summer holidays (Strel et al., 2004b).

Motivation for participation in sport

Primary school children nowadays, regardless of gender, list the same reasons for participating in sport as they did 20 years ago (Strel et al., 2004a, b): it is good for health, improves one's fitness level, and develops abilities (Petkovšek & Strel,1985; Strel et al., 2004a, b). There is also no disparity between the genders for the higher placed reasons, however, it can be seen that in general the different genders have different reasons for participating in sport (Strel et al, 2004a).

These differences can be observed by applying a factorial analysis of 35 reasons. Similar factors applied for both genders and the biggest differences might be seen in extrinsic motivation. For boys, this is manifested as participation in sports for the purpose of achieving a certain status (popularity, contact with girls, money and other benefits) and, for girls, as a way of achieving a better external appearance (Strel et al, 2004a).

A comparison with other findings (Petkovšek & Strel, 1985) which used similar methods demonstrates big changes in the motivational dimension of primary school children in two directions (Strel et al., 2004a):

- Motivation is becoming identical regardless of gender.

- There is less extrinsic motivation when children expect outside benefits from participating in sports activity, and a greater intrinsic motivation which is characteristic of the popularity of a sports activity and its direct effects.

Uncertainties about traditional values in the ranking of reasons have been eliminated by findings concerning the free-time sports activities of children and youth, since more frequent participation in sport, in particular aerobic activities, has been noticed (Jurak et al., 2002a, b, c; Strel et al., 2004a). Children today are more enlightened about the importance of sports as a way of life. Apart from school and parents, the media has an important role in this. Starc (2003) found that a sporting way of life is becoming a fashion trend for young people precisely as a result of the media's influence.

Intrinsic reasons of well-being, in relation to the process of searching for one's own identity in adolescence, could result in a reduced interest in motor activities and an increase in the passive way of spending of one's free time. This represents a period that calls for the attention of experts.

Consumption of the mass media and use of modern technology

The mass media mirrors the image of society; however, adverse effects are also becoming more apparent, implying that society is becoming an image of the mass media. The media influences our habits and lifestyles, sets value norms and concentrates on specific problems of society. Many researchers argue that the growing use and importance of new media will replace the use of traditional media forms.

The findings of different Slovenian researchers (Erjavec, 1999; Nadoh, 2001; Jeriček, 2001; Jurak et al., 2002a, b, c; Strel et al., 2004a) can be expressed in several conclusions.

Use of media. Slovenian children spend most of their time on electronic media; however, they still use written media (18.5 % of free time). The most frequently used medium is television. Youth in Slovenia watch TV between 14 and 36 hours a week, depending on age, day, season, gender, education of parents, parents watching TV etc. The time spent in front of a TV has decreased in the last decade, whereas the use of new media has increased (see Tab. 4).

Tab. 4:   Percentage of 11 to 14-year-old children in Slovenia with access to new media in comparison to access to TV, and daily usage of modern media in comparison with TV during summer holidays (Erjavec, 1999; Nadoh, 2001; Strel et al., 2004a)

Medium	Access (in %)		Daily usage (in minutes)		
	At home	In own room	total	boys	girls
TV	98	28	153	145	162
Electronic or computer games	80	40	92	126	54
Mobile phone – for talking and sending SMS	82	82	62	47	79
Videotapes or DVD			59	62	55
Internet	47	20	42	44	41
Other activities on a computer	81*	40*	36	38	35

* Access to a computer

Access to media. Youth in Slovenia have very easy access to new media (see Table 12). With the exception of mobile phones, access depends on the education of one's parents. Boys have more frequent access at home to electronic games than girls and also play them more often. Access to computers and mobile phones differs according to age, as older children have more frequent access than younger children. Internet and mobile phones are more easily accessible in bigger towns. TV remains the easiest to access as every Slovenian household owns one. Boys more frequently have a TV in their rooms, whereas the age of children does not make a difference.

Use of media according to age.

• Slovenian children start watching TV usually at the age of 2 or 3. The amount of time watching TV increases up until the age of 11 (4-5 hours a day) and then drops to 2-3 hours a day. Younger children (aged 7-10 years) watch TV most frequently between 4pm and 9pm, after they return from school. Older children participate in more out-of-school activities and watch TV later in the day, after dinner. Despite having more free time, young people watch less TV during summer holidays, on average two-and-a-half hours, with smaller differences in various age groups.

- Reading declines with age. 30 % of children read regularly at the age of 7, only 8.6 % do so at the age of 14.

- Frequency of the use of electronic and computer games declines with age, the use of Internet increases up to the age of 17. Creative work on a computer increases significantly up until the age of 9 and then remains at the same level.

- Frequency of the use of mobile phones increases with age. By the end of primary school, children use mobile phones for more than 80 minutes a day.

Frequency of media use differs according to school-free days.

- Watching of TV increases significantly on the weekend. 19 % of primary school children regularly watch TV in the weekend until 11pm and 10 % after midnight. Children of parents who watch TV more often spend more time in front of TV themselves. Young people watch two-and-a-half hours of TV a day during their summer holidays. Watching of TV slightly increases with age during holidays.

- Approximately a quarter of children play computer games or use computers and the Internet one or more times a week. Children who use a computer everyday use it even longer over the weekend. During summer holidays almost half of young people on an average spend less than an hour per day using a computer.

- The use of mobile phones has the opposite tendency. The use of this medium is experiencing the biggest increase; however its use drops significantly at the weekend.

Use of media according to gender.

- Findings on the frequency of watching TV are slightly controversial. During the school year boys spend more time in front of TV than girls. During holidays, there is bigger percentage of primary school girls watching TV, whereas there are no differences between genders for secondary school pupils.

- Boys use a computer more often, however, both genders use a computer for school equally. It seems that boys are more drawn to playing computer games.

- The percentage of girls who read is twice the level for boys.

- Girls use mobile phones more often than boys.

Use of media according to the education of one's parents. Children whose parents have a higher education spend less time watching TV and more time in front of a computer. The use of mobile phones does not depend on the education of one's parents.

Use of media and academic results. Children with worse academic results watch TV, videotapes and DVDs more often; they also play electronic and computer games more often and more frequently use mobile phones. Children with better academic results use the Internet more often in search of information. The existence of a reverse correlation can be assumed, e.g. the use of such media influences academic results and vice versa.

Individual versus group use of media. Young people in Slovenia use the new media and mostly watch TV on their own, followed by the use of media within groups of friends. Individual use of media is in particular typical for boys and is also dependent on the individual medium and age (see other findings).

Purpose of using new media. Young people in Slovenia perceive and divide media into two opposing groups: entertaining and informative media. Computer games are most frequently played out of boredom and in reflection of the need for amusement and relaxation. Computers and the Internet are being used as a way of finding new information. Young people talk on mobile phones and send SMS messages when they feel lonely and use it as a way of different and limitless communication. Books are perceived as a boring medium and are being read less often or simply not at all.

Use of media and sports activity. Young people who watch TV more often are less sportingly active. Surprisingly, there is a positive correlation between the use of a computer and sports activities, which could be explained by the education of one's parents: the children of parents with a higher education do more work on a computer and are also more sportingly active. The use of mobile phones does not have any influence on sports activity.

Social environment

Children aged 12 to 15 learn most about the factors with an effect on health in their family circle and at school. Of the factors listed (body weight, alcohol, smoking, drugs, physical activity, nutrition, sport activity), children are informed most about sport. Young people rate the mass media surprisingly low as a source of information about health factors (Strel et al., 2004a).

On several occasions, researchers in Slovenia have detected the strong effect of the social environment on participation in sport; among the parameters of social status the educational and cultural status of one's parents has the most important impact on children's participation in sport. Particularly important are the level of education of one's parents and consequently their financial situation, belonging to a certain social class, and the sports activity of one's parents (Doupona, 1996; Jurak et al., 2003a; Strel et al., 2004a; Kovač et al., 2005). Parents influence their children's behaviour through the examples they set, and their wishes and demands in combination with their financial possibilities. Parents either encourage children to actively spend their free time or they turn them away from sports activities. The latest findings here (Kovač et al., 2005) reveal strong chances of developing sport for children and youth in Slovenia since more than 95 % of parents claim they would direct their children to sport if they expressed the desire to participate.

Another important change in Slovenian society is a significant increase in the number of sportingly active women, compared to men (see Table 5). Kovač et al. (2005) state several possible reasons for this: the many new programmes that target women; greater media promotion of sports activities and healthy life styles; fashion, which dictates the baring of a suitably shaped body and a more casual dress code; women's enhanced self-confidence, as expressed through their external appearance and attempts at extending their youth into later years; efforts of the health system to promote the importance of motor activities for health and vitality; and more free time.

Tab. 5: Sportingly active men and women – comparison between 1973, 2000 and 2003 (Kovač et al., 2005)

	1973	2000	2003
Sportingly active men	52,4 %	55,9 %	56,4 %
Sportingly active women	31,2 %	36,8 %	48,0 %
Gender differences	21,2 %	19,1 %	8,4 %

Women's more frequent participation in sport also has an effect on mothers' opinions about the importance of PE (Doupona, 1996; Strel et al., 2004a), which is often a crucial factor in children's participation in sport. Doupona (1996) also found that women in Slovenia play a dominant role in the formation of the pattern of a family's sports activity. Therefore, the development of sport for women affects the sport of children and youth significantly and generally the active use of young people's free time.

Girls show similar tendencies to women (Strel, et al., 2004a); however, changes in contents are also noticed for this age group and the sports activities of boys and girls are becoming more similar (Jurak et al., 2003b) than they used to be years ago (Strel et al., 1993). This is in line with the finding that boys and girls today have more similar reasons for participating in sport than in the past (Strel et al., 2004b).

Conclusions

As a result of these findings and practical experience, several activities, which are more precisely described on our web side, are recommended.

* Improvement in the quality of physical education for children aged 7-11 years.
* Improved quality of diet at home and at school.
* Reduction of the unpleasant factors of everyday school life, such as long periods of sitting, poor ventilation, disturbance, noise, and dehydration.
* Education for understanding sport.
* Emphasis on endurance sports activities.
* Encouragement of socialization.
* Encouragement of competitiveness in girls.
* Manuals for parents about their children's sports exercising.
* Possibilities for women's participation in sport and the systematic monitoring of women's sport.
* Balanced sports media.
* Possibilities for future successful programs.

References

Cole, T., & Rolland Chachera, M. F. (2002). Measurement and definition. In W. Burniat, T. Cole, I. Lissau, & E. Poskitt (Eds.), *Child and Adolescent Obesity* (pp.1-22). Cambridge: Press syndicate of the University of Cambridge.

Doupona, M. (1996). *Socialno demografska struktura mater in očetov šoloobveznih otrok in njihov odnos do športa.* Unpublished doctoral dissertation, Ljubljana: Fakulteta za šport.

Erjavec, K. (1999). Raziskava: Mladi in mediji. In K. Erjavec & Z. Volčič (Eds.), *Odraščanje z mediji* (pp. 119-136). Ljubljana: Zveza prijateljev mladine Slovenije.

Gabrijelčič Blenkuš, M. (2001). Nekatere prehranjevalne navade ljubljanskih srednješolcev s poudarkom na razliki med spoloma. *Zdravstveno varstvo, 40* (Supplement), 135-143.

Jeriček, H. (2001). Internet, mladi in zasvojenost. In B. Lobnikar & J. Žurej (Eds.), *Raziskovalno delo podiplomskih študentov v Sloveniji – Novo tisočletje: družboslovje in humanistika.* (pp. 95-105). Ljubljana: Društvo mladih raziskovalcev Slovenije.

Jurak, G., & Kovač, M. (2002). *Analiza znanja plavanja v šolskem letu 2001/02.* Retrieved September 25, 2002, from www.sportmladih.net.

Jurak, G., Kovač, M., & Strel, J. (2002a). Differences in spending summer holidays of Slovenian children and youth in different periods of schooling. *International Journal of Physical Education, 39*(2), 34-43.

Jurak, G., Kovač, M., & Strel, J. (2002b). How Slovene primary school pupils spend their summer holidays. *Kinesiologia Slovenica, 8*(2), 35-43.

Jurak, G., Kovač, M., & Strel, J. (2002c). Spending of summer holidays of Slovenian secondary school children. *Acta Universitatis Carolinae, Kinanthropologica, 38*(1), 51-66.

Jurak, G., Kovač, M., Strel, J., Majerič, M., Starc, G., Filipčič, T. et al. (2003a). *Sports activities of Slovenian children and young people during their summer holidays.* Ljubljana: University of Ljubljana, Faculty of Sport.

Jurak, G., Kovač, M., Strel, J., Starc, G., Majerič, M., Filipčič, T. et al. (2003b). Gender differences of Slovenian children and youth in spending summer holidays. *Finnish Sports and Exercise Medicine, The International XVII Puijo Symposium special issue.* Retrieved September 20, 2003, from http://ffp.uku. fi/cgi-bin/edueditor/presenter. pl?slideshow_id=102&slide_id=1029&language_id=1

Kovač, M. (2001). Physical education. In A. Barle Lakota, M. Gajgar & M. Turk Škraba (Eds.), *The development of education. National report of the Republic of Slovenia by Ministry of education, science and sport* (pp. 89-92). Ljubljana: Ministry of Education, Science and Sport.

Kovač, M. (2003). Assessment of physical education at the end of the nine-year primary school. In A. Cankar (Ed.), *Assessment in Physical education in Alps Adriatic countries* (pp. 104-114). Ljubljana: The National Education Institute.

Kovač, M., Jurak, G., Strel, J. & Bednarik, J. (2003). Comparison of motor development of boys and girls aged 11-17. *Journal of Human Kinetics, 10*, 63-75.

Kovač, M., Starc, G., & Doupona, M., (2005). *Šport in nacionalna identifikacija Slovencev.* Ljubljana: Fakulteta za šport, Inštitut ta kineziologijo.

Kropej, V. L., Škof, B. & Milić, R. (2002). Achievement of VO_2 plateau in children. In D. Milovanović & F. Prot (Eds.), *3rd International scientific conference Kinesiology: New perspectives. Proceedings book.* (pp. 511-514). Zagreb: Faculty of kinesiology, University of Zagreb.

Nadoh, J. (2001). *Uporaba novih medijev pri slovenskih mladih.* Unpublished bachelor's thesis, Ljubljana: Fakulteta za družbene vede.

Petkovšek, M. & Strel, J. (1985). *Vpliv šolskega okolja na dinamiko razvoja športne motiviranosti učenk in učencev osnovnih šol v SR Sloveniji.* Ljubljana: Univerza Edvarda Kardelja, Fakulteta za telesno kulturo, Ištitut za kineziologijo.

Petrović, K., Ambrožič, F., Bednarik, J., Berčič, H., Sila B. & Doupona Topič, M. (2001). Športnorekreativna dejavnost v Sloveniji 2000. *Šport, 49* (3), 1-48.

Starc, G. (2003). Bolj razkazovanje kot tekmovanje: mag. Gregor Starc o fenomenu telesa v sodobnem športu. *Delo*, 4-6.

Strel, J. (1976). *Spremembe relacij med nekaterimi antropometričnimi in motoričnimi karakteristikami v obdobju od 11. do 15. leta.* Unpublished master's thesis, Ljubljana: Visoka šola za telesno kulturo, Inštitut za kineziologijo.

Strel, J., Novak, H., Pisanski, M., Mesarič, V. & Štihec, J. (1993). *Obremenjenost učencev z delom za šolo in stanje gibalnih sposobnosti in morfoloških značilnosti.* Ljubljana: Fakulteta za šport.

Strel, J., Kovač, M., Štihec, J., Kondrič, M., Tušak, M., Leskošek, B. et al. (1996). *Analiza razvojnih trendov motoričnih sposobnosti in morfoloških značilnosti in relaciji obeh s psihološkimi in sociološkimi dimenzijami slovenskih otrok in mladine med 7.-18. letom starosti v obdobju 1970 - 1983 -1993. Zaključno poročilo.* Ljubljana: Fakulteta za šport, Inštitut za kineziologijo.

Strel, J., Ambrožič, F., Kondroč, M., Kovač, M., Leskošek, B., Štihec, J. et al. (1997). *Sports educational chart.* Ljubljana: Ministry of Education and Sport.

Strel, J., Kovač, M., Jurak, G., Bednarik, J. & Leskošek, B. (2001). Comparison of physical
    development of school children between 1990 and 2000 on the basis of the data
    obtained from the sports educational chart. *Anthropological notebook, 7* (1), 11-32.
Strel, J., Kovač, M., Jurak, G. & Bednarik, J. (2003). Gender differences of Slovenian school
    children in physical and motor development in the period from 1990 to 2000. *Finnish
    Sports and Exercise Medicine, The International XVII Puijo Symposium special issue.*
    Retrieved September 20, 2003, from http://ffp.uku. fi/cgi-bin/edueditor/presenter.
    pl?slideshow_id=101&slide_id=1012&language_id=1
Strel, J., Kovač, M., Jurak, G., Starc, G., Bučar, M., Emberšič, D. et al. (2004a). *Analiza
    razvojnih trendov motoričnih sposobnosti in morfoloških značilnosti ter povezav obeh
    z drugimi bio-psiho-socialnimi razsežnostmi slovenskih otrok in mladine med 6. - 18.
    letom v obdobju 1970 - 1983 - 1993 - 2003. Delno raziskovalno poročilo.* Manuscript
    submitted for publication.
Strel, J., Kovač, M. & Jurak, G. (2004b). *Study on young people's lifestyle and sedentariness
    and the role of sport in the context of education and as a means of restoring the
    balance. Case of Slovenia.* Retrieved June 30, 2004, from http://www.sp.uni-
    lj.si/didaktika/english.htm.
Škof, B. & Milić, R. (2002). Delež energijskih sistemov pri teku na 600 in 2400 metrov pri
    otrocih različne starosti. *Šport, 50* (3), 17-23.
Štemberger, V. (2003). *Kakovost športne vzgoje v prvem vzgojno-izobraževalnem obdobju
    devetletne osnovne šole.* Unpublished doctoral dissertation, Ljubljana: Univerza v
    Ljubljani, Pedagoška fakulteta.
Šturm, J. & Strel, J. (1985). *Primerjava nekaterih motoričnih in morfoloških parametrov v
    osnovnih šolah SR Slovenije v obdobju 1970/71-83. Zaključno poročilo.* Ljubljana:
    FTK, Inštitut za kineziologijo.

Chapter 14:
Determinants and correlates of physical activity among European children and adolescents

Risto Telama, Heimo Nupponen & Lauri Laakso

Introduction

Maintaining and increasing the physical activity among young people is one of the most important aims of physical education and sport policy. A crucial question is, how can children's physical activity be maintained and increased and the decline of activity be diminished or prevented. In order to enhance the habitual physical activity of young people it is important to know the factors which correlate with physical activity and which promote or prevent participation in physical activities. The information about correlates and determinants of physical activity is also important when planning physical activity interventions.

Only a part of the factors which are related to the physical activity of young people are that kinds of determinants which let speak about causal relationship. Gender, age and environmental factors belong to these determinants .Also parent's physical activity and support can be called determinants, although it is possible that children's active sport participation activate parents. Many personal variables which are related with physical activity, like perceived competence, goal orientation, and BMI can be both determinants or outcomes of physical activity. Therefore we prefer to use the term correlate instead of determinant. We share the opinion that information about relationships between correlates and physical activity is pedagogically important regardless of the nature of relationship, causal or reversible.

The correlates of physical activity have been categorised in many ways. Because children's and adolescents' physical activity is in the focus of this report we emphasise socialisation into sport and use a sport socialisation model as a framework when grouping the correlates. According to the old model the important factors in socialisation into sport are personal attributes (biological, psychological and social), significant others (family members, peers, teachers, coaches) and socialisation situations in various social and physical environments (McPherson, Curtis & Loy, 1989). Actually this model includes most of the factors listed in the reviews of determinant studies, such as demographic and biological, psychological, behavioural, social and cultural, and physical environment factors (Sallis, Prochaska & Taylor, 2000).Also characteristics of physical activity has been mentioned which remind us that that the correlates may be different concerning different activities (Buckworth & Dishman, 2002). Many good reviews of correlates of youth physical activity have been published before. Our contribution tries to emphasise a European perspective on this topic. This means that our review ignores many important studies carried out outside Europe. As a basic source of information we have used international comparative studies always when possible.

Individual attributes

Individual attributes here are age, gender, body composition (e.g. BMI), and psychological characteristics, such as self-esteem and competence. The age and gender differences in physical activity (declining with age; boys more active than girls) are well documented in numerous studies in most European countries. The new information may concern possible cross-cultural differences in relationships. Gender difference has a strong cultural background and a great variation between European countries in the gender difference has been documented. A ratio telling how many sport participating girls compared to participating boys varied from 81 in Norway to 37 in Spain among 15-year-olds (Telama, Kannas & Tynjälä, 1995). A certain trend showing diminishing of gender difference in sport participation during past decades is apparent at least in Northern countries (De Knop, Engström & Skirstad, 1996). A nation wide survey 12-, 15- and 18-year-old boys and girls implemented in Finland every second year since 1977 shows a remarkable increase in girls' participation in organised sport and thus, diminishing of gender difference (Laakso, Nupponen & Rimpelä, 2006). Nowadays in age of 15 and 18 Finnish girls are more active than boys when the frequency of physical activity is regarded, but boys still participate more than girls in organised sport and in vigorous physical activity (Laakso & al. 2006; Telama & Yang, 2000).

According to WHO' Health behaviour in School-aged Children (HBSC) study there is a great cross-cultural variation also in age differences, Austria, Scotland and Wales representing countries of big differences and France, Netherlands and Spain being small difference countries (Roberts, Tynjälä & Komkov, 2004). Also age-gender interaction has been found in physical activity so that the decline is steeper among girls than boys in many countries (Roberts, Tynjälä & Komkov, 2004). However in Finland the physical activity of boys declines more than that of girls leading to the situation mentioned before that girls are as active or more active than boys at age 15 and later (Telama & Yang, 2000). Another interesting age-related change found among Finnish boys is some kind of polarisation of physical activity which means that by age the number of inactive boys increases but at the same time increases the number of highly active (frequent vigorous activity) boys (Telama & Yang, 2000). The same change has been found in a smaller degree between ages 12 and 15 in Czech and German boys (Telama, Naul, Nupponen et al., 2002). Also age-related changes may depend of the type physical activity. A study from Portugal reports significant decrease in unstructured physical activity but no age differences in formal, organised activity (Mota & Esculcas, 2002). An important trend during past decades regarding age and sport participation is the decrease of age of beginners in sport (De Knop, Engström & Sirstad, 1996). The fact that even pre-school children participate in organised sport evidently has connections to the determinants of sport participation, e.g. influence of parents and family.

Physical activity has been seen as a means to prevent overweight at young age. On the other hand overweight can be barrier of participation in physical activity. However, a general finding is that the correlation between physical activity and measures of fatness, e.g. BMI or skin fold, is very low (Physical activity and health, 1996).Results of a comparative European study showed non significant correlation between physical activity index and BMI based on measured weight and height in four countries (Belgium, Czech R., Estonia, and Finland) and very low negative significant correlation in Germany. The result was the same concerning participation competitive sport and BMI (Telama & al., 2002). The result of a Czech study supports the poor relationship between physical activity and BMI (Skalifk, Frömel, Sigmund et al., 2001). A French study reported significant relationship between skin fold and sport participation among boys. An extensive Finnish study also reported a significant relationship between physical activity and skin fold while the correlation of BMI with physical activity was zero in most cases (Yang 1997; Yang, Telama & Leskinen, 2000). The evidence is rather scarce but it seems that skin fold is more reliable and valid measure of obesity than BMI. More results are needed about the relationship of heavier obesity with physical activity and participation. In general, the evidence available about the relationship between overweight and physical activity let conclude that overweight or mild obesity do not limit or prevent very mush participation in physical activity and sports.

Psychological attributes, particularly those connected to self concept and self-esteem have been found to be important predictors of motivation for physical activity and thus predictors of physical activity (De Bourdeaudhuij, 1998). On the other hand they are characteristics which may develop in physical activity and therefore they can also be outcomes of physical activity. Social-cognitive theories of motivation emphasise the importance of self-perceptions. For example, the Deci and Ryan's self-determination theory (1991) points out to three elements: perceived competence, perceived autonomy and social relatedness. Perceived physical competence measured through Lintunen's scale

(1987) correlated with physical activity index moderately high in five European countries coefficients varying from 0.36 to 0.47 among boys and from 0.40 to 0.52 among girls. Correlations between perceived physical competence and participation in competitions were about the same size. (Telama et al., 2002). The consistency of the moderately high correlations in five countries (Belgium, Czech, Estonia, Finland and Germany) indicates that perceived competence is an important correlate of physical activity in different cultural surroundings. This is supported by the survey of many German studies (Brettschneider, 2003). Also many other European studies have shown the relationship between physical activity and variables related to self-concept, such as self-efficacy in overcoming barriers (Loucaides, 2004), perceived sport competence and physical self-worth (Raudsepp, Liblik & Hannus, 2002), and self-worth (Trew Scully, Kremeral. et al., 1999). In addition perceived physical competence has been found to be positively related with physical activity intentions (Lintunen, Valkonen, Leskinen et al., 1999; Biddle & al., 1999). German studies have revealed gender specific relationships between self concept and physical activity. Among boys fitness and sport or athletic competence have been connected with a positive self image while among girls mainly attractiveness of body is important for self-worth (Brettschneider, 2003).

Perceived competence plays also an important role in the achievement goal theory. Demonstration of competence and the criteria of competence evaluation are important dimensions of motivation (Nicholls, 1989; Roberts, 2001). Especially task oriented goal orientation, which is based on self-referenced evaluation of success and competence, has been found to be positively related with many kinds of motivational factors. There is less results concerning the correlation between goal orientation and physical activity. In a European comparative study task orientation correlated significantly with both physical activity index and participation in competitions among boys in five countries coefficients being 0.27 – 0.40 for activity index and 0.20 – 0.32 for competitions. Also among girls the relationships were significant in four countries ($r = 0.25 – 0.31$) but not in Czech Republic The result regarding participation in competition was similar but correlations were smaller. Correlations of ego orientation with physical activity were low positive or zero. Also perceived health had low significant correlation with physical activity among boys in fifc countries and among girls in three countries (Telama & al. 2002).

According to Harter's theory (1990) competence supports more the self-worth if the competence area, e.g. sport, is important for the individual. The results of European comparative study show that importance of being good in sports has a moderately high correlation with physical activity. Correlations were among boys 0.40 – 0.53 and among girls 0.32 – 0.50. Also importance of being fit correlated significantly in both genders (Telama et al. 2002).

Significant others and family as socialisation environment

Family is a very important institution regarding socialisation in physical activity and sports in many meanings. Family members, parents and siblings, have an important role as significant others in particular for children. In late childhood and in adolescence the peers become important socialising agents. Family also offers the first socialisation situations and environment, which are affected by the socio-economic status of family. Family carries out psychological encouragement and gives social support in one hand, and offers economical opportunities and concrete aid, on the other hand. Bourdieu (1978) has introduced the concepts of cultural and economical capital of family referring to these different influences of family on children's physical activity. The whole process how family is involved in children's sport socialisation is very complicated because cultural and economical capital evidently correlate and because children's sport participation may influence the family life and may socialise also parents into sports (Vanhalakka-Ruoho, 1981; 1990).

Parents' and other family members' attitudes of and participation in physical activity is one expression of cultural capital of family which influences children's physical activity. According to the review of determinants of physical activity the results concerning the correlation between father's and children's physical activity were inconsistent showing more no relationship results than positive correlations (Sallis & al., 2000). This review was based on mainly American studies. An over-all analysis of Results from ten European countries (WHO's HBSC study) in 1985-1986 showed significant but very low correlation between father's, mother's, elder brother's and elder sister's physical activity and children's (10 – 16 years) physical activity. There were some evidence about same sex family member influence. The relationship between number of sport participating family members and children's physical activity was calculated in every ten counties and the relationship was significant in all countries (Wold & Anderssen, 1992). A European comparative study in 1995 also showed consistently low-moderate correlations between father's physical activity and children (12 and 15 years.) physical activity in five countries Also mother's physical activity correlated significantly children's physical activity but a lower level. No clear sex-specific (father – boy, mother – girl) influence was found in this analysis. (Telama & al, 2002). The HBSC study has revealed a great cross-cultural variation in fathers' and mothers' physical activity between European countries Finland being a country were more students than in any other country said that their fathers and mothers participate while in Poland and Spain the number of those children were smallest (King & Coles, 1992).

Many studies in European countries support the concept that of parents' and siblings' physical activity correlates with children's and adolescents' physical activity, for example in France (Deflandre Lorant, Gavarry et al., 2001), Estonia

(Raudsepp & Viira, 2000) England (Shopshire & Carrol, 1997), and Finland (Telama & al. 1994; Yang & al 1996). Some of these studies have supported the same-sex influence but all studies counting the result is not consistent. Some results indicate that the influence of parents is more important for children's participation in organised sport than for physical activity in general. It has also shown that the influence of parents may be different in the different phases of sport socialisation. Parents' support and encouragement may be important already at the first phase of socialisation, during the "sampling years" , when young people are trying many sport disciplines, but it becomes more important in "specialising years" (Macphail & Kirk, 2006). The same paper also discussed the problem of parents' over-involvement in their children's sport when their influence may be negative showing e.g. pressure toward children.

The influence of parents and other family members in children's social learning can be explained in many ways. Parents may show acceptance and social support, provide models, express expectations, strengthen children's behaviour by rewarding and, and control their behaviour giving detailed instructions (Woolger & Power, 1993). As intervening variables in parents' influence may be children' individual attributes, such as perceived competence, and other self perceptions, enjoyment and motivation which are reinforced by parents' encouragement and support. The HBSC survey 1986 revealed that in those countries where fathers participated physical activity they also encouraged children to participate (King & Coles, 1992).

In addition to family members, peers are important significant others. The over-all analyses of HBSC data of ten European countries showed that sport participating best friend was a good predictor of adolescents' physical activity, better than sport participating family members (Wold & Andersen, 1992). The peer influence was supported by a more recent HBSC data from the years 2001-2002. Number of same sex and opposite sex friends correlated significantly with physical activity among boys and girls. Also number of evening meetings with friends correlated with physical activity (Setterbulte & Matos, 2004). An interesting finding from 1986 HBSS data was that while there was remarkable variance in the number of young people whose parents participated physical activity in European countries, the variation in the number of those who had sport participating best friend was rather small (King & Coles, 1992). The importance of peers and friends in particular for the physical activity of young people is also supported by a German study showing that majority of young people participate in sport with a friend or in friend group (Gogol, Kurz & Menze-Sonneck, 2003).

The results regarding peer influence emphasise the fact that physical activity and sport participation is to a great extent a social activity. This is supported by the finding from a study where the use of time was compared between those who spent lot of time for physical activity and those who used little time to physical activity. The main difference between these two groups was in the time used in other social activities, i.e. the time spent on physical activity was mainly taken from other social activities (Telama, Silvennoinen & Vuolle, 1986).

Socio-economic status of family as socialisation situation and environment

Socio-economic status of family represents both cultural and economic capital of home which means factors enhancing social learning and socialisation in one hand and factors enabling to participate in different activities regardless of expenses. The influence of family's socioeconomic status is supported by the fact that parents' physical activity, an important socialising factor, correlates with it (Brownson & al., 2000; Wold & Hendry, 1998: Yang & al. 1999). Physical activity and sport participation of young people have been found to be related with parents' socioeconomic status in many studies but not quite consistently. For example the review by Sallis & al. (2000) lists several studies, mainly in USA, reporting no relationship. In addition to possible cross-cultural differences the relationship may also depend on method of measuring socio-economic status. The most common indicators of family's socioeconomic status have been occupational status of parents, education of parents, and indicators of family affluence or wealth. In some countries the method has been to divide children to those who are eligible for free school meal and those who are not.

In the HBSC survey 1987-1988 three measures of family's socioeconomic status were used. Family affluence scale (FAS) included number of cars own by family, own bedroom for the child, and number of holiday trips of family. The wealth of family was measure by asking young people "how well off they thought their families were on a five-point rating scale. The third measure was fathers and mothers occupational status. The results of ten European countries showed significant but very low ($0.05 - 0.10$) correlation in four and medium ($0.10 - 0.20$) correlation in four countries, and no correlation in Norway between FAS and young people's physical activity at least twice a week. Family wealth had low significant correlation with physical activity in six countries and medium correlation in two countries, and no correlation in Norway and Hungary. Father's occupational status had significant relationship with physical activity only in four countries, in two countries very weak and in two countries medium relationship (Mullan & Currie, 2000). The results show rather great differences in the relationships between the different measures of socio-economic status supporting the idea that the affluence and wealth of family is more important determinant of children's physical activity than the social status defined by father's occupation.

The importance of Family affluence for children's physical activity was supported by the results of a recent HBSC survey. In the 2001-2002 FAS was measured again. The number of computers at home had been added to affluence scale. FAS, correlated significantly with young people's physical activity at least 60 min. during 4 – 7 days in 22 European countries among boys. Countries reporting no correlation were Austria, Germany, Lithuania, Malta, Poland and Ukraine. Among girls the relationship was significant in all other countries but not in Malta neither Switzerland.

Many studies in various European countries have reported results about the positive relationship between family's socioeconomic status and children's physical activity and sport participation in Estonia (Raudsepp & Viira 2000), in Sweden (Barnekow-Bergkvist, 1998), in Scotland (Hendry, 1996), in UK (Duncan & al., 2002), in Portugal (Santos, 2004), in Finland (Tammelin & al. 2003; Laakso & Telama, 1981, Yang & al, 1996). Although HBSC study showed that family affluence did not correlate with German boys' physical activity, a recent review of German research lets understand that socioeconomic status influence participation in physical activity also in Germany (Thiel & Cachay, 2003)

What family's socioeconomic status means regarding socialisation environment of children's physical activity depends on the history and cultural background of the country. A Turkish study reported a negative relationship between parents' education and 11 – 14-year-old girls' physical activity (Kocak & al., 2002). The authors discuss the results stating that sport and leisure time activities are not part of the lifestyle of the majority of Turkish population, especially in Turkish women, and therefore modelling of sport and physical activity for girls may be particularly rare in Turkey.

There has been great changes in European societies during past decades. Some of the countries has changed from centralised socialistic system to open market societies, and in all countries influence of business market and economical competition has become more prominent. Also lifestyles and leisure time activities have adopted new forms, contents and meanings. The world of sport and physical activities is also changing all the time which can be seen in numerous new sport disciplines and activities which are to be chosen by more and more people. At the same time in many countries the number of people participating in physical activity has increased. It could be expected that these changes would affect also the socialisation situations and environments of physical activity. There has been discussions about possible levelling of socioeconomic differences in physical activity but very little or no research evidence to our knowledge has been published. Many recent European studies give evidence for the conclusion that socioeconomic status of family still influences the physical activity of young people in many European countries.

This is also supported by the Finnish Adolescent Health and Lifestyle Study which has surveyed 12-, 15- and 18-year-old boys' and girls' health habits, physical activity included, in nation wide samples since 1977 every second year. The survey has included also father's education. The results during 28 years from 1977 to 2005 showed significant relationship between father's education and children's physical activity, and there is no notable change in this relationship during 28 years (Laakso & al., unpubl.). Regardless the great changes in society, living conditions and sport culture the social inequality in physical activity and sport participations has been unchanged.

Family structure is also associated with sport participation of children. Children and adolescents in nuclear families participate more in sports than young people in other families, for example, single parent families (Laakso & al., in press). At least part of this relationship is probably explained by the socioeconomic status of family.

Physical environment

Physical activity needs always some place and space and often also equipments in order to be carried out. It can be done at home, for example, gymnastics, but most often it is realised outside home and needs therefore an appropriate environment and conditions. Variables which have been found to be related with physical activity are access to built facilities and access to natural facilities. Variables which have been studied but which have been not related with physical activity are neighbourhood safety, functionality of environment (foot paths, shops), appeal of environment (Buckworth & Dishman, 2002; Giles-Corti & Donovan, 2002; Sallis & al., 2000). These kinds of environmental variables have not studied much among children and adolescents. The distance to facilities may be important barrier of physical activity for children but it is often compensated by car transportation by parents, which may explain a non significant relationship between children's physical activity and the proximity of sport installations (Deflandre & al., 2001).

Environmental factor sometimes connected with physical activity and sport participation is urbanisation level of residence area. It has been found that the physical activity and sport participation is at higher level in urban than rural environment at least in Germany (Brettschneider, 1996) and in Finland (Telama & al., 1994). The probable explanation for the higher activity level in urban environment is better access to different facilities and more possibilities to participate in organises sport. What means a rural environment in Finland may differ from what it is in Germany. But also in Finland due to relatively late urbanisation process the situations and opportunities have changed during the past decades. In 1969 the physical activity level of adolescents was higher in rural than in urban communities (Telama, 1970). In Finland also interaction between gender and environment has been found so that boys' physical activity and sport participation is more dependent on urban environment than girls' participation (Yang & al, 2003; Telama & al, 2005).

Seasonal variation connected with meteorological conditions is a factor which influence physical activity in European countries and in particular in Nordic countries although rather little research data is available. Especially in Nordic countries the seasons mainly influence the type of physical activity but also season differences have been found in physical activity in general. The time spent playing outdoors is longer in summer than in winter among pre-school age children, and also 9–12-year-old children spend more time in physical activity during spring-summer time than fall-winter time in Finland (Nupponen & al., 2005). That season may influence also in other European countries has been shown by the results from a Portuguese study reporting that boys and girls in all age groups participated less in physical activity during fall-winter than spring-summer season. This concerned both organised and unorganised physical activity (Santos & al., 2005). In Finland the seasonal variation in the physical activity of school children was not found in 1969 (Telama, 1970). It may mean that the great changes in sport culture and life styles have weakened the adaptation to the seasonal variation and especially to winter conditions because a trend seems to be that physical activity happens more and more in constructed facilities, and if possible, indoors.

Summarising discussion

Ignoring the influence of gender and age which have been found to be universal correlates of young people's physical activity the psychological attributes seem to be most important correlates of children's and adolescents' physical activity. The key term is self and self perceptions. How a young people perceive oneself and one's body in physical activity is very important to motivation for and intention to participate. Actually this has been known in sport psychology already rather long time. What could be a new contribution of this kind review, is to show how consistent this relationship is in different cultures independent of the economical status, educational system, level and types of physical activity of each country. This should also be an important educational message to school physical education, youth sport institutions and families. The positive self concept predicts participation in physical activity and self concept can be developed in activity.

The review of recent European studies supported the concept that family is important institution for the physical activity of young people. In terms introduced by Bourdieou (1978) the family is important both due to its cultural and economic capital which means psychological and social support as some kind of social heritage in one hand, and concrete opportunities to participate on the other hand. It can be expected that when children begin to participate in organised sport younger and younger family maintain or even increases it's importance at least regarding organised sports. Regardless the many changes in European countries there still exists inequality in physical activity and sport participation of young people due to different socioeconomic background of families.

The influence of family members is rather strong and consistently found in many European countries showing, however, big variation between countries according to physical activity of family members. The same gender influence was found in many countries but not consistently. However, peer influence appeared to be stronger than the influence of family members indicating the social character of young people's physical activity and sport participation

Determinants and correlates of children's and adolescents' physical activity have been studied rather much also in Europe. The most studies have focused in on or two correlates in each study. Because it has been found that determinants and correlate may interact, multi-disciplinary studies and multivariable analyses are recommend in order to produce new information about the factors enhancing or limiting physical activity among young people.

References

Aarnio, M., Winter, T., Kujala, U. & Kaprio, J. (2002). Associations of health related behaviour, social relationships, and helath status with persistent activity and inactivity: a study of Finnish adolescent twins. *British Journal of Sports Medicine, 36,* 360-364

Baxter, J. & Maffuli, N. (2003). Parental influence on sport participation in elite young athletes. *Journal of Sports Medicine and Fitness, 43 (2),* 250-255

Barnekow-Bergkvist, M., Hedberg, G., Janlert, U. & Jansson E. (1998). Prediction of physical fitness and physical activity level in adulthood by performance and physical activity in adolescence – An 18-year follow-up study. *Scandinavian Journal of Medicine and Science in Sport, 8,* 299-308.

Biddle, S. J. H., Sood, I. & Chatzisarantis, N. (1999). Predicting physical activity intentions using a goal perspectives approach: a study of Hungarian youth. *Scandinavian Journal of Medicine & Science in Sport,* 353-357.

Biddle, S., Corely, T. & Stensel, D. (2004). Health-enhancing physical activity and sedentary behaviour in children and adolescents. *Journal of Sport Sciences, 22 (8),* 679-701.

Bourdieu, P. (1978). Sport and social class. *Social Science Information, 17 (6),* 819-840.

Brettschneider, W-D. (1996). Youth sport in Germany. In P. De Knop, L-M. Engström, B. Skirstad & M. R. Weiss (Eds.). *Worldwide trends in youth sport* (pp. 139-151). Champaign Ill. Human Kinetics.

Brettschneider, W-D. (2003). Sportliche Aktivität und jugendliche Selbstkonzeptentwicklug. In W. Schmidt, I. Hartman-Tews & W-D. Brettschneider (Eds.). *Erster Deutscher Kinder- und Jugendsportbericht* (pp. 211-233). Schorndorf: Verlag Karl Hoffmann.

Buckworth, J. & Dishman, R. K. (2002). Determinants of exercise and physical activity. In J. Buckworth (Ed.). *Exercise Psychology* (pp. 191-209). Champaign Ill, Human Kinetics.

De Bourdeaudhuij, I. (1998). Behavioural factors associated with physical activity in young people. In S. Biddle, J. Sallis & N. Cavill (Eds.), *Young and active, young people and health-enhancing physical activity – evidence and implications* (pp. 98-118). London: Health Education Authority.

Deci, E. L. & Ryan, R. N. (1991). A motivational approach to self: Integration in personality. In R. Dienstbier (Ed.), *Nebraska symposium on motivation* (pp. 237-288). Lincoln: University of Nebraska Press.

Deflandre, A., Lorant, J., Gavarry, O. & Falgairette, G. (2001). Determinants of physical activity and sports activities in French school children. *Perceptual and Motor Skills, 92,* 399-414.

De Knop, P., Engström, L-M. & Sirstad, B. (1996). World-wide trends in youth sport. In P. De Knop, L-M. Engström, B. Skirstad & M.R. Weiss (Eds.). *World-wide trends in youth sport* (pp. 276-281). Champaign, Ill. Human Kinetics.

Duncan, M., Woodfield, L., Al-Nakeeb, Y. & Nevill, A. (2002). The impact of socio-economic status on the physical activity levels of British secondary school children. *European Journal of Physical Education, 7,* 30-44

Giles-Corti, B. & Donovan R. J. (2002). The relative influence of individual, social and physical environment determinants of physical activity. *Social Science & Medicine, 54,* 1793-1812.

Gogol, A., Kurz, D. & Menze-Sonneck A. (2003). Sportengagements Jugendlicher in Westdeutschland. In W. Schmidt, I. Hartman-Tews & W-D. Brettschneider (Eds.), *Erster Deutscher Kinder- und Jugendsportbericht* (pp. 211-233). Schorndorf: Verlag Karl Hofmann.

Harter, S. (1990). Causes, correlates, and the functional role of global self-worth: A life-span perspective. In R. J. Sternberg & J. Kolligian (Eds.), *Competence considered* (pp. 67-97). New York: Vail-Ballou.

Hendry, L. B. & Love, J. G. (1996). Youth sport in Scotland. In P. De Knop, L-M. Engström, B. Skirstad & M R. Weiss (Eds.), Worldwide trends in youth sport (pp. 204-221). Chapign Ill. Human Kinetics.

Holstein, B., Parry-Langdon, N., Zambon, A., Currie, C. & Roberts C. (2004). Socioeconomic inequality and health. In C. Currie & al. (Eds), Young people's health in context, Health Behaviour in School-aged Children (HBSC) study: international report from the 2001/2002 survey (pp. 165-172). Copenhagen, WHO, Health Policy for Children and Adolescents no 4.

Kay, T. (2000). Sporting excellence: a family affair. *European Physical Education Review, 6 (2),* 15-169

King, A. & Coles, B. (1992). The health of Canada's youth, views and behaviours of 11-, 13- and 15-year-olds from 11 countries. Canada: Minister of Supply and Services Canada.

Kocak, S. Harris, M. Isler, A. K. & Cicek, S. (2002). Physical activity level, sport participation, and parental education level in Turkish junior high school students. *Pediatric Exercise Science, 14,* 147-154.

Laakso, K. & Telama, R. (1981). Sport participation of Finnish youth as a function of age and schooling. *Sportwissenschaft, 11 (1),* 28-45.

Laakso, L. Nupponen, H., Rimpelä, A. & Telama, R. (2006). Suomalaisten nuorten liikunta, katsaus nykytilaan, trendeihin ja ennusteisiin. (Physical activity of Finnish adolescents, a review of present situation, trends and predictions). *Liikunta ja tiede, 2,* xx-xx.

Laakso, L., Nupponen, H., Koivusilta, L., Rinpelä, A. & Telama, R. (2005, in press). *Leisure time physical activity of Finnish young people.* Proceedings of AIESEP World Congress, Lisbon, 17 – 20 November 2005.

Laakso, L., Nupponen, H., Rimpelä, A. & Telama, R. (Unpublished manuscript). *28-year trends in youth physical activity and its social background.*

Lintunen, T. (1987). Perceived physical competence scale for children. *Scandinavian Journal of Sport Sciences, 9 (2),* 57-64.

Lintunen, T., Valkonen, A., Leskinen, E., & Biddle S. J. H. (1999). Predicting physical activity intentions using a goal perspectives approach: a study of Finnish youth. Scandinavian Journal of Medicine & Science in Sport, 344-352.

Loucaides, C. A. (2004). Correlates of physical activity in a Cypriot sample of sixth-grade children. *Pediatric Exercise Science, 16 (1),* 25-36

Macphail, A. & Kirk, D. (2006). Young peoples's socialisation in sport: experiencing the specialising phase. *Leisure Studies, 25 (1),* 57-74.

McPherson, B. D., Curtis, J. E. & Loy, J. W. (1989). The social significance of sport: an introduction to the sociology of sport. Champign: Human Kinetics Books.

Mota, J. & Esculcas, C. (2002). Leisure-time physical activity behaviour: Structured and unstructured choices according to sex, age and level of physical activity. *International Journal of Behavioural medicine, 9 (2),* 11-121.

Mota, J. & Silva, G. (1999). Adolescents'physical activity: association with socio-economic status and parental participation among a Portuguese sample. *Sport, Education and Society, 4 (2),* 193-199.

Mullan, E. & Currie, C. (2000). Socioeconomic inequalities in adolescent health. In C. Currie, K. Hurrelman, W. Settertobulte, R. Smith & J. Todd (Eds.), *Health and health behaviour among young people* (pp. 65-72). Copenhagen: WHO Policy Series, Health policy for children and adolescents.

Nicholls, J. G. (1989). *The competitive ethos and democratic education.* Cambridge, MA: Harvard University Press.

Nupponen, H., Halme, T. & Parkkisenniemi, S. (2005). Arjen oma liikunta lasten liikunnan perusta. *Liikunta ja tiede, 42 (4),* 4-9.

U.S. Department of Health and Human Services (1996). Physical Activity and Health: A report of the surgeon general. Atlanta, GA: Centers for Disease Control.

Raudsepp, L., Liblik, R. & Hannus, A. (2002). Children's and adolescents' physical self-perceptions as related to moderate to vigorous physical activity and physical fitness. *Pediatric Exercise Science, 14,* 97-106.

Raudsepp, L. & Viira, R. (2000). Influence of parents' and siblings' physical activity on activity levels of adolescents. *European Journal of Physical Education, 5,* 169-178.

Raudsepp, L. & Viira, R. (2000). Socio-cultural correlates of physical activity in adolescents. *Pediatric Exercise Science, 12,* 51-60.

Roberts, G. C. (2001). Understanding the dynamics of motivation in physical activity: the influence of achievement goals on motivational processes. In G. C. Roberts (Ed.), Advances in motivation in sport and exercise (pp. 1-50). Champaign IL: Human Kinetics.

Roberts, C., Tynjälä, J. & Komkov, A. (2004). Physical activity. In C. Currie & al. (Eds.), *Young people's health in context, Health Behaviour in School-aged Children (HBSC) study: international report from the 2001/2002 survey* (pp. 90-97). Copenhagen: WHO, Health Policy for Children and Adolescents no 4.

278   R. Telama, H. Nupponen & L. Laakso

Sallis, J. F. (2000). Age-related decline in physical activity: synthesis of human and animal studies. *Medicine & Science in Sports & Exercise, 32 (9)*,1598-1600.

Sallis, J., Prochaska, J. J. & Taylor, W. (2000). A review of correlates of physical activity of children and adolescents. *Medicine & Science in Sports & Exercise , 32 (5)*,963-975.

Santos, M. P. (2004). The relationship between socioeconomic status and adolescents' organised and nonorganised activities. *Pediatric Exercise Science, 16 (3)*, 210-218

Santos, M. P., Matos, M. & Mota, J. (2005). Seasonal variations in Portuguese adolescents in organised and unorganised physical activities. *Pediatric Exercise Science, 17 (4)*.

Settertobulte, W. & Matos, M. (2004). Peers and health. In C. Currie & al (Eds.), *Young people's health in context. Health Behaviour in School-aged Children (HBSC) study: international report from the 2001/2002 survey* (pp. 178-183). Copenhagen: WHO, Health Policy for Children and Adolescents.

Shropshire, J. & Carrol, B. (1997). Family variables and children's physical activity: Influence of parental exercise and socio-economic status. *Sport, Education and Society 2 (1)*, 95-116.

Skalifk, K., Frömel, K., Sigmund, E., Vasendove, J. & Wirdheim, E. (2001). Weeksly physical activity in secondary school students: a comparative probe into Czech, Polish and Swedish conditions. *Gymnica (abstract), 31 (1)*, 21-26.

Tammelin, T., Näyhä, S., Laitinen, J., Rintamäki, H. & Järvelin, R.-M. (2003). Physical activity and social status in adolescence as predictors of physical inactivity in adulthood. *Preventive Medicine, 37*, 375-381.

Telama R. (1970). *Oppikoululaisten fyysinen aktiivisuus ja liikuntaharrastukset I, Kuvaileva osa (Secondary school pupils' physical activity and leisure-time sports; descriptive part, In Finnish with English titles of pictures and tables).* Jyväskylä: Kasvatustieteiden tutkimuslaitoksen julkaisuja.

Telama, R., Kannas, L. & Tynjälä, J. (1995). Comparative and international studies in physical activity and sports: a Scandinavian perspective. In B. Svoboda & A. Rychtecky (Eds.), *Physical activity for life: East and West, South and North* (pp. 324-336). Prague: Meyer & Meyer Verlag.

Telama, R., Naul, R., Nupponen, H., Rychtecky, A. & Vuolle, P. (2002). *Physical fitness, sporting lifestyles and Olympic ideals: Cross-cultural studies on youth sport in Europe.* Schorndorf: Verlag Karl Hofmann.

Telama, R., Laakso, L. & Yang, X. (1994). Physical activity and participation in sports of young people in Finland. *Scandinavian Journal of Medicine & Science in Sports, 4,* 65-74

Telama, R., Silvennoinen, M. & Vuolle, P. (1986). Kouluikäisten liikuntakäyttäytyminen (Physical activity in school age) In P. Vuolle, R, Telama & L. Laakso (Eds.), *Näin suomalaiset liikkuvat (Physical activity of Finnish population)* (pp. 51-66). Jyväskylä: Reports of Physical Culture and health.

Telama, R. & Yang, X. (2000). Decline of physical activity from youth to young adulthood in Finland. *Medicine & Science in Sports & Exercise 32 (9),* 1617-1622.

Telama, R. Nupponen, H. & Piéron, M. (2005). Physical activity among young people in the context of lifestyle. *European Review of Physical Education, 11 (2)*,115-137.

Thiel, A. & Cachay, K. (2003). Soziale Ungleichheit im Sport. In W. Schmidt, I. Hartmann-Tews & W.-D. Brettschneider (Eds.), *Erster Deutscher Kinder- und Jugendsportbericht* (217-295). Schorndorf: Verlag Karl Hoffmann.

Trew, K., Scully, D., Kremer, J. & Ogle, S. (1999). Sport, leisure and perceived self-competence among male and female adolescents. *European Physical Education Review, 5 (1)*, 53-73.

Vanhalakka-Ruoho, M. (1990). The ecological view in studying children's sport. In R. Telama, L. Laakso, M. Piéron, I Ruoppila & V. Vihko (Eds.). *Physical education and life-long physical activity* (pp. 185-193). Jyväskylä: Reports of Physical Culture and Health 73.

Wold, B. & Anderssen, N. (1992). Health promotion aspects of family and peer influences on sport participation. *International Journal of Sport Psychology, 23,* 343-359.

Wold, B. & Hendry, L. (1998). Social and environmental factors associated with physical activity of young people. In S. Biddle, J. Sallis & N. Cavill (Eds.) *Young and Active?: Young People and Health Enhancing Physical Activity: Evidence and Implications.* London, England: Health Education Authority.

Woolger, C. & Power, T. (1993). Parent and sport socialization: Views from the achievement literature. *Journal of Sport Behaviour, 16 (3),* 171-189

Yang, X. (1997). A multidisciplinary analysis of physical activity, sport participation and dropping out among young Finns. Jyväskylä: LIKES Research Center for Sport and Health Sciences, Research Reports on Sport Health 103.

Yang, X., Telama, R. & Laakso, L. (1996). Parents' physical activity, socioeconomic status and education as predictors of physical activity and sport among children and youths – a 12-year follow-up study. *International Review for Sociology of Sport, 31 (3),* 273-294.

Yang, X., Telama, R., Leino, M. & Viikari, J. (1999). Factors explaining physical activity of young adults: importance of early socialisation. *Scandinavian Journal of Medicine and Science in Sport, 31,* 273-294.

Yang, X., Telama, R. & Leskinen, E. (2000). Testing a multidisciplinary model of socialisation into physical activity: a 6-year follow-up study. *European Journal of Physical Education, 5,* 67-87

Yang, X., Telama, R. Laakso, L. & Viikari, J: (2003). Children's and adolescents' physical activity in relation with living environment, parents' physical activity, age and gender. *Acta Kinesiologica Universitatis Tartuensis, 8,* 61-88.

Chapter 15:
Obesity, physical activity patterns and sedentary lifestyles of young people in Austria, Germany and Switzerland

Wolf-Dietrich Brettschneider, Roland Naul, Andrea Bünnemann & Dirk Hoffmann

Introduction

The object of this review is to provide an overall picture of the younger generations in three countries of central Europe: Austria, Germany and Switzerland. The second and third chapters of this review deal with children's and adolescents' state of health with regard to overweight and obesity, fitness, and motor abilities. The fourth and fifth chapters focus on young people's lifestyles, which are dominated by sedentary activities (i.e. media-related activities such as viewing television or playing with computers) but also influenced by sport and physical activity. Finally, chapter 6 will identify those factors and determinants that occasion both the physical activity and sedentary behaviour of the young people in these three countries.

National and international databases (such as SPOLIT, SPOFOR, SPOMEDIA, PSYNDEX, and PUBMED) were exhaustively explored in order to identify studies pertaining to the key topics of this review. In addition, the internet was searched for references to scientific experts in the various subject areas so that the authors could contact these experts for additional insights into relevant data.

Because of the limited number of representative national studies in the countries under review, our study considers mainly regional and local surveys and investigations. The inclusion of these more local and regional investigations made possible an approximate assessment of trends within the different subject areas reviewed in this paper. The different operational definitions and measurement techniques used do introduce the problem of comparability. Nonetheless, we have attempted to describe each topic on the basis of existing studies of children and adolescents to the three countries.

Prevalence of overweight and obesity

Germany

Currently available data on overweight and obesity among children and adolescents in Germany are inconsistent, and even very diffuse. The review showed that rates of prevalence of overweight and obesity vary between 5 % and 30 % (Table 1). On the one hand, these discrepancies are due to sample characteristics. On the other hand, overweight and obesity among children and adolescents are described on the basis of different reference systems, ultimately resulting in highly variable findings. Whereas an internationally accepted reference system exists to determine the Body Mass Index (BMI) of adults, there is no uniform and standardised solution for children and adolescents. To illustrate this problem, a number of studies on overweight and obesity during childhood are discussed below.

The authors from the German Nutrition Society (DGE) who conducted a nationwide survey for the Federal Ministry of Health and the Federal Ministry of Nutrition, Agriculture and Forestry in 1998/1999 have doubts about their own results because they applied the reference system of Rolland-Cachera et al. (1982; 1991) to determine the BMI. This reference system is recommended by the European Childhood Obesity Group (ECOG), but is based on studies conducted many years ago and thus may be no longer representative. For example, in response to increasing average height over the last few years, one must question whether respectively 16.4 % and 11.3 % of all 6 to 8-year-olds are truly obese and overweight, or whether these children are simply taller and therefore heavier than the children from the original database (DGE, 2000).

Increasingly, data are presented according to Cole's reference system. This system was based on six national studies and is supported by the Childhood Group of the International Obesity Task Force (IOFT) (Kromeyer-Hauschild et al., 2001). According to Cole's reference system, several studies show a 15 % prevalence rate among German children and adolescents (Böhm, Friese, Greil & Lüdecke, 2002; Kalies, Lenz & von Kries, 2002). An overweight prevalence of 16 % among 7 to 11-year-olds was calculated by Wabitsch, who applied anthropometric data from 32,429 children and adolescents aged between 1 and 17 for an international comparison. Cole's reference system does appear relevant in the context of international comparisons, but the absence of German children from the original database questions to what extent the system may be representative for German children.

To describe the situation of German children and adolescents, the "National Task Force against Obesity in Infancy and Adolescence" (AGA) recommends the classification system of Kromeyer-Hauschild et al. (2001) as reference system. This system was used by the Jena research team led by Kromeyer-Hauschild (Kromeyer-Hauschild et al. 2001), in the Kiel Obesity Prevention Study (KOPS) (Spethmann, Mast, Langnäse, Danielzik & Müller, 2002) and in North Rhine-Westphalia's (NRW's) Provincial Health Report (MFJFG, 2002) (Table 1).

Tab. 1.   Prevalence of overweight and obesity among children (%) in Germany according to different surveys and reference systems

Survey	Year	Gender	Overweight	Obesity	Total	Reference System
Jena 7- to 14-year-olds	1975	♂	3.1	0.9	4.0	Kromeyer-Hausschild
		♀	2.5	0.8	3.3	
		both	2.8	0.9	3.7	
	1985	♂	2.9	0.8	3.7	
		♀	2.4	0.4	2.8	
		both	2.7	0.6	3.3	
	1995	♂	**4.5**	**2.4**	**6.9**	
		♀	**6.2**	**0.8**	**7.0**	
		both	**5.4**	**1.6**	**7.0**	
KOPS 6- to 7-year-olds	1996	♂	-	-	6.6	Kromeyer-Hausschild
		♀	-	-	9.2	
		both	-	-	7.9	
	2000	♂	-	-	**13.7**	
		♀	-	-	**18.9**	
		both	-	-	**16.3**	
NRW 5- to 6-year-olds	2002	♂	-	4.8	-	Kromeyer-Hausschild
		♀	-	4.4	-	
		both	-	4.6	-	
Brandenburg 6-year-olds	1994	♂	9.4	3.6	13.0	Cole
		♀	12.9	4.6	17.5	
		both	11.2	4.1	15.3	
	1999	♂	**9.4**	**4.9**	**14.3**	
		♀	**12.0**	**4.9**	**16.9**	
		both	**10.7**	**4.9**	**15.6**	
Bavaria 5- to 6-year-olds	1987	♂	7.6	1.5	9.1	Cole
		♀	9.5	2.1	11.6	
		both	8.6	1.8	10.4	
	1997	♂	**11.0**	**2.8**	**13.8**	
		♀	**13.6**	**2.8**	**16.4**	
		both	**12.3**	**2.8**	**15.1**	
Wabitsch 7- to 11-year-olds	1995	both	-	-	**16.0**	Cole
DGE 6- to under- 8- year-olds	1998/99	both	**11.3**	**16.4**	**27.7**	Rolland-Cachera

Whereas NRW's Provincial Health Report reports only the prevalence of overweight, KOPS gives an account of the prevalence of both overweight and obesity. Among Kiel's 6-year-olds, 13.7 % of the boys and 18.9 % of the girls have an increased body weight (Spethmann et al., 2002). Data from the Jena study, which was conducted for 7- to 14-year-olds nearly ten years ago (1995), show an overall prevalence rate of overweight and obesity of 7 %.

As regards the prevalence of overweight and obesity during adolescence the results are similar: the data vary between 6 and 22 % and are not representative (Table 2).

Tab. 2. Prevalence of overweight and obesity among adolescents (%) in Germany according to different surveys and reference systems

Survey	Year	Gender	Overweight	Obesity	Total	Reference System
HBSC 11- to15 -year-olds	**2001/02**	♂	**6.0**	**2.4**	**8.4**	Kromeyer-Hausschild
		♀	**3.3**	**1.7**	**5.0**	
		both	**4.6**	**2.1**	**6.7**	
Osnabrück 13- to15 -year-olds	**1985-1999**	♂	**15.1**	**5.1**	**20.2**	Kromeyer-Hausschild
		♀	**15.9**	**7.6**	**23.5**	
Hamburg 13- to15 -year-olds	**1991-1998**	♂	**13.8**	**5.2**	**19.0**	Kromeyer-Hausschild
		♀	**15.5**	**6.4**	**21.9**	
		both	**14.6**	**5.8**	**20.5**	
Brandenburg 16-year-olds	1995	♂	13.2	3.7	16.9	Cole
		♀	13.0	3.2	16.2	
		both	13.1	3.4	16.5	
	1999	♂	**15.1**	**4.7**	**19.8**	
		♀	**14.7**	**4.9**	**19.6**	
		both	**14.9**	**4.8**	**19.7**	
Wabitsch 14- to 17-year-olds	**1995**	♂				Cole
		♀				
		both			**13.0**	
DGE 12- to under-17-year-olds	**2002**	♂	-	-	-	Rolland-Cachera
		♀	-	-	-	
		both	**9.5**	**6.9**	**16.4**	

Generally speaking, overweight and obesity increase during childhood and decrease during adolescence. However, with respect to gender, no generalisations can be drawn from the examined German studies: the prevalence of overweight and obesity is neither consistently higher nor consistently lower for boys or girls.

Data regarding temporal shifts in the prevalence of overweight and obesity are ambiguous. Yet existing data do indicate changes over the last few years or decades. The majority of longitudinal surveys conclude that the number of overweight children and adolescents has increased (Table 1). According to the Jena survey, the prevalence of overweight and obesity among children has doubled from 3.3 % to 7.0 % over a period of ten years. The KOPS study reported a doubling during a four-year time span (1996: 7.9 %; 2000: 16.3 %). A Bavarian study showed that the prevalence of overweight and obesity increased by 4.7 % over a ten-year period (from 10.4 % to 15.1 %) (Kalies et al., 2002). Finally, the authors of the Nutrition Report discussed an important increase in the prevalence of overweight and obesity in the age group of 6 to 10-year-olds (DGE, 2000).

According to a recent study representative for Germany, the prevalence of overweight among the young generation is 15.3 % and the prevalence of obesity is 6.3 %, with no difference between boys and girls (Robert Koch Institute, 2006). About 10 % to 20 % of Germany's younger generation is estimated to be severely affected by health problems calling for longer-term intervention or treatment (Sygusch et al., 2003; Hurrelmann, 2000; Palentien, 2003).

These objective data do not correspond with children's and adolescents' subjective perception of their state of health: 3 % of children between the ages of 6 and 12 and 5 % of adolescents consider themselves severely affected by health problems (Deusinger, 2002; Kolip, Nordlohne & Hurrelmann, 1995). 82.5 % of the interviewees evaluate their state of health to be excellent or good (Ravens-Sieberer, 2003).

The fundamental causes for changes in the disease spectrum – particularly with respect to overweight and obesity – and these disturbing figures are to be sought in altered lifestyles. Four areas of life that are particularly important explanatory variables for the prevalence of overweight and obesity are family, sport and leisure time, nutrition, and education and information (Wabitsch, 2004). Factors such as media consumption, sport, physical activity, and nutrition, children's and adolescents' origins and parental homes are crucial parameters for overweight and obesity. For example, children of immigrants and children from lower social strata are more frequently overweight than children of German origin and from higher social strata (Wabitsch, 2004; Müller, 2003, Sygusch, Brehm & Ungerer-Röhrich, 2003), and children's body weights can be predicted from their parents' body weights.

Switzerland

Considering the figures for overweight and obesity in Swiss children and young people given in Tables 3 and 4 we see that between 5.5 % and 24 % of adolescents and between 13 % and 34 % of children are overweight, and between 0.6 % and 2.7 % of adolescents and between 1.6 % and 16.4 % of children are obese. (Buddenberg-Fischer, 2000, 2002; Zimmermann, Hess, Hurrel, 2000; Debus, 2002; Eichholzer et al., 1999; Huwiler, Stephan, Katharine, 2004; Ledergerber, Bächlin, 2004; Woringer, Schütz, 2004; Currie et al., 2004). This wide range of values is partially due to the different definitions of overweight and obesity used in the various reference systems, and to sampling (sex, age, region – the question of representativity) and methodological differences. The following sections will allow a more detailed analysis of the selected studies.

Tab. 3:   Prevalence of overweight and obesity among adolescents in Switzerland according to different surveys and reference systems

Survey	Year	Gender	Overweight	Obesity	Total	Reference System
Switzerland 15- to 24-year-olds	1992/93	♂	11.8	1.1	-	WHO references
		♀	6.1	0.7	-	
		both	8.9	0.9	-	
Canton Zurich 14- to 19-year-olds	1993-1996	♂	22.6	-	-	Swiss references
		♀	22.0	-	-	
City of Zurich 14½ year-olds	1994	both	18.0	-	-	Cole
	2002	both	22.0	-	-	
City of Basel 9th school year	1976/77	♂	7.0	-	-	Swiss references
		♀	10.0	-	-	
	2002/03	♂	24.0	-	-	
		♀	20.0	-	-	
City of Lausanne 11½- 16-year-olds	1985-1996 logitudinal	♂	17.6	2.3	-	Cole
		♀	14.0	2.7	-	
Switzerland 13-year-olds	2001/02	♂	7,8	1.9	-	WHO references
		♀	5.6	0.6	-	
15-year-olds		♂	10.2	1.2	-	
		♀	5.5	1.2	-	

A national survey conducted in 1996 recorded the weight and height (without shoes and wearing light summer clothing) of a representative random sample of 595 Swiss children aged from 6 to 12 and calculated their BMI (Zimmermann, Hess, Hurrel, 2000, Debus, 2002). These BMIs were compared with different reference percentiles, taking into account the cut-off points recommended for defining overweight and obesity in each country. Depending on the reference values that were used, the prevalence of obesity varied between 9.7 and 16.1 % and the prevalence of overweight between 21.7 and 34.2 %. There were no significant differences in the prevalence of overweight and obesity for boys and girls. The American reference data showed the highest prevalence of overweight (27.4 %) and obesity (16.3 %) among 6-8-year-old boys; significantly more girls than boys were obese among 11-12-year-olds (10.3 % compared to 7.5 %).

Tab. 4:   Prevalence of overweight and obesity among children in Switzerland according to different surveys and reference systems

Survey	Year	Gender	Overweight	Obesity	Total	Reference System
City of Zurich 7-year-olds	**1994**	**both**	**16.0**	3.4	-	Cole
	2002	**both**	**17.0**		-	
10-year-olds	**1994**	**both**	**16.0**	4.3	-	
	2002	**both**	**19.0**		-	
Switzerland 6- to 8-year-olds		♂	27.2	16.3	-	NHCS-references
		♀	27.2	12.6	-	
9- to 10-year-olds		♂	19.2	5.6	-	
		♀	24.6	7.8	-	
11- to 12-year-olds	**1996**	♂	23.0	7.5	-	
		♀	21.8	10.3	-	
6- to 12-year-olds		♂	34.1	17.2	-	Swiss references
		♀	34.3	15.0	-	
		both	**34.2**	**16.1**	-	
6- to 12-year-olds		♂	31.9	16.4	-	French references
		♀	33.8	15.2	-	
		both	**32.8**	**15.8**	-	
City of Basel Kindergarten	**1976/77**	♂	9.0	-	-	Swiss references
		♀	10.0	-	-	
	2002/03	♂	13.0	-	-	
		♀	16.0	-	-	
3rd school year	**1976/77**	♂	7.0	-	-	
		♀	11.0	-	-	
	2002/03	♂	26.0	-	-	
		♀	26.0	-	-	
City of Lausanne 5- to 11½-year-olds	**1985-1996 logitudinal**	♂	13.5	1.7	-	Cole
		♀	14.0	2.7	-	

Between 1993 and 1996 Buddenberg carried out a survey of young people in the canton Zurich (Buddenberg-Fischer, 2000, 2002). A total of almost 2300 14-19-year-old boys and girls were interviewed, weighed and measured (clothed but without shoes). Their BMI values were compared with the randomised calibration references for Switzerland. Young people whose BMI was below the 15th percentile were classified as underweight, those between the 15th and 85th percentile were classified as normal, and those whose BMI was beyond the 85th percentile as overweight. For the surveyed Zurich adolescents the results showed 69.4 % of the girls and 67.6 % of the boys to be of normal weight, 8.6 % and 9.8 % respectively to be underweight and 22 % and 22.6 % respectively to be overweight. Neither sex nor age had any influence on the classifications, but the survey did find some correlation with the young people's social status. More young girls of higher social status were underweight and more young girls with lower social status were overweight. A higher percentage of obese boys were from lower social status.

Another study compared the results of two longitudinal studies (Woringer, Schütz, 1998). The purpose of this comparison was to calculate the percentiles of a group of 1203 children and young people born in the year 1980, who were monitored from their 5th to 16th year. The data were compared with the findings of longitudinal study carried out by Prader and Largo on 413 children born in 1954-56 in the canton Zurich. Both studies are representative of their respective areas. The percentiles were calculated using Cole's method from values for weight and height measured by school doctors. Comparing the results we see a deviation between the percentiles of the two comparative studies of approximately zero for the third percentile (cf. figures 1 and 2), increasing progressively with age up to 2 BMI units for the 50th percentile (one BMI unit

Fig. 1:   Differences in the BMI percentiles for boys after Woringer-Schütz (children born in 1980) and the Prader-Largo study (children born in 1954-56) (Woringer, Schütz, 2004)

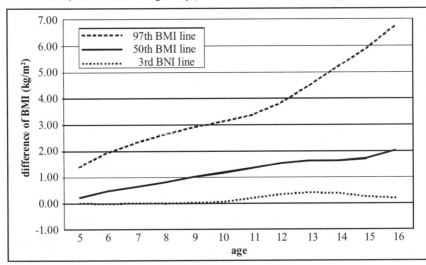

Fig. 2:   Differences in BMI percentiles for girls after Woringer-Schütz (children born in 1980) and the Prader-Largo study (children born in 1954-56) (Woringer, Schütz, 2004)

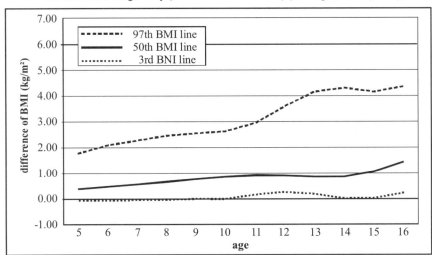

corresponds to 3 kg body weight). For the girls the increase is not quite so steep as for the boys. For the 97th percentile the visible deviation increases from the 5th year up to the 11th, where it stabilises for the girls at 4.3 BMI units while continuing to increase for the boys until the 15th year to a value of 6.8 units. The percentage of girls who are overweight remains constant at 14 % throughout the age range; for the boys it is 13.5 % for 5-11½-year-olds and 17.6 % for 11½-16-year-olds. The proportion of obese children is 2.7 % for the girls and between 1.7 and 2.3 % for the boys in the two specified age groups. Overall this study shows that there has been considerable change over the surveyed period of 25 years, particularly for the boys.

Considering the overall picture – despite all the methodological differences in the ways the data were gathered – one has to conclude that overweight and obesity represent an increasing health risk for Swiss children and young people.

There is no difference between boys and girls as regards overweight; young people from lower social classes seem to be overrepresented.

Austria

For Austria there only a few studies on the prevalence of overweight and obesity of children and adolescents.

According to the available data, between 9.0 % and 19.0 % of children are overweight and between 2 % and 8.8 % are obese. Amongst Austrian adolescents, 6 % to 41.9 % are overweight and 1 % to 11 % are obese (Elmadfa et al., 2003;

BM für Soziale Sicherheit und Generationen, 2002; Widhalm & Dietrich, 2003, 2004; Currie et al., 2004; Waldherr & Rollet, 2001; ÖBIG, 2006; Altern mit Zukunft, 2006) (see Table 5 & 6).

Overweight and obesity are more prevalent in children (10–12-years-old); in all age groups the values for boys are higher than for girls. Particularly high prevalences of overweight and obesity were found among Viennese apprentices, especially females.

Tab. 6:　Prevalence of overweight and obesity in children in Austria according to different surveys and reference systems

Survey	Year	Gender	Overweight	Obesity	Total	Reference System
Austria 3- to 6 -year-olds	-	♂	**10.0**	**6.0**	-	Kromeyer-Hausschild
		♀	**10.0**	**3.0**	-	
Lower Austria 7- to 10 -year-olds	-	♂	**11.0**	**5.0**	-	Kromeyer-Hausschild
		♀	**10.0**	**4.0**	-	
Austria 11-year-olds	2001	♂	**11.0**	**2.0**	-	Cole
		♀	**9.0**	**2.0**	-	
Vienna 10- to 12-year-olds	2002/03	both	**19.5**	**8.8**	-	Kromeyer-Hausschild

Tab. 6:　Prevalence of overweight and obesity in youth in Austria according to different surveys and reference systems

Survey	Year	Gender	Overweight	Obesity	Total	Reference System
Austria 15- to 18 -year-old trainees	-	♂	**13.0**	**11.0**	-	Kromeyer-Hausschild
		♀	**6.0**	**4.0**	-	
Austria 13-year-olds	2001	♂	**13.0**	**2.0**	-	Cole
		♀	**9.0**	**1.0**	-	
15-year-olds		♂	**9.0**	**4.0**	-	
		♀	**7.0**	**1.0**	-	
Vienna 13- to 15-year-olds	2002/03	both	**14.3**	**7.4**	-	Kromeyer-Hausschild
Vienna 15- to 19-year-old trainees	1996-2000	♂	**28.8**	**5.4**	-	Schlaf & Pudel
		♀	**41.9**	**3.7**	-	
Austria 18-year-olds recruits	2002	♂	**14.8**	**5.3**	-	-

Besides the differences in the prevalence of overweight and obesity Austria is said to exhibit geographical differences. In the eastern states (Styria, Burgenland, Vienna, Lower Austria) the proportion of overweight children and young people between the ages of 6 and 18 is higher than in the western states. Rieder and Widhalm/Dietrich report a correlation between the prevalence of overweight and obesity in Austrian children and young people and their parents' social class and standard of education: a higher proportion of children belonging to lower social classes (working class, lower middle class) and children of parents with a poor standard of education are overweight or obese.

The Austrian data on children and adolescents display methodological weaknesses and limitations, i.e. lack of representativity. Variations in data assessment – self-reported versus measured – and different classifications make it inadvisable to draw far-reaching conclusions.

Physical fitness and motor abilities

Germany

Representative studies on fitness and motor abilities in children and adolescents are rare in Germany.

Based on recent reviews (Dordel,2000a, 2000b; Gaschler,1999, 2000, 2001), a meta-analysis (Bös, 2003) aggregated and analysed more than 20 German studies covering more than 10,000 children and adolescents between the ages of 4 and 15. Data assessment was difficult due to the fact that there are no standardised tests that are representative for Germany and the studies did not use the same evaluation criteria. Nonetheless, it can be stated that a significant proportion of Germany's young generation shows noticeable motor deficits (Bös, 2003).

Considering German studies on temporal shifts of motor abilities among children and adolescents, one may conclude that there has been a decrease in motor abilities (Crasselt, 1991; Crasselt, Forchel & Stemmler, 1985; Schott, 2000; Rusch & Irrgang, 2002; WIAD, 2000; Kirchem, 1998; Gaschler & Heinecke, 1990). In addition, some studies on young Germans' physical fitness and motor performance were conducted using international test batteries and items, which enabled us to compare German findings with data from other EU countries (Naul 1997; Naul et al. 2003; Telama 2002).

The meta-analysis of Bös (2003) attempted to draw conclusions about temporal shifts in motor ability and the development of children and adolescents. The meta-analysis aggregated and examined as much data as possible from identical test items – German studies as well as other European studies from the last about 40 years. In this way the meta-analysis included data for several 100,000 male and female children and adolescents between the age of 6 and 17. The mean values for 1975 and 2000 show that young Germans' motor ability decreased during the last quarter of the twentieth century, and that this decrease has been quite extreme. On average, the decrease in motor ability is approximately 10 to 15 % (Bös, 2003). This decrease is most obvious with respect to endurance tests and forward-bend tests for the assessment of flexibility. A change in ability is also apparent with respect to 20m runs, which show children and adolescents of the early twenty-first century to be less efficient than those of the 1980s. Differences between the cohorts are smaller with respect to standing long-jumps. The only test that is possibly associated with an increase in ability from 1975 to 2000 is the muscular endurance test involving sit-ups. In contrast to the results for the other test exercises, ability changes in sit-up exercises were not statistically significant.

As in the case of children's and adolescents' changed state of health, causes for a steady decline of motor ability are thought to be due to changed lifestyles in an altered social environment. Most likely, one primary reason for the deterioration in motor skills is the lack of physical activity in everyday life. In addition, it should be noted that differences with respect to a decreasing overall coordination are more pronounced in children from urban areas than in those from rural areas (Dordel, 2000a). At the present time it is impossible to make any differentiated statements about the importance of characteristics influencing motor ability (e.g., age, gender, socialisation characteristics) due to the aforementioned deficiencies in the data (Bös, 2003).

Switzerland

In 1996/7 Michaud et al.(1999) investigated the fitness parameters of 3,450 young people from the canton Waadt. The EUROFIT test served as an appropriate instrument. The results can be summarised as follows:

- Girls show better results for flexibility (sit and reach) whereas boys achieve better performance for strength (standing broad jump).

- The values for stamina (the 20m endurance shuttle run test/Leger test) decline continually with increasing age (cf. figure 3). At all ages the values for girls were lower than for boys and indicate a significant difference between the sexes.

- The effect of puberty on strength and stamina is more expressed for boys than for girls.

- The different levels of performance recorded vary from test to test. In some cases there are only slight differences in performance in the various age groups (e.g. sit and reach), while the measurements of strength and stamina differ increasingly with increasing age, particularly for the boys.

It does not seem appropriate to derive a possible trend in the development of children's and young people's fitness and motor performance from a single study, particularly one that is not nationally representative, but the negative tendency shown by the studied parameters seems undeniable. In this context we can cite a report compiled from the annual examinations of 30,000 Swiss recruits (Hüttenmoser, 2002): in 1988, the young men called up at age 18/19 needed 4.9 seconds to climb a 5m pole; in 2001 the average time was 5.73 seconds. This indicates a loss of performance of 17 % over a period of 13 years.

Fig. 3:   Calculated values of VO$_2$max, broken down by age and gender (Michaud et al., 1999)

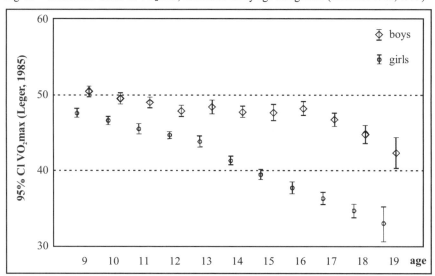

Austria

A national representative survey carried out in Austria ("Clever & Fit" study, Sandmayer, 1994) recorded the levels of motor performance of Austrian schoolchildren. The participants were 67,000 girls and boys between the 11 and 14 from regular schools and sports schools (extended elementary schools specialising in skiing and/or other sports). The level of motor performance was assessed by using a battery of standardised motor tests.

In addition to these motor tests the study included four tests of muscle function intended to establish muscular dysbalance. These included muscles in the following groups: groin (m. iliopsoas), upper thigh (mm. ischiocrurales), pectorals (m. pectoralis major), femoral extensors (m. rectus femoris), buttocks (m. glutaeus maximus), thoracic (m. erector trunci), abdomen (m. rectus abdominis) and shoulder-blade fixators (m. serratus anterior and m. rhomboideus).

The results of these tests are given below. The results for regular schools are shown first, and these are then compared these with the results from specialist sports schools.

20m sprint (speed)

On the basis of a 20m sprint, the action speed of Austrian boys was found to improve between the 10th and 14th year by about 8 % (0.32s). Most of this improvement took place between the 12th and 14th year. This result is in accordance with expectations, because the increased strength due to male puberty has a positive influence on speed. The development of speed levels in girls is extremely negative: the mean difference between 11-year-old and 14-year-old girls was 1.3 %, which is not statistically significant. This means that girls' motoric speed levels stagnate from the 11th year. The difference between boys and girls at age 11 is 1.7 %, but this increases to around 8 % by age 14.

Standing broad jump (strength)

Boys' jumping strength increased between their 10th and 14th year on average by 17 %, while girls' strength increased by an average of barely 6 % over the same period. There are two probable reasons for this difference in the sexes' development of strength: firstly, the hormonal changes during male puberty, and secondly, the girls' physical inactivity. While the difference in jumping strength between boys and girls at age 10 is only 2 %, it is already over 13 % at age 14.

8 min run (stamina)

The results for stamina, which are so important for the proper functioning of the cardio-vascular system, are similar to those for coordination. The 8-minute run showed that boys' stamina improves only by around 8 % between their 10th and 14th year. Since this improvement can primarily be attributed to the longer stride afforded by the body's longitudinal growth at this age, we can assume that the functionality of the cardio-vascular system is not markedly developed during this period. Girls' level of stamina is poorly developed: the level of performance of 14-year-olds is almost identical to that of 10-year-olds.

Girls' motor development must be judged particularly deficient. A large proportion of the tested motoric abilities begin to stagnate as early as their 11th year. In areas such as coordination and stamina, which are so important for health, the performance already begins to deteriorate from their 12th year.

An analysis of the data for 12-year-old boys and girls (at regular schools) with respect to their domicile shows that the performance of those from the westernmost states (Vorarlberg, Tyrol, Upper Austria and Salzburg) is significantly better than those from the east (Lower Austria, Styria, Carinthia, Vienna and Burgenland). It is particularly remarkable that this tendency can be observed even for 11-year-old and 13-14-year-old boys and girls. These geographical tendencies are also reported for the prevalence of overweight and obesity in Austrian young people (see chapter 2) and there may be a correlation between these results – a high prevalence of overweight and obesity and a low level of physical fitness.

We also see clear differences in young people's motoric performance in the comparison between urban and rural areas. Those young people in all four age groups who live in towns and cities with populations between 30,000 and 100,000 exhibit the best performance parameters. The lowest performance is achieved by young people who live in towns and villages with fewer than 2,000 people and those who inhabit cities with populations of over one million (Vienna).

Lifestyles of today's young generation

Germany

Due to the great number of options and activities available these days, children and adolescents now have the opportunity to live quite differentiated lifestyles. The Euronet project 1992 investigated how young people utilise their time (Alsaker & Flammer, 1999a) by collecting data about both necessary and leisure activities of adolescents from twelve different countries, including 267 German 14 and 16-year-olds. For the German adolescents (Flammer, Alsaker & Noack, 1999; Alsaker & Flammer, 1999b), it was found that 18 hours per day are utilised for necessary activities, leaving a little more than five hours per day for leisure time activities (three quarters of an hour are used for 'other activities' and were not further specified) (Table 7).

When one considers necessary activities from the aspect of physical activity or sedentariness, results show that at least 92.6 % (16.7 hours) of necessary daily activities are sedentary. Indeed, since some of the necessary activities cannot be clearly classified as either active or inactive the time involved in sedentary activities is even higher for some adolescents. For example, the time involved in travelling to school (i.e. a little less than one hour) cannot be clearly classified because it was not differentiated according to pedestrians and cyclists versus those that are taken to school by bus or car. In comparison to necessary activities, leisure activities are characterised by somewhat less inactivity (75.3 %). Of the 3.9 hours of sedentary leisure activities almost two hours are devoted to viewing television. Regardless of the means whereby adolescents get to school, results from this study indicate that German adolescents spend less than two hours each day on physically demanding activities such as sport, music, or physical labour. More specifically, adolescents apportion less than one hour per day to sport – the only activity that actually stimulates the cardiovascular system. For the remainder of the day adolescents pursue activities that demand rather too little from the human body, which was formerly the main instrument for 'hunting and gathering'.

Tab. 7. Daily activities (% and hours per day) of German adolescents (data based on the Euronet project 1992: Flammer et al., 1999 and Alsaker & Flammer, 1999b).

Necessary Activities 18 hours/day			Leisure Activities 5.2 hours/day	
Inactive	Active	Not Determinable	Inactive	Active
Sleeping Personal hygiene Eating School Homework	Working Shopping	Way to school	Reading Watching TV Hanging around with friends Dating	Playing music Doing sport Working
92.6% (16.7 hrs.)	2.7% (0.5 hrs.)	4.8% (0.9 hrs.)	75.3% (3.9 hrs.)	24.7% (1.3 hrs.)
all in all				
Less than 2 hours of physical activity per day; Less than 1 hour of sport per day				

In addition to the television as a classical medium, newer technologies have become central elements in the life of the young generation. Access to media and entertainment electronics is growing as more households and, in particular, children and adolescents themselves, own electronic devices.

Two recent longer-term studies that were representative for Germany – „Kinder und Medien" (KIM; Children and Media) (Feierabend & Klingler, 2003b, 2003c, 2004) and „Jugend, Informationen, (Multi-)Media" (JIM; Adolescence, Information, (Multi)Media) (Feierabend & Klingler, 2002, 2003a) – dealt rigorously with the media behaviour of children and adolescents, respectively. The population of the KIM study is composed of roughly seven million German-speaking children between the ages of 6 and 13, as well as their mothers or mother-equivalents. The population of the JIM study is composed of the nearly six-million German adolescents between the ages of 12 and 19. Both were longitudinal studies and have been conducted annually by the Medienpäda-gogischen Forschungsverbund Südwest (Media-Pedagogical Research Group Southwest) since 1998 (MPFS 1998, 2000a, 2000b, 2000c, 2001, 2002a, 2002b, 2003a,2003b, 2004, 2005).

As illustrated in Figure 4, television was far and away the most popular medium used by adolescents throughout the course of the investigated period. About 93 % of the adolescents and 98 % of the children view television every day or several times per week (MPFS, 2002b, 2003a, 2004, 2005). Almost no changes have occurred in the amount of television viewing since the study was first conducted in 1998. After television, audio media are the most important media, used particularly by adolescents. However, while the use of audio media has remained relatively stable between 1998 and 2002, it declined for the first time in 2003. For example, while 93 % of the adolescents listened to music (e.g., via CD) every day or several times per week in 2002, this number declined to only 89 % in 2003. Similarly, the use of the radio declined from 86 % in 2002 to 77 % in 2003. Children do not use audio media as much as adolescents. However, as in the case of the adolescents, audio media are the second and third most popular media among children (CD use: 81 % in 2003; radio use: 69 % in 2003). The importance of the newspaper as an information medium has also declined over the study period. While 59 % of the adolescents read the newspaper every day or several times per week in 1998, only 49 % did so in 2003.

Fig. 4.   Media use (daily or several days per week) by adolescents, 1998-2005 (based on MPFS data).

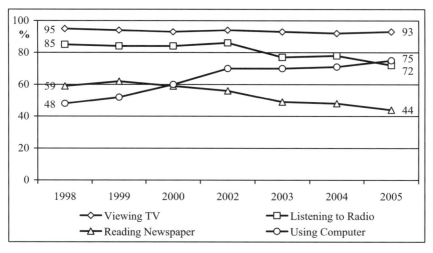

It is possible that the decline in newspaper and audio media use is associated with the enormous increase in the importance of computers over the last few years. For example, in 1998, only about half (48 %) of the adolescents used a computer every day or several times per week, and 20 % had no interest at all in this rather modern medium. By 2005, the number of adolescent computer users had increased to 75 %, and the number of non-users declined to a mere 3 %. As shown in Figure 3, this constant increase in computer use was paralleled by a constant decrease in newspaper use, with the computer displacing the newspaper to a lower importance ranking for the first time in 2000, and the gap between the use of the two media becoming increasingly larger (approximately 21 %). Similarly, the difference between computer and radio use has become fairly small by 2003 (approximately 7 % more radio use).

The KIM and JIM studies also examined the extent to which children and adolescents engage in sport. As shown in Figure 3, somewhere between 60 and 70 % of the adolescents pursued sporting activities every day or several times per week between 1998 and 2003. However, while sport was more popular than computer use throughout most of the study period, it appears that computer use is now replacing sport in popularity: in 2003, 67 % of the adolescents engaged in sport and 70 % used computers every day or several times per week. Children use computers less frequently than adolescents. However, even among children, an enormous increase in computer use can be observed: in 1999, only 34 % of the children used computers on a daily basis or at least several times per week; by 2002 this number had increased to 53 % (MPFS, 2000c, 2002b, 2004).

As the preceding discussion and the illustration indicate, there appears to be a major shift in media use among children and adolescents, with the use of computers increasing at the expense of traditional media such as radio, CDs, and newspapers. It is possible that this shift is due to the fact that modern computers can perform a number of operations, including the playing of music and providing information (e.g., news) through the internet. The only medium that remains entirely unaffected by these changes is television.

In general terms, it can be noted that TV viewing time varies according to both gender and age, for example, boys and older children view more television than girls and younger children. In addition to these variations there are differences depending on region of origin and socio-economic stratum (Feierabend & Klingler, 2003c). Children that grew up in the former German Democratic Republic (eastern Germany) view 32 minutes more television per day than children from the former Federal Republic of Germany (western Germany). Children from lower social strata view more television than children from higher social strata. Another strong factor influencing the extent of TV consumption among children and adolescents is the consumption behaviour of the parents themselves. Accordingly, parents' behaviour appears to have an important role model effect on their own children. Furthermore, overweight children watch more television than non-overweight ones, and 'Hauptschüler'[1] spent more time in front of the television than 'Gymnasiasten'[1]. Aside from the quantity of television consumption, the quality of programs

---

[1] The traditional German school system is characterized by early and selective assignment to different tracks of secondary school types. 'Hauptschüler' visit the 'Hauptschule' as the lower educational track. 'Gymnasiasten' visit the 'Gymnasium' as the upper track. The middle track is called 'Realschule'. Their students are named 'Realschüler'.

viewed is of significance. About 55 % of the programs viewed by 3 to 13-year-old German children falls into the category fiction (e.g., primarily cartoons but also comedies such as sitcoms, suspense films, and daily soap operas), which basically does not stimulate cognitive abilities at all. Children spend another 14 % of the television viewing time watching entertainment shows (e.g. game shows, talk shows). To the same degree, children invest their leisure time in educational programs. The remainder of the time passes in the viewing of sport shows (3 %), and an inordinately large portion of time in the viewing of commercials (12 %) (Feierabend & Klingler, 2004).

Switzerland

A study by the research service of the Swiss public broadcasting organisation SGR SSR idee suisse (SGR SSR, MD/SW, 2004) provides information about the daily activity habits of adolescents in Switzerland. A representative sample of 499 adults with children were interviewed and asked about details of their children's day-to-day routine during the week and at weekends, and about their media consumption and media access.

In general we can say that the children's schedules and the time they spent on their various daily activities (eating, sleeping, playing, school, etc.) differed between the various language regions. We can observe differences both between their weekday routine (see Table 8) and that for weekends, between the sexes, and also between younger children (7-10-year-olds) and teenagers (11-14-year-olds) (SGR SSR, MD/SW, 2004).

Tab. 8:   Average daily activity times (in minutes) for Swiss children aged 7-14 in the context of their activity fields on weekdays (based on SGR SSR, MD/SW, 2004)

	German Swiss	French Swiss	Italien Swiss
Activities at home			
Sleeping	601	613	592
Eating	83	98	76
Homework	74	73	76
Doing work at home, helping in the household	60	67	49
Leisure time at home	155	132	151
Activities outside home			
School	325	335	349
Way to school	64	61	56
Playing outside, hanging around with friends	160	159	153
Doing sport, playing music	101	90	113

If we consider the children's overall daily routine without reference to individual activity fields then we find predominately similarities between the language regions. Firstly, these include the fact that markedly more time is spent at home at weekends (between 17.40 and 18.34 hours) than on weekdays (between 16.08 and 16.39 hours). It is also the case that in all three language regions 7-10-year-olds spend considerably more time at home than do 11-14-year-olds. The regions also agree in that over 80 % of the investigated individuals were at home over the midday period.

From the available data it is not possible to determine the ratio of active time to inactive time in these daily periods because we have no precise information about the detailed contents of the activity profile relating to the questions 'Leisure time at home', 'Way to school', 'Playing outside, hanging around with friends' or 'Doing sport, playing music'. In this context, if we look at the statements made to the same study regarding Swiss adolescents' daily use of media (see Table 9) then we are forced to conclude that the greater proportion of their leisure activities are characterised by the use of audio-visual media, and are therefore quite possibly of a sedentary nature.

Tab. 9: Daily media consumption in minutes of 9-16-year-old Swiss children in 1997 (average of all interviewees) and of 7-14-year-old children in 2003 (average of all parental interviewees) (Süss, Giordani, 2000; SGR SSR, MD/SW, 2004)

Media	German Swiss		French Swiss		Italian Swiss	
	1997	2003	1997	2003	1997	2003
Watching TV	81	92	102	92	85	123
Listening to radio	81	81	51	62	85	68
Listening to CDs/ records (1997) +MDs/MP3/LPs (2003)	100	78	81	78	94	82
Digital video games	28		46		19	
Computer games	23	49	35	69	21	39
Playing Game Boy	20		26		14	
Watching videos	24	-	33	-	26	-
Computer	12	-	12	-	15	
Internet	2	80	1	55	7	63
Reading comics	11		22		19	
Reading books	29	40	24	39	27	54
Reading magazines	12		8		10	
Reading newspapers	7		5		10	
Average total time of media consumption	455	420	461	395	453	429

Since Switzerland is a multi-lingual country its available media are not uniform but differentiated according to the local language, and most users do choose the media available in their mother tongue (Rathgeb, 1998; Süss, Giordani, 2000). In addition to a number of regional investigations on children's and young people's use of media there are only a few representative national study on this topic (e. g. Süss, Giordani, 2000; SGR SSR, MD/SW, 2004) and these will principally be referred to in the following discussion.

Television and audio media occupy the highest proportion of the children's media consumption in both studies; this applies to all three parts of the country. Computer-related media take second place; in 1997 this mainly consists of playing games, in 2003 of using the Internet. The smallest amount of time is occupied by printed media and it appears that this is declining still further (cf. Table 9). In all parts of the country the average total time the surveyed children spent on media is around 7.5 hours in 1997, and around 6.55 hours in 2003. This change may be due on the recorded investigation into the use of different media in 1997 and 2003. For example, in 2003 there are no reported data on computer usage or watching videos.

There were marked individual discrepancies in the preference for media consumption between the three language regions of Switzerland. In French-speaking Switzerland, more television is watched in 1997; in Italian-speaking Switzerland in 2003. More computer games are played by French-speaking Switzerland in both studies and in 2003 the preference for print media is higher in Italian-speaking Switzerland than in other parts. (Süss, Giordani, 2000; SGR SSR, MD/SW, 2004)

The different prevalence of media consumption in Switzerland's various language regions was also established in 1997 in an earlier study by Begert/Steinmahn.

In view of the heterogeneous data and different survey methods used it is not possible to clearly state whether media consumption overall has increased or decreased between the two survey periods – there may merely have been a regrouping between preferences for individual media. We can recognise a clear reduction in preferences for certain media (e.g. printed media) while television and the internet both show increased preferences.

The consumption of individual media must also be viewed not only in the context of unrestricted access – i.e. not subject to parental control – but also with reference to the availability of those media. Only 68 % of adolescents in Swiss households have free access to a television, and only 59 % have free access to a computer, whereas for radio and audio media the figures are over 90 %. We can also state that the more numerously individual media are available the greater is the likelihood of uncontrolled access (SGR SSR, MD/SW, 2004).

Austria

In Austria, most of the available information about the media consumption of Austrian children and young people is supplied by national surveys or derived from surveys carried out in the individual federal states (cf. Austrian Institute for Family Research, 1998; Austrian Federal Ministry for Social Security, and Generations, 1999; Dür, Marvlag, 2002; Austrian Federal Ministry for Social Security, Generations and Consumer Protection, 2003).

There are only a few records offering precise times for individual media consumption for Austria. Most publications offer personal percentage preferences for media use (cf. Austrian Institute for Family Research, 1998; Austrian Federal Ministry for Social Security, and Generations, 1999; Dür, Marvlag, 2002; Austrian Federal Ministry for Social Security, Generations and Consumer Protection, 2003). Most young Austrian boys and girls can barely imagine life without radio and television – they have become classic everyday media. Regardless of their age, sex and level of education, most young Austrians have integrated radio and TV into their daily assortment of media. In 1992 the average television consumption on weekdays was 103.7 minutes for 10 to 14-year-olds and 114.1 minutes for 15 to 18-year-olds. At weekends the average daily television consumption for 10 to 14-year-olds increases to 173.4 minutes, and for 15 to 18-year-olds to 157.9 minutes (Austrian Institute for Family Research, 1998).

Mobile communication is already a firmly established factor in the lives of 14-19-year-olds. Most of them own their own mobile phone and there is no detectable difference between the sexes in this respect. Telephoning as a leisure pursuit plays a far greater role for girls than for boys and occupies correspondingly more time. There are, however, no detectable sex-specific differences in boys and girls' usage of newer forms of communications technology (SMS, e-mail, chatting) (Austrian Federal Ministry for Social Security, and Generations, 1999; Austrian Federal Ministry for Social Security, Generations and Consumer Protection, 2003).

As regards the leisure-oriented use of computers and the Internet, 14-19-year-olds are not aware of any sex-specific differences in usage, but for the over 20s the distinction is still very much entrenched. If we believe young people's own estimates of their usage there is almost no difference between boys and girls, but if we compare the absolute frequency of daily computer and Internet usage we see that the proportion of boys is still markedly higher (Austrian Federal Ministry for Social Security, and Generations, 1999; Austrian Federal Ministry for Social Security, Generations and Consumer Protection, 2003).

Young people's sport culture and physical activity patterns

Young people's involvement in physical activities includes compulsory PE lessons at school and extra-curricular activities either as a part of the voluntary school based PE programme or as part of voluntary participation in organised sport club activities. In addition, in Germany as well as in Austria and Switzerland modern types of informal physical activities e.g. running, biking, rollerblading etc. are becoming more popular and more frequently practised in recent years.

The status of physical education at school

Germany

Current surveys on young people's lifestyles in Germany provide the background against which all actions and efforts in PE and school sport have to be evaluated:

- 15 % overweight boys and girls (90th percentile) and 6.3 % obese young people (97th percentile) (KIGGS, 2006).

- The physical inactivity in the daily lives of young people is constantly growing; it cannot be compensated by their high participation in organised and informal sporting activities.

- Almost 1/3 of elementary school children are no longer able to swim.

- The level of motor abilities has declined by 10-15 % in the course of the last 25 years.

As to the situation in physical education and school sport in Germany the data are drawn from the first representative national study SPRINT (DSB, 2006).

Concerning the time allocated to school PE the results of the study show a wide gap between curricula and reality. The three hours per week suggested in the curriculum are not the norm, but rather the exception. On average one out of four lessons does not take place.

In general, teachers who give PE lessons in school have a qualified degree – with the primary school as an exception. Here 49 % of teachers teaching PE have no specific education in our subject matter.

The quality of sport facilities is satisfactory. As to the state of the buildings, equipment, safety, hygiene and attractiveness, the votes of pupils, teachers and principals are very similar.

Almost two thirds of all pupils consider PE lessons – with low differences between the genders – to be important or very important. And so do their parents. Concerning young people's perception of the quality of PE lessons the evaluation scale of the pupils presents a positive picture. They want to be physically challenged and long for achievement, relaxation and, above all, fun. They are interested in those activities that support fitness and health and can be applied in their leisure time outside school.

Pupils feel more comfortable in PE lesson than in other subjects and in school in general and the findings show the important role of PE and sport programmes in creating a positive school climate.

Against the background of the problems and challenges faced by the young generation the importance of school PE and its valuable contribution to an active and healthy lifestyle is obvious.

Switzerland

There is no available information regarding the extent to which Swiss young people can or actually do avail themselves of sports activities provided by their schools, there is merely a record of how well individual cantons have complied with and continue to comply with the statutory provision of three hours compulsory school sport per week (Lamprecht/Murer/Stamm, 2000; Lamprecht/ Stamm, 2004, 2006). We can therefore establish that in 1994 and again in 2000 about four fifths of Swiss cantons complied with the statutory requirement. From 2000 on, however, a large proportion of cantons made use of a more flexible statute that permitted them to include sports days and sports camps in the obligatory minimum. This increased "flexibility" particularly affects the upper school (from year seven) and those pupils who have already completed their compulsory schooling (from year ten).

Youth+Sport (J+S) is the confederation's central furtherance programme for sport for children and young people from 10 to 20 (Lamprecht/Stamm, 2004, 2006). J+S is extra-curricular and subsidiary, and organises its events together with cantons, clubs and other sports institutions. Until 1994 it was available only to young people from their 14th year; since the minimum age was reduced to 10 in 1995 an average of 500,000 boys and about 350,000 girls have participated in J+S events. In 2004 750,000 children and adolescents have participated in the events. That is more or less half of all Swiss 10 to 19-year-olds. The events in football had the most participants (21.9 %), followed by snow sports (18.5 %), sports camp activities & trekking (11.4 %), gymnastics (7.7 %) and tennis (4.8 %). In the most recent years, more girls than boys are involved in J+S events, the age group from 11 to 13 years has the highest involvement and the involvement of girls declines with age. (Lamprecht/ Stamm, 2004, 2006)

Austria

In 2001 the Austrian Federal Ministry of Education, Science and Culture prescribed the following curricular provision for sport at the various levels: in elementary schools from 2 to 3 hours, for lower secondary schools (HS), academic secondary schools (AHS) and upper secondary schools from 3 to 4 hours compulsory physical education per week, but it is possible to deviate from these figures. The survey carried out by Redl/Gerhartl in 2003, which interviewed boys in the 8th to 10th class, found that between 22.6 % and 21.7 % of academic secondary schools and upper secondary schools offer 3 hours compulsory physical education per week. Of the boys interviewed, 86 % do not wish to change the amount of physical education they receive or have more hours of compulsory or voluntary physical activity, but boys do express such a wish significantly more often than girls. The desire for more sport is more frequently expressed in schools with a good sporting infrastructure than in schools whose sporting infrastructure is perceived as poor. Only 16.2 % of boys and girls state that sports lessons are cancelled several times per week or month.

All Austrian schools are required to help to correct the deficiencies of any girls and boys with a poorly developed motoric base. Voluntary physical education courses are constrained to pursue only two objectives – to encourage less well performing girls and boys and to systematically compensate for school stress: only if the "school partnership committee" (similar to a parent-teacher association) has expressly stated that these activities are not required may any other content be included (Austrian Federal Ministry of Education, Science and Culture, 2001a).

In the school year 1999/2000, about 44 % of Austrian schools offered one or more voluntary physical education courses. Most held only one course and most voluntary physical education classes were continued throughout the school year (Austrian Federal Ministry of Education, Science and Culture, 2001a). Voluntary physical education is generally carried out in multi-class groups.

From 1991 the number of voluntary physical education classes first rose, then dropped sharply for the school year 1995/96, and subsequently rose again. The numbers of schoolchildren participating in such classes show a similar tendency, but far fewer girls and boys at medium-level and higher-level technical and vocational upper secondary schools participate in voluntary physical education, and the numbers are decreasing still further (Austrian Federal Ministry of Education, Science and Culture, 2001a). The survey carried out by Redl/Gerhartl in 2003 also reports that the distribution of additional sports lessons depends on the level and type of school.

In the school year 1999/2000 a total of 138,514 children and young people, 58,858 girls (42.5 %) and 79,656 boys (57.5 %), attended voluntary physical education classes (Austrian Federal Ministry of Education, Science and Culture, 2001a). That figure represents about 23 % of the schoolchildren surveyed (606,235). The survey carried out by Redl/Gerhartl in 2003 arrived at a similar figure for participating boys (28 %). Of the 6,329 voluntary physical education classes (an umbrella term for more than 20 types of sport) 20 % are devoted to football, with a total of 26,205 participants (23,536 boys and 2,669 girls). Volleyball is the subject of 13.6 % of all voluntary physical education classes. Less widely disseminated sports that are nonetheless quite frequently the subject of voluntary physical education classes include "trendy" sports such as circus games, juggling, and acrobatics (28 voluntary classes, in 26th place with 0.5 %, 577 girls and boys) and "games/sport/fun" (25 voluntary classes, in 27th place with 0.4 %, 515 girls and boys). Activities intended to improve posture (123 voluntary classes, in 15th place with 2 %), condition ("fitness" with 148 voluntary classes, in 12th place with 2.3 %, 1928 girls and 1417 boys) or motopedagogy (movement education) (34 voluntary classes, in 24th place with 0.6 %) are encountered much less frequently than one might expect, in view of the expressly stated purpose of this "voluntary physical education" (Austrian Federal Ministry of Education, Science and Culture, 2001a).

"Sports weeks" or "project weeks with the emphasis on sport" are school events lasting longer than a single day. During the school year 1999/2000 one or more sports weeks were held in 2691 schools (Austrian Federal Ministry of Education, Science and Culture, 2001b) amounting to a total of 6630 sports weeks altogether, 11 % more than in the school year 1996/97 (i.e. 779 more than 5851). A total of 282,336 boys and girls participated in sports weeks during 1999/2000, approximately 27 % of the 1,058,191 boys and girls whose school timetables would have permitted them to attend these events had they wished to, slightly lower than in 1996/97 (288,754, about 28 %).

Under "summer sports weeks" (conducted by all kinds of organisations) we see that about 19 % of the events offered only one type of sport (600 of 3169). These are swimming weeks and hiking weeks (principally held by elementary schools and extended elementary schools). School sports and physical education events that offered more than one type of sport generally concentrated on tennis with horse-riding (and other sports), sailing with tennis, or windsurfing with sailing. If we consider the frequency of individual sports in summer sports weeks we find tennis at the very top of the list with 11 %, alongside swimming, and hiking in third place, undoubtedly due to its great significance in elementary schools.

Participation in organised club sports and informal 'peer sport'

Germany

In addition to questions about PE, the participation in organised and informal sport are of interest. However, questions about the degree to which German children and adolescents participate in either organised or informal sport can not be answered for all of Germany and for all age groups (Gogoll, Kurz & Menze-Sonneck, 2003). Five studies are to be mentioned that examined adolescents' participation in sport outside of PE:

- 1978 (Study area: Hesse; Number of subjects: 3600; Age of subjects: 12-18), (Sack, 1980);

- 1987 (Study area: NRW; Number of subjects: 4079; Age of subjects: 14-18), (Baur & Brettschneider, 1994; Brettschneider & Bräutigam, 1990);

- 1992 (Study area: NRW; Number of subjects: 2425; Age of subjects: 12-19) (Brinkhoff, 1998; Kurz, Sack, Brinkhoff, 1996; Menze-Sonneck, 1998; Sygusch, 2000);

- 1995 (Study area: NRW; Number of subjects: 1656; Age of subjects: 12-19) (Endrikat, 2001; Gogoll, 2003; Kurz & Tietjens, 2000; Tietjens, 2001; Menze-Sonneck, 2002); and

- 1998 to 2000 (Study area: NRW; Number of subjects: 1565 (544[2]); Age of subjects: 12-18) (Brettschneider & Kleine, 2002).

In summary, it can be noted that – in addition to the required PE lessons in school – 88 % of the adolescents do engage in sport regularly at least once per week. On average, participation in sport during leisure time has its peak around the age of 12. When compared to earlier years we see that this peak has shifted towards younger ages: in 1978, it was around the age of 14 (Sack, 1980). Throughout their youth, male adolescents, 'Gymnasiasten', and adolescents from higher social strata engage in more sport on average than female adolescents, 'Hauptschüler', and adolescents from lower social strata. Furthermore, the degree of physical activity among parents influences that of their children. If parents are inactive, their children are also more frequently inactive (Graf et al., 2003).

With regard to the social settings for young Germans' physical activities we can differentiate seven categories (Gogoll et al., 2003):

- Sports club;

- Partially public corporations: youth centre, school for extramural studies;

---

[2] Case number for the longitudinal study

- Voluntary groups in PE: PE association, sport study groups;

- Commercial facilities: gym, dance school, ballet school, horseback riding school, martial arts school, tennis centre;

- Unorganised municipal facilities: swimming pool, ice rink, athletics ground, half pipe

- Familiar surroundings: at home, in the yard and garden

- Other settings without sport-specific exclusivity: street, school yard, parking lot, nature.

Figure 6 shows how adolescents' regular athletic activity is distributed among those settings. Among the organised facilities, the municipal sports club has an outstanding position, with 47 % of the adolescents engaging in sport there at least once per week. Only sport in settings without sport-specific exclusivity appears more important (52 %). There are gender differences with respect to the use of the different settings described above. Boys tend to favour clubs, unorganised municipal facilities, and PE study groups. Girls tend to favour sport in familiar surroundings and at commercial facilities. However, these findings from NRW cannot simply be generalised for other regions in Germany. Apparently, the distribution of sport among different settings largely depends on the options available and the infrastructure in a given location.

Fig. 6:   Sport participation (at least once per week) in different settings (%) (Kurz & Tietjens, 2000, p.394, in Gogoll et al., 2003, modified)

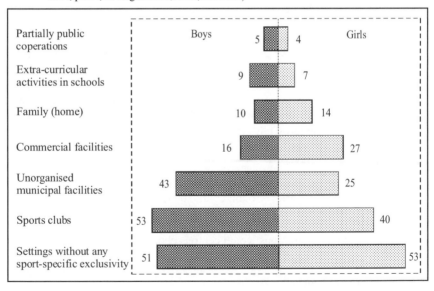

Informal 'peer sport' activities

The sport that adolescents play during their leisure time – outside of school and sports clubs – is comparatively poorly researched. There is some data in existence relating to preferred forms of sport or sport activities, which will be described separately according to gender. According to these data, traditional forms of sport have great appeal despite the broadening of the array of forms of sport (Brettschneider & Kleine, 2002). Among male adolescents, soccer assumes a dominant rank (47 %) in the top-ten list of favourite informal sport activities. Other forms of sports, such as basketball (10 %), cycling (9 %) and swimming (8 %) are less preferred. Among the girls, there is no favoured form of sport. Instead five forms of sports, all of which aim at improving fitness, are close in popularity: cycling (17 %), swimming (14 %), inline-skating, skate-boarding, roller-skating (14 %), jogging (12 %) and horseback riding (12 %). Considering the amount of participation in leisure time sport among adolescents, it can be concluded that adolescents are also committed to sport outside of schools and sports clubs. Depending on operational definitions and sample characteristics, 69 % (study 1992) or 86 % (study 1998-2000) of adolescents play sport at least once per week outside of schools and clubs. Male and younger adolescents are more frequently athletically active during their leisure time than female and older adolescents. Adolescents report choosing informal sport due to a lack of "right options" in sports clubs, as well as a desire to play sport without social control by adults and to organise their athletic commitment in a flexible fashion (Brettschneider & Kleine, 2002).

Differentiating the adolescents with regards to the contents of specialisation, it turns out that nearly two thirds (65 %) of the male adolescent who are sport club members primarily train for competitions and are members of a competitive team. Even most female club members are oriented towards competition. However, in contrast to the boys, many of the girls also pursue leisure time sport. Overall, 80 % of all adolescents – at least in NRW – are members of a sports club for an average of more than eight years until they reach age 19 (Kurz & Sonneck, 1996). During this time, adolescents go to a sports club on average twice per week and for a total of about five hours per week (Gogoll et al., 2003). Until graduation from high school, most adolescents in NRW have played more sports in clubs than in school (Kurz & Sonneck, 1996).

While the growth rate of sports clubs in western Germany was around 8 % between 1991 and 2001, the growth rate in eastern Germany was around 55 %. During the same period, the growth rate with respect to adolescent membership was approximately 78 % in eastern Germany, while in western Germany the rate was only around 19 %. However, in addition, the time invested in sport activities is shorter among the smaller number of children and adolescents that play sport in eastern Germany than it is among the larger number of children and adolescents that play sport in western Germany (Kurz & Tietjens, 2000); no precise data are available regarding this issue. Overall, the average membership duration among eastern German adolescents is between five and seven years, but the eastern German adolescents are more loyal to one club than the western German adolescents.

Switzerland

A survey of the numbers of children who belong to sports clubs (Lamprecht/ Stamm, 1997) shows that girls achieve a similar level of membership to boys only in the under-10 age group (cf. Table 6). As the children get older more boys join or belong to sports clubs while the figure for girls declines (Lamprecht/Stamm, 1997; Jeker/Lamprecht/Stierlin, 2005).

Fig. 6:   Level of young people's membership of sports clubs, by sex (in %) (Lamprecht/Stamm, 1997)

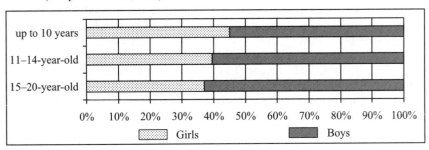

The rate of fluctuation for young club members increases markedly with age, but in all three age groups there are more joining than leaving (Table 4). The 15-20-year-olds also have the highest leaving rate of any age groups in Swiss sports clubs.

Tab. 4:   Joining and leaving in the last five years, by age (percentage of affected clubs) (Lamprecht/Stamm, 1997)

	Clear increase	Almost no change	Clear decrease
Children up to age 10	35.5	59.8	4.7
Young people ages 11-14	31.9	57.9	10.2
Young people ages15-20	23.3	58.9	17.8

The survey by Michaud et al. in 1999 came to a similar conclusion. When asked about their activity in sports clubs, between 61 % and 75 % of girls and between 61 % and 85 % of boys, depending on their school grade, stated that they belonged to a sports club. The level of membership markedly declines between children's 13th and 14th year, more for girls than for boys. A statistical analysis also established that for adolescents the level of membership in organised sports correlates positively with their participation in informal sporting activities. This applies to both sexes (Michaud et al., 1999).

Neverless, today more children and adolescents are currently involved in organised sport than ever before. (Jeker/Lamprecht/Stierlin, 2005)

Austria

As they get older, an increasing proportion of children and young people belong to no clubs at all, as various Austrian studies have shown. Whereas rather more than one third of 10-year-olds do not belong to any clubs (Nagl, 1993), the proportion for 14-15-year-olds rises to about half, increasing to over 60 % for 16-17-year-olds (Fessl + Gfk, 1990; Austrian Institute for Youth Studies, 1989). The trend showed by this rather old data is confirmed by results given in the Health Report for Vienna 2002 (Magistrate of the City of Vienna, 2002), which assumes only 16 % sports club membership for 14-24-year-olds. The low proportion of children and young people in clubs is reflected in results obtained by Redl/Gerhartl in 2003, who speak of an "increasing individualisation" of the leisure sports activities of boys between the 8th and 10th classes. The report quotes 65 % of the surveyed girls and boys as preferring to engage in exercise and sport "alone", while 30 % preferred their sports "in a group".

Conclusions

Factors that influence behaviour and lifestyles have already been mentioned in the various sections above. In order to specify more exactly the factors and determinants that foster the forms of participation in sport and physical activity as well as sedentary activities, and also for purposes of clarification, these factors and determinants are assigned to four different levels of analysis marking the socialisation process (Lerner & Busch-Rossnagel, 1981).

Psychological determinants

On the first level – the level of the individual – individual competences and self-concept appear to be of importance for participation in club-organised sports. According to one study (Brettschneider & Kleine, 2002), a high positive self-esteem, a stable emotional self-concept, high social competence, positive self-assessment of motor abilities, and positive physical appearance encourage club membership. If these characteristics are less positive or absent, adolescents tend to leave the club or do not even join it. If adolescents have the personal goal to increase their performance and success in sport or the goal to play sport in the community to feel socially accepted and to experience support from the group, then adolescents increasingly join sports clubs. The goal of physical and mental fitness also facilitates this commitment to clubs. However, if commitment in a sports club represents shortage of time and stress for an individual, then in the long run, that individual will turn his or her back on the club.

Social determinants

On the level of social interactions, parents and siblings are particularly important because both are crucial determinants for the leisure time organisation of children and adolescents. In addition, persons such as teachers, trainers, and youth workers exert an influence; social inequalities and the residential surroundings are also of significance.

Parental home and siblings

While there are no studies with respect to the influence of siblings, parental influence is frequently the focus of researchers looking for causes. From existing studies, it can be concluded that parents generally serve as role models with respect to both consumption behaviour and degree of physical activity. Children of parents that view a lot of television also spend a lot of time in front of the television (Feierabend & Klinger, 2003c). Likewise, children of inactive parents tend to be more frequently inactive, while children of athletically ambitious parents also tend to be enthusiastic about sport (Graf et al., 2003).

School teachers, coaches in clubs, youth workers and other persons

There are no empirical findings with respect to the question of how much teachers, trainers, and youth workers sustainably foster the participation in sport or not, or encourage or discourage children to be active. However, trainers appear to have an influence on the participation in sports clubs, whereby the role-model effect of trainers grows with increasing sport competence, stricter leadership, and a higher degree of orientation towards efficiency. If their trainer functions as a role model, children and adolescents less frequently leave the sports club (Brinkhoff, 1998) and instead remain loyal to it.

Social inequalities

One-sided differences can be noted with respect to gender. It is the boys that both view more television (Feierabend & Klingler, 2003c) and play more sport (Gogoll et al., 2003). Only with respect to computer use are the gender differences nearly negligible, with a slightly more frequent use among the boys (Feierabend & Klingler, 2003a).

Regarding lifestyle facets such as sport or physical activity and media consumption, there are significant differences according to the socio-economic stratum. On one side, children from higher social strata have shorter television viewing times than children from lower social strata (Feierabend & Klingler,

2003c). On the other hand, children from higher social strata play on average more sport than children from lower social strata (Gogoll et al., 2003).

Germany has one special feature with respect to social inequalities because the reunification between the East and West happened only 15 years ago. If one separates children into eastern and western German children, two conclusions can be drawn: firstly, that children that grew up in the former DDR view more television than children from the former FRG (Feierabend & Klingler, 2003c); and secondly, that eastern German children play much less sport than western German children.

Residential surroundings

Particularly for children but also for adolescents, the residential surroundings represent the area in which the young generation can be physically active. There are no representative studies that concern themselves with the residential surroundings of the young generation. However, the development of car traffic, which has negative consequences for children and adolescents, can be described (Limbourg, Flade & Schönharting, 2000). Individual passenger traffic has increased from 48.6 % (1980) to 52.7 % (1996) during a period of 16 years. Stated differently: whereas in 1960, there were four children per car, the relationship is now reversed. Depending on geographic location there are three to four cars per child. Germany is among the most motorised countries in the world, which brings several negative consequences for children's lives. Firstly, traffic accidents are the most frequent cause of death in childhood. Furthermore, the risk of accidents limits children's independent mobility (Limbourg et al., 2000). Diverse local studies that compared the outdoor activities of children between different residential areas (rural communities to large towns) confirm this limited mobility (Engelbert, 1986; Flade, 1994; Fölling-Albers & Hopf, 1995; Deutsches Jugendinstitut, 1992). The larger the town and the accompanying increase in traffic load, the shorter the time that children play with their peers on the street. The possibilities for play and exercise on the road have markedly decreased for children in Germany (Limbourg, 2003).

Organisational and institutional determinants

On the third analytical level are organisations and institutions that foster or hamper physical activity among the young generation.

Access to appropriate exercise/sport settings

The existence and the usability of attractive sport settings is a major factor for the sporting and physical activity among children and adolescents. While one may speak of an all-inclusive sport infrastructure in western Germany and adolescents characterise sports clubs as easily accessible (Brettschneider &

Kleine, 2002), 15 years after the reunification, one still finds a lack of sport facilities in eastern Germany (Baur & Braun, 2000). This lack is not only limited to DIN-standardised sport facilities but also to facilities for informal sport activities. Furthermore, the condition of streets in many places does not facilitate a use for sport activities. Despite the greater percentage increase of informal sport opportunities in eastern Germany, eastern German children and adolescents still do not have as much access to informal sport settings, municipal sport options, commercial sport facilities, and sports clubs as western German children and adolescents. This is particularly true for rural areas (Baur & Burrmann, 2000). The smaller number of children participating in sport in eastern Germany is particularly attributable to the currently unsatisfactory sport infrastructure.

Transport

The everyday activity of children and adolescents is also determined by the modes of transport they use to travel, e.g., to school. In one study (Flade & Limbourg, 1997), which was conducted in six larger towns, the bicycle was the most frequently used means of transport among the 10 to 15-year-olds in everyday life. On average, nearly every third route (34 %) is covered by bicycle. Only every fourth route (25 %) is walked on foot. The remaining 41 % of the routes are covered in motorised vehicles, either as passengers in public transport (28 %) or, but less frequently so, in cars. A comparison between children from rural and urban areas shows that the former use public transport much more frequently than the latter. No difference between children from rural and urban areas could be detected with respect to transport by car. Another investigation considers the different means of transportation not from the perspective of individual ways, but from the perspective of the time that is spent in road traffic (Funk & Faßmann, 2002). According to this study, children and adolescents are en route for an average of about one hour per day, primarily as passengers in cars (31 % of the entire participation duration in traffic) and as pedestrians (29 %). Cycling only makes up about 12 % of the time spent in traffic.

Societal historical determinants

Demographic developments

Considering general demographic developments, it can be assumed that children have fewer playmates in their surroundings today than they did several years ago. In the 1950s, one could still speak of an age 'pyramid.' However, today, the shape of the corresponding graph for Germany's ageing society resembles more closely a 'mushroom'. Humans live longer due to improved medical support; at the same time, the birth-rate has declined to only about 1.4 children per woman over the last few decades (Federal Statistical Office of Germany, 2003). Within merely two years, the decline in birth-rate resulted in a decrease of the number of children of ages 1 to 15 from 12.8 million (2000) to 12.4 million (2002) (Federal Statistical Office of Germany, 2004). Stated differently, the number of children between 1 and 15 years of age decreased by 400,000 or 3 % during a mere two-year period.

Values and norms

The values and norms of today's young generation are no longer comparable to those of past young generations. Considering that society is changing, the evaluation of the lives of adolescents results in ambiguous conclusions (Brettschneider, 2003b). Adolescents today have good hopes in modernisation but are also the group at risk of modernisation. Therefore, the „Inflation am Wertehimmel" ("inflation of the value system"; Deutsche Shell, 2000) of today's adolescents is not to be interpreted as a deterioration of values, but rather as a loss of intra-personal durability and super-individual validity. Adolescents find themselves confronted with the tasks of carefully estimating ambiguous expectations of the future and examining life plans for chances and risks. In this manner, adolescents become flexible designers of their own lives, the guidelines of which adolescents have to sketch alone. Following the trend in the development of values, the results of the fourteenth and most recent Shell youth study show an increasingly pragmatic attitude among adolescents (Deutsche Shell, 2002). According to the study, adolescents of both genders embrace a success and performance-oriented society, paired with a re-orientation from social and ecological commitment to economically dominated thinking and behaviour. The priorities of young people shift from reaching ideological goals of societal reform to personally mastering specific and practical problems (Deutsche Shell, 2002). In the private area, there is furthermore the hedonistic wish to enjoy life (Noelle-Neumann & Petersen, 2001).

Advertisement and promotion of physical/sedentary activities and fast food/healthy food

Considering announcement and advertisement mechanisms for sport and physical activity or sedentariness on the one hand, and healthy or unhealthy food products on the other hand, commercials brought to all homes by means of television are particularly important. A study on the most frequently advertised child-specific products (Baacke, Sander, Vollbrecht & Kommer, 1999) resulted in a list of 16 commercials. Eight of these commercials advertised toys, whose use are associated with physical inactivity. Another four commercials advertise sugar-containing sweets. The remaining four products (e.g., toothpaste) are not associated with either physical activity/inactivity or nutrition. Not a single product in the list encouraged physical activity or healthy nutritional habits. Another analysis, which concentrated specifically on food commercials, yielded the same result: the most frequently advertised nutritional products are sweets such as chocolate bars and candy (Diehl, 1998). Regarding the effects of television commercials, it is generally concluded that such commercials stimulate the buying behaviour of children and adolescents (Glogauer, 1999; Baacke et al., 1999).

To promote physical activity – particularly in the form of sport – the *Deutsche Sportbund* (DSB; German Sports Federation started a nationwide campaign projected to run for at least four years, entitled *"Sport tut Deutschland gut"* (Sport is good for Germany") in 2004. As advertising media the DSB uses posters, television commercials, a big series of advertisements in the *"Bild am Sonntag"*, further smaller advertisements in other newspapers, and a newsletter that is sent to all 88,000 gymnastics and sports clubs in Germany (DSB-Presse, 2002).

Appearance of mass media and modern technology

While the media television, radio, and CD already had their broad distribution one or two decades ago, the extensive appearance of computers, mobile phones, and also digital video games is still young. As previously illustrated in Section 5.2, the ownership of computers among adolescents increased from 35 % to 47 % during a five-year time span. The increase in digital video games in children's rooms is also unmistakable (1998: 23 %; 2002: 35 %). But it is mobile phones that have experienced the most marked increase during the five-year period, with an increase of 74 % (1998: 8 %; 2002: 82 %) (Feierabend & Klingler, 2003a). The use of all media, both older and newer forms, is associated with physical inactivity. And with this increase in media, the daily time adolescents spend on sedentary activities will also increase.

References

Alsaker, F. D. & Flammer, A. (Eds.) (1999a). *The Adolescent Experience – European and American Adolescents in the 1990s*. Mahwah: Lawrence Erlbaum Associates.
Alsaker, F. D. & Flammer, A. (1999b). Time Use by Adolescents in an International Perspective. II: The Case of Necessary Activities. In F. D. Alsaker & A. Flammer (Eds.), *The Adolescent Experience – European and American Adolescents in the 1990s* (pp. 61-83). Mahwah: Lawrence Erlbaum Associates.
AMZ (Hrsg.) (2006). *Erster Österreichischer Adipositasbericht 2006. Grundlage für Zukünftige Handlungsfelder: Kinder, Jugendliche, Erwachsene*. www.adipositas-austria.org/pdf/3031_AMZ_Adipositas_3108_final.pdf
Baacke, D., Sander, U., Vollbrecht, R. & Kommer, S. (1999). *Zielgruppe Kind: Kindliche Lebenswelt und Werbeinszenierungen*. Opladen: Leske + Budrich.

Baur, J. & Braun, S. (2000). *Freiwilliges Engagement und Partizipation in ostdeutschen Sportvereinen. Eine empirische Analyse zum Institutionentransfer.* Köln: Sport und Buch Strauß.

Baur, J. & Brettschneider, W.-D. (1994). *Der Sportverein und seine Jugendlichen.* Aachen: Meyer & Meyer.

Baur, J. & Burrmann, U. (2000). *Unerforschtes Land. Jugendsport in ländlichen Regionen.* Aachen: Meyer & Meyer.

Böhm, A., Friese, E., Greil, H. & Lüdecke, K. (2002). Körperliche Entwicklung und Übergewicht bei Kindern und Jugendlichen – Eine Analyse von Daten aus ärztlichen Reihenuntersuchungen des Öffentlichen Gesundheitsdienstes im Land Brandenburg. *Monatsschrift Kinderheilkunde, 150,* 48-57.

Bös, K. (2003). Motorische Leistungsfähigkeit von Kindern und Jugendlichen. In W. Schmidt, I. Hartmann-Tews & W.-D. Brettschneider (Eds.), *Erster Deutscher Kinder- und Jugendsportbericht* (pp. 85-107). Schorndorf: Hofmann.

Brettschneider, W.-D. & Kleine, T. (2002). *Jugendarbeit im Sportverein. Anspruch und Wirklichkeit.* Schorndorf: Hofmann.

Brettschneider, W.-D. & Bräutigam, M. (1990). *Sport in der Alltagswelt von Jugendlichen.* Frechen: Ritterbach.

Brettschneider, W.-D. (2003b). Jugend, Jugendliche und ihre Lebenssituation. In W. Schmidt, I. Hartmann-Tews & W.-D. Brettschneider (Eds.), *Erster Deutscher Kinder- und Jugendsportbericht* (pp. 43-61). Schorndorf: Hofmann.

Brinkhoff, K.-P. (1998). *Sport und Sozialisation im Jugendalter. Entwicklung, soziale Unterstützung und Gesundheit.* Weinheim, München: Juventa.

Buddeberg-Fischer, B., Gnam, G., Klaghofer, R., Buddeberg, K. (1998). Störung des Essverhaltens bei Jugendlichen als Risiko für die Entwicklung einer Anorexie oder Bulimie. In Bundesamt für Gesundheit (Ed.), 4. *Schweizerischer Ernährungsbericht,* Bern, 290-305.

Buddeberg-Fischer, B. (2002). Körpergewicht, Körpererleben und Essverhalten von Jugendlichen. In Institut für Sozial- und Präventivmedizin der Universität Zürich (Eds.). *Die Gesundheit Jugendlicher im Kanton Zürich.* Bundesministerium für Bildung, Wissenschaft und Kultur (Hrsg.) (2001a). *Unverbindliche Übungen Bewegung & Sport. Zur Situation der unverbindlichen Übungen mit bewegungserziehlichem Schwerpunkt an österreichischen Schulen. Bericht zum Schuljahr 1999/2000.* Wien.

Bundesministerium für Bildung, Wissenschaft und Kultur (Hrsg.) (2001b). *Sportwochen. Zur Situation der unverbindlichen Übungen mit bewegungserziehlichem Schwerpunkt an österreichischen Schulen. Bericht zum Schuljahr 1999/2000.* Wien.

Bundesministerium für soziale Sicherheit und Generationen (Hrsg.) (1999). *3. Bericht zur Lage der Jugend in Österreich.* Wien.

Bundesministerium für soziale Sicherheit und Generationen (Hrsg.) (2002). *Gesundheit und Gesundheitsverhalten bei Kindern und Jugendlichen. Bericht zur Gesundheit der 11-, 13- und 15-Jährigen in Österreich. Aufbereitung der Daten des 6. WHO-HBSC-Surveys 2001.* Wien.

Bundesministerium für soziale Sicherheit und Generationen und Konsumentenschutz (Hrsg.) (2003). *4. Bericht zur Lage der Jugend in Österreich.* Wien.

Crasselt, W. (1998). Entwicklung der körperlich-sportlichen Leistungsfähigkeit von Kindern und Jugendlichen im Zeitraum von 1981-1991. In J. Rostock & K. Zimmermann (Eds.), *Bericht zum Kolloquium „Theorie und Empirie sportmotorischer Fähigkeiten* (pp. 50-59). Chemnitz: Institutsbericht.

Crasselt, W., Forchel, I. & Stemmler, R. (1985). *Zur körperlichen Entwicklung der Schuljugend in der Deutschen Demokratischen Republik.* Leipzig: Ambrosius Barth.

Currie, C., Roberts, C., Morgan, A., Smith, R., Settertobulte, W., Samdal, O., Barnekow Rassmussen, V. (eds) (2004). *Young people's health in context. Health Behaviour in School-aged Children (HBSC) study: international report from the 2001/2002 survey. Health Policy for children and adolescent; No. 4.* WHO.

Debus, J.-M. (2002). Adipositas im Kindesalter: Tägliches Brot des Pädiaters? *Paediatrica, Vol. 13, No. 1*, 9-13.

Deusinger, I. M. (2002). *Wohlbefinden bei Kindern, Jugendlichen und Erwachsenen: Gesundheit aus medizinischer und psychologischer Sicht.* Göttingen: Hogrefe.

Deutsche Shell (Ed.) (2000). Jugend 2000. 13. Shell Jugendstudie (Volume 1 and 2). Opladen: Leske + Budrich.

Deutsche Shell (Ed.) (2002). Jugend 2002. Zwischen pragmatischem Idealismus und robustem Materialismus. Frankfurt a. M.: Fischer.

Deutsches Jugendinstitut (Ed.) (1992). *Was tun Kinder am Nachmittag? Ergebnisse einer empirischen Studie zur mittleren Kindheit.* München: Verlag Deutsches Jugendinstitut.

DGE (Deutsche Gesellschaft für Ernährung e.V.; Ed.) (2000). *Ernährungsbericht 2000.* Frankfurt am Main: Heinrich.

Diehl, J. M. (1998). Fernsehwerbung für Süßes. Botschaften und Auswirkungen. *Verbraucherdienst, 43* (4), 425-429.

Dordel, S. (2000a). Kindheit heute: Veränderte Lebensbedingungen = reduzierte motorische Leistungsfähigkeit? *Sportunterricht, 49* (11), 340-349.

Dordel, S., Drees, C. & Liebel, A. (2000b). Motorische Auffälligkeiten in der Eingangsklasse der Grundschule. *Haltung und Bewegung, 20* (3), 5-16.

DSB (2006). *DSB-SPRINT-Studie. Eine Untersuchung zur Situation des Schulsports in Deutschland.* Aachen: Meyer & Meyer.

DSB-Presse (2002, April 16). Der Sport wirkt positiv in alle Bereich des Lebens. DSB-Kampagne „Sport tut Deutschland gut" vom Bundespräsidenten gestartet.

Dür, W., Marvlag, K. (2002). *Gesundheit und Gesundheitsverhalten bei Kindern und Jugendlichen. Bericht zur Gesundheit der 11-, 13- und 15-Jährigen in Österreich.* Wien.

Eichholzer, M., Lüthy, J., Gutzwiller, F. (1999). Epidemologie des Übergewichts in der Schweiz: Resultate der Schweizerischen Gesundheitsbefragung 1992/93. *Schweizer Medizinische Wochenzeitschrift, 129*, 353-361.

Elmadfa et al., (2003). *Austrian Nutrition Report.* Wien

Endrikat, K. (2001). *Jugend, Identität und sportliches Engagement.* Lengerich: Pabst.

Engelbert, A. (1986). *Kinderalltag und Familienumwelt.* Frankfurt: Campus.

Feierabend, S. & Klingler, W. (2002). Medien- und Themeninteressen Jugendlicher. Ergebnisse der JIM-Studie 2001 zum Medienumgang Zwölf- bis 19-Jähriger. *Media Perspektiven, 1*, 9-21.

Feierabend, S. & Klingler, W. (2003a). Medienverhalten Jugendlicher in Deutschland. Fünf Jahre JIM-Studie Jugend, Information, (Multi-)Media. *Media Perspektiven, 10*, 450-462.

Feierabend, S. & Klingler, W. (2003b). Kinder und Medien 2002. Ergebnisse der Studie KIM 2002 zum Medienumgang Sechs- bis 13-Jähriger in Deutschland. *Media Perspektiven, 6*, 278-289.

Feierabend, S. & Klingler, W. (2003c). Was Kinder sehen. Eine Analyse der Fernsehnutzung von Drei- bis 13-Jährigen 2002. *Media Perspektiven, 4*, 167-179.

Feierabend, S. & Klingler, W. (2004). Was Kinder sehen. Eine Analyse der Fernsehnutzung Drei- bis 13-Jähriger 2003. *Media Perspektiven, 4*, 151-162.

Fessel + Gfk (1990). *Jugendstudie 1990 "Jugendkarte"*. Wien.

Flade, A. (1994). Effekte des Straßenverkehrs auf das Wohnen. In A. Flade (Ed.), *Mobilitätsverhalten. Bedingungen und Veränderungsmöglichkeiten aus umweltpsychologischer Sicht* (pp. 155-169). Weinheim: Psychologie Verlags Union.

Flade, A. & Limbourg, M. (1997). Das Hineinwachsen in die motorisierte Gesellschaft. Darmstadt, Essen: Universität Gesamthochschule Essen.

Flammer, A., Alsaker, F. D. & Noack, P. (1999). Time Use by Adolescents in an International Perspective. The Case of Leisure Activities. In F. D. Alsaker & A. Flammer (Eds.), *The Adolescent Experience – European and American Adolescents in the 1990s* (pp. 33-60). Mahwah: Lawrence Erlbaum Associates.

Fölling-Albers, M. & Hopf, A. (1995). *Auf dem Weg vom Kleinkind zum Schulkind – eine Langzeitstudie zum Aufwachsen in verschiedenen Lebensräumen*. Opladen: Leske + Budrich.

Funk, W. & Fassmann, H. (2002). Beteiligung, Verhalten und Sicherheit von Kindern und Jugendlichen im Straßenverkehr. *Berichte der Bundesanstalt für Straßenwesen, Unterreihe „ Mensch und Sicherheit, Heft M 138*.

Gaschler, P. (1999). Motorik von Kindern und Jugendlichen heute – Eine Generation von „Weicheiern, Schlaffis und Desinteressierten"? (Teil 1). *Haltung und Bewegung, 19* (3), 5-16.

Gaschler, P. (2000). Motorik von Kindern und Jugendlichen heute – Eine Generation von „Weicheiern, Schlaffis und Desinteressierten"? (Teil 2). *Haltung und Bewegung, 20* (1), 5-16.

Gaschler, P. (2001). Motorik von Kindern und Jugendlichen heute – Eine Generation von „Weicheiern, Schlaffis und Desinteressierten"? (Teil 3). *Haltung und Bewegung, 21* (1), 5-17.

Glogauer, W. (1999). Wir essen und trinken uns dick und krank vor dem Bildschirm. In W. Glogauer (Ed.), *Die neuen Medien machen uns krank. Gesundheitliche Schäden durch die Medien-Nutzung bei Kindern, Jugendlichen und Erwachsenen* (pp. 75-83). Weinheim: Beltz.

Gogoll, A. (2003). *Belasteter Geist – Gefährdeter Körper. Sport, Stress und Gesundheit im Kindes- und Jugendalter*. Schorndorf: Hofmann.

Gogoll, A., Kurz, D. & Menze-Sonneck, A. (2003). Sportengagements Jugendlicher in Westdeutschland. In W. Schmidt, I. Hartmann-Tews & W.-D. Brettschneider (Eds.), *Erster Deutscher Kinder- und Jugendsportbericht* (pp. 145-165). Schorndorf: Hofmann.

Graf, C, Koch, B., Dordel, S., Coburger, S., Christ, H. Lehmacher, W. et al. (2003). Prävention von Adipositas durch körperliche Aktivität – eine familiäre Aufgabe. *Deutsches Ärzteblatt, 100* (47), A3110-A3114.

Hurrelmann, K. (2000). *Gesundheitssoziologie. Eine Einführung in sozialwissenschaftliche Theorien von Krankheitsprävention und Gesundheitsförderung*. Weinheim/München: Juventa.

Hüttenmoser, M. (2002). *Und es bewegt sich noch! Bewegungsmangel bei Kindern: Ursachen, Folgen, Massnahmen*. Vortrag von Marco Hüttenmoser anlässlich der Medienorientierung am 1. November 2002 im Kornhausforum in Bern

Huwiler, S., Stephan, Ch., Katharine, T.-S. (2004). Time Trends in prevalence of overweight and obesity in an urban schoolpopulation: Zürich 1994 – 2002. *European Journal of Paediatri (2004), 163: R20*.

Jeker, M.; Lamprecht, M.; Stierlin, A. (2005) *Sportvereine haben eine Zukunft – wir tun etwas dafür! Unterlagen für die Sommerkonferenz 2005 der kant. J+S.-Verantwortlichen in Basel.* Bundesamt für Sport. Magglingen.

Kalies, H., Lenz, J. & von Kries, R. (2002). Prevalence of overweight and obesity and trends in body mass index in German pre-school children, 1982-1997. *International Journal of Obesity, 26* (9), 1211-1217.

Kirchem, A. (1998). *Werden unsere Kinder schwächer?* Essen: Projektbericht.

Kolip, P., Nordlohne, E. & Hurrelmann, K. (1995). Der Jugendgesundheitssurvey 1993. In P. Kolip, K. Hurrelmann & P.-E. Schnabel (Eds.), *Jugend und Gesundheit. Interventionsfelder und Präventionsbereiche* (pp. 25-48). Weinheim/München: Juventa.

Kromeyer-Hauschild, K., Wabitsch, M., Kunze, D., Geller, F., Geiß, H. C., Hesse, V., et al. (2001). Perzentile für den Body-Mass-Index für das Kindes- und Jugendalter unter Heranziehung verschiedener deutscher Stichproben. *Monatsschrift Kinderheilkunde, 149,* 8, 807-818.

Kurz, D., Sack, H.-G. & Brinkhoff, K.-P. (1996). *Kindheit, Jugend und Sport in Nordrhein-Westfalen. Der Sportverein und seine Leistungen. Eine repräsentative Befragung der nordrhein-westfälischen Jugend.* Düsseldorf: Moll.

Kurz, D. & Sonneck, P. (1996). Die Vereinsmitglieder – Formen und Bedingungen der Bindung an den Sportverein. In Ministerium für Stadtentwicklung, Kultur und Sport des Landes Nordrhein-Westfalen (Ed.), *Kindheit, Jugend und Sport in Nordrhein-Westfalen. Der Sportverein und seine Leistungen. Eine repräsentative Befragung der nordrhein-westfälischen Jugend* (pp. 75-160). Düsseldorf: Satz & Druck GmbH.

Kurz, D. & Tietjens, M. (2000). *Das Sport- und Vereinsengagement der Jugendlichen. Ergebnisse einer repräsentativen Studie in Brandenburg und Nordrhein-Westfalen.* Sportwissenschaft, 30 (4), 384-407.

Lamprecht, M., Stamm, H. (1997). *Die Situation der Sportvereine in der Schweiz. Kurzbericht.* Zürich

Lamprecht, M., Stamm, H. (2004). *Observatorium Sport und Bewegung Schweiz. Zwischenbericht Februar 2004.* Zürich

Lamprecht, M., Stamm, H. (2006). *Observatorium Sport und Bewegung Schweiz. Zwischenbericht August 2006.* Zürich

Lamprecht, M., Murer, K., Stamm, H. (2000). *Obligatorischer Schulsport und das Bewegungsverhalten von Jugendlichen.* Forschungsbericht. ETH. Zürich.

Ledergerber, M., Bächlin, A. (2003). Fast jedes vierte Basler Schulkind ist übergewichtig. *Basler Schulblatt 12/2003,* 15-16.

Lerner, R. M. & Busch-Rossnagel, N. A. (Eds.) (1981). Individuals as producers of their development. A life-span perspective. New York: Academic Press.

Limbourg, M. (2003) Kinder sicher unterwegs. Verkehrs- und Mobilitätserziehung mit den Schwerpunkten „Sicherheitserziehung und Unfallprävention". In R. Siller (Ed.), *Kinder unterwegs – Schule macht mobil. Verkehrs- und Mobilitätserziehung in der Schule.* Donauwörth: Auer Verlag.

Limbourg, M., Flade, A. & Schönharting, J. (2000). *Mobilität im Kindes- und Jugendalter.* Opladen: Leske + Budrich.

Magistrate of the City of Vienna, (Hrsg.) (2002). *Wiener Jugendgesundheitsbericht 2002.* Wien.

Menze-Sonneck, A. (1998). *Mädchen und junge Frauen im Sportverein: Sportkarrieren und Fluktuation im Turnen.* Schorndorf: Hofmann.

Menze-Sonneck, A. (2002). Zwischen Einfalt und Vielfalt. Die Sportvereinskarrieren weiblicher und männlicher Jugendlicher in Brandenburg und Nordrhein-Westfalen. *Sportwissenschaft, 32*, 147-169.

Michaud, P.-A., Narring, F., Caudereray, M., Cavadini, C. (1999). Sports activity, physical fitness of 9- to 19-year-old teenagers in the canton of Vaud (Switzerland). *Schweizer Medizinische Wochenschrift, 129*, 691-699

MPFS (Medienpädagogischer Forschungsverbund Südwest) (1998). *JIM' 98. Jugend, Information, (Multi-)Media. Basisuntersuchung zum Medienumgang 12- bis 19jähriger in Deutschland.* Retrieved February 12, 2004, from http://www.mpfs.de/studien/jim/JIM98.pdf

MPFS (Medienpädagogischer Forschungsverbund Südwest) (2000a). *JIM 99/2000. Jugend, Information, (Multi-) Media. Basisuntersuchung zum Medienumgang 12- bis 19jähriger in Deutschland.* Retrieved February 12, 2004, from http://www.mpfs.de/studien/jim/Jim99Down.pdf

MPFS (Medienpädagogischer Forschungsverbund Südwest) (2000b). *JIM 2000. Jugend, Information, (Multi-) Media. Basisuntersuchung zum Medienumgang 12- bis 19jähriger in Deutschland.* Retrieved February 12, 2004, from http://www.mpfs.de/studien/jim/JIM2000.pdf

MPFS (Medienpädagogischer Forschungsverbund Südwest) (2000c). *Kinder und Medien – KIM ,99. Basisuntersuchung zum Medienumgang 6- bis 13jähriger in Deutschland.* Retrieved May 26, 2004, from http://www.mpfs.de/studien/kim/KIM99.pdf

MPFS (Medienpädagogischer Forschungsverbund Südwest) (2001). *KIM-Studie 2000. Kinder und Medien. Computer und Internet. Basisuntersuchung zum Medienumgang 6- bis 13jähriger in Deutschland.* Retrieved May 26, 2004, from http://www.mpfs.de/studien/kim/KIM2000.pdf

MPFS (Medienpädagogischer Forschungsverbund Südwest) (2002a). *JIM 2001. Jugend, Information, (Multi-) Media. Basisuntersuchung zum Medienumgang 12- bis 19jähriger in Deutschland.* Retrieved February 12, 2004, from http://www.mpfs.de/studien/jim/JIM2001.pdf

MPFS (Medienpädagogischer Forschungsverbund Südwest) (2002b). *KIM 2002. PC und Internet. Basisuntersuchung zum Medienumgang 6- bis 13jähriger in Deutschland.* Retrieved May 26, 2004, from http://www.mpfs.de/studien/kim/KIM2002.pdf

MPFS (Medienpädagogischer Forschungsverbund Südwest) (2003a). *JIM 2002. Jugend, Information, (Multi-) Media. Basisuntersuchung zum Medienumgang 12- bis 19jähriger in Deutschland.* Retrieved February 12, 2004, from http://www.mpfs.de/studien/jim/JIM2002.pdf

MPFS (Medienpädagogischer Forschungsverbund Südwest) (2003b). *KIM-Studie 2003. Kinder und Medien.* Retrieved May 26, 2004, from http://www.mpfs.de/studien/kim/KIM03-pm.pdf

MPFS (Medienpädagogischer Forschungsverbund Südwest) (2004). *JIM 2003. Jugend, Information, (Multi-) Media. Basisuntersuchung zum Medienumgang 12- bis 19jähriger in Deutschland.* Retrieved June 2, 2004, from http://www.mpfs.de/studien/jim/jim03.pdf

MPFS (Medienpädagogischer Forschungsverbund Südwest) (2005). *JIM 2004. Jugend, Information, (Multi-) Media. Basisuntersuchung zum Medienumgang 12- bis 19jähriger in Deutschland.* Retrieved June 2, 2005, from http://www.mpfs.de/studien/jim/jim03.pdf

322 W.-D. Brettschneider, R. Naul, A. Bünemann & D. Hoffmann

Müller, M. J. (2003). *Übergewicht bei Kindern und Jugendlichen – Urachen und Möglichkeiten der Prävention.* Retrieved March 11, 2004, from http://www.bll-online.de/downloads/mueller.pdf

Nagl, R. (1993). Der Freundeskreis und das Freizeitverhalten Zehnjähriger. In: Katholische Jungschar Österreichs (Hrsg.): *Bericht zur Lage der Kinder 1993.* Wien. 87-97.

Naul, R. Rychtecky, A. & Telama, R. (1997). Physical Fitness and Active Lifestyle of Czech, Finnish and German Youth. *Acta Universitas Carolina - Kineantrophologica, 33, 2,* 5-15

Naul, R., Hoffmann, D., Telama, R. & Nupponen, H. (2003). PISA-Schock auch im Schulsport? Wie fit sind deutsche und finnische Jugendliche? *Sportunterricht 54 (2003),* 137-141.

Noelle-Neumann, E. & Petersen, T. (2001). Zeitenwende. Der Wertewandel 30 Jahre später. Aus Politik und Zeitgeschichte. *Das Parlament, 51* (29, supplement), 15-23.

Österreichisches Institut für Familienforschung (Hrsg.) (1998). *Was machen Kinder, Frauen und Männer, Mütter und Väter mit ihrer Zeit? Familienbezogene Auswertung der Zeitbudgeterhebung 1992.* Materialiensammlungen, Heft 6. Wien.

Österreichisches Institut für Jugendkunde (Hrsg.) (1989). *Verbandliche Jugendarbeit in Österreich.* Wien.

Palentien, C. (2003). Kinder und Jugendliche. In B. Badura, R. Busse, R. Leidl, H. Raspe, J. Siegrist & U. Walter (Eds.), *Public Health. Gesundheit und Gesundheitswesen* (pp. 636-641). München: Urban & Fischer.

Rathgeb, J. (1998). Medienlandschaft Schweiz. In: Bonfadelli, H., Hättenschwiler, W. (Hrsg.): *Einführung in die Publizistikwissenschaft.* Diskussionspunkt Nr. 27,3. Zürich.

Ravens-Sieberer, U. Thomas, C. & Erhart, M. (2003). Körperliche, psychische und soziale Gesundheit von Jugendlichen. In K. Hurrelmann, A. Klocke, W. Melzer & U. Ravens-Sieberer (Eds.), *Jugendgesundheitssurvey. Internationale Vergleichsstudie im Auftrag der Weltgesundheitsorganisation WHO* (pp. 19-98). Weinheim and Munich: Juventa.

Robert Koch Institute (2006). Symposium zur Studie zur Gesundheit von Kindern und Jugendlichen in Deutschland.Bundesgesundheitsbl – Gesundheitsforsch – Gesundheitsschutz 49 (2006), 1051-1052.

Rolland-Cachera, M. F., Cole, T. J., Sempé, M., Tichet, J., Rossignol, C. & Charraud, A. (1991). Body Mass Index variations: centiles from birth to 87 years. *European Journal of Clinical Nutrition, 45,* 13-21.

Rolland-Cachera, M. F. Sempé, M., Guilloud-Bataille, M. Patois, E., Péquignot-Guggenbuhl, F. & Fautrad, V. (1982). Adiposity indices in children. *American Journal of Clinical Nutrition, 36,* 178-184.

Rusch, H. & Irrgang, W. (2002). Aufschwung oder Abschwung? Verändert sich die körperliche Leistungsfähigkeit von Kindern und Jugendlichen oder nicht? *Haltung und Bewegung, 22* (2), 5-10.

Sack, H.-G. (1980). *Die Fluktuation Jugendlicher im Sportverein.* 2 Bände. Marburg: Philipps-Universität.

Sandmayer, A. (2004). *Das motorische Leistungsniveau der österreichischen Schuljugend.* Meyer & Meyer. Aachen.

SGR SSR, MD/SW, (Hrsg.)(2004). *Die Mediennutzung von Kindern in der Schweiz – gemessen und erfragt. Eine Untersuchung zum Medienverhalten sowie zu Radiointeressen und -motiven von sieben bis vierzehnjährigen Kindern.* Repro-Center SRG SSR. Bern.

Spethmann, C., Mast, M., Langnäse, K., Danielzik, S. & Müller, M. J. (2002). Entwicklung des Ernährungszustandes präpubertärer Kinder – Erste Ergebnisse der 4-Jahres-

Nachuntersuchungen der Kiel Obesity Prevention Study (KOPS). *Aktuelle Ernährungsmedizin, 27*, S352-S353.

Statistisches Bundesamt (2003). *In the spotlight. Population of Germany today and tomorrow. 2002 – 2050.* Wiesbaden.

Statistisches Bundesamt(2004). *Bevölkerung.* Retrieved July 13, 2004, from http://www.destatis.de/basis/d/bevoe/bevoetab5.php

Süss, D., Giordani, G. (2000). Sprachregionale und kulturelle Aspekte der Mediennutzung von Schweizer Kindern. *MedienPädagogik, 34.* www.medienpaed.com

Sygusch, R. (2000). *Sportliche Aktivität und subjektive Gesundheitskonzepte. Eine Studie zum Erleben von Körper und Gesundheit bei jugendlichen Sportlern.* Schorndorf: Hofmann.

Sygusch, R., Brehm, W. & Ungerer-Röhrich, U. (2003). Gesundheit und körperliche Aktivität bei Kindern und Jugendlichen. In W. Schmidt, I. Hartmann-Tews & W.-D. Brettschneider (Eds.), *Erster Deutscher Kinder- und Jugendsportbericht* (pp. 63-84). Schorndorf: Hofmann.

Telama, R., Naul, R., Nupponen, H., Rychtecky, A. & Vuolle, P. (2002) *Physical fitness, sporting lifestyles, and Olympic ideals: cross-cultural studies on youth sports in Europe.* Schorndorf: Karl Hofmann.

Tietjens, M. (2001). *Sportliches Engagement und sozialer Rückhalt im Jugendalter. Eine repräsentative Surveystudie in Brandenburg und Nordrhein-Westfalen.* Lengerich: Pabst.

Wabitsch, M. (2004). Kinder und Jugendliche mit Adipositas in Deutschland. Aufruf zum Handeln. *Bundesgesundheitsblatt – Gesundheitsforschung – Gesundheitsschutz, 47,* 251-255.

Waldherr, K.; Rollet, B. (2001). Geundheit von Lehrlingen in Wien – Ergebnisse einer repräsentativen Studie. Statistische Mitteilungen zur Gesundheit in Wien 2001/1. Magistratsabteilung für Angelegenheiten der Landessanitätsdirektion, Dezernat II – Gesundheitsplanung (Hrsg.), Wien.

WHO (1989). WHO-MONICA project: Risk factors. *International Journal of Epidemiology, 18* (Suppl. 1), 46-55.

WIAD (Ed.) (2000). *Bewegungsstatus von Kindern und Jugendlichen in Deutschland.* Bonn: Forschungsbericht im Auftrag des DSB und der AOK.

Widhalm, K., Dietrich, S. (2003). Adipositas Prävalenzstudie aus Wien – Ein gesundheitliches Problem? *Akt Ernähr Med 2003;28,* 343.

Widhalm, K., Dietrich, S. (2004). Prävalenz von Übergewicht/Adipositas bei 10-15-jährigen Wiener SchülerInnen. *Akt Ernähr Med 2004;29,* 303.

Woringer, V., Schütz, Y. (1998). What is the evolutionen of body mass index (BMI) in Swiss children from five to sixteen years, measured one decade apart. *International Journal of Obesity, 22,* 209.

Woringer, V., Schütz, Y. (2004). Übergewicht in der Schweiz. Percentilen des Body Mass-Indexes (BMI) von Kindern und Jugendlichen aus Lausanne mit Jahrgang 1980 – Abweichungen von der schweizerischen Normen von 1955. *Paediatrica, Vol. 15 (3),* 45-49.

Zimmermann, M.B., Hess, S.Y., Hurell, R.F. (2000). A national study of the prevalence of overweight and obesity in 6-12y-old Swiss children: Body mass index, body-weight perceptions and goals. *European Journal of Clinical Nutrition, 54,* 568-572.

SPORT SCIENCES INTERNATIONAL

Edited by Herbert Haag, Dieter Hackfort, Ken Hardman, Manfred Lämmer,
Roland Naul, Maurice Pieron, George H. Sage, Daryl Siedentop, Robert W. Schutz

Vol.   1   Dieter Hackfort (Ed.): Psycho-Social Issues and Interventions in Elite Sports. 1994.

Vol.   2   Roland Naul (Ed.): Contemporary Studies in the National Olympic Games Movement.
           1997.

Vol.   3   Herbert Haag / Gerald Haag in cooperation with Birte Kaulitz: From Physical Fitness to
           Motor Competence. Aims – Content – Methods – Evaluation. 2000.

Vol.   4   Wolf-Dietrich Brettschneider / Roland Naul (eds.): Obesity in Europe. Young people's phy-
           sical activity and sedentary lifestyles. 2007.

www.peterlang.de

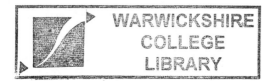